Digestive Diseases

The Latest in Diagnosis and Treatment of Gastrointestinal Disorders

Formerly "Survey of Digestive Diseases"
Founded in 1983 by T.S.N. Chen and R.K. Zetterman
Former Editor: S.R. Achem (1993–2000)

KARGER

Printed in Germany on acid-free and non-aging paper (ISO 9706) by Stückle Druck, Ettenheim

Digestive Diseases

KARGER

E-Mail karger@karger.com
www.karger.com

The Journal Home Page is available at:
www.karger.com/ddi

Guidelines for Authors

Digestive Diseases

Aims and Scope

Digestive Diseases publishes original reports and review articles that describe the most recent advances in diagnostic methods and treatment options for diseases of the gastrointestinal tract and the hepato-pancreato-biliary system. The journal also covers related topics such as microbiota, nutrition and probiotics, endoscopy and imaging. Providing information about the latest clinical evidence and their application in patient care, *Digestive Diseases* is an invaluable source of information for clinicians, specialists and physicians-in-training.

Submission

Manuscripts written in English are considered and should be submitted online at

www.karger.com/ddi

All manuscripts must be accompanied by a cover letter. Assurance should be given in the cover letter that the manuscript is not under simultaneous consideration by any other publication. In the cover letter, the authors should declare their potential conflicts of interest and provide a statement on authorship.

Manuscript Types

Original Papers
Submitted manuscripts should be fully documented reports of original clinical research. Basic research is considered if the study shows a translational aspect and may lead to practical clinical applications: for instance a promising new treatment or diagnosis tool.
Original articles should not exceed 4,000 words, excluding up to 6 tables or figures and up to 60 references.

Review Articles
The maximum length of a Review article should be 3,500 words including abstract and discussion, excluding figure legends and references.

Systematic Review and Meta-Analysis
We strongly encourage authors to comply with the Preferred Reporting Items for Systematic Reviews and Meta-Analyses (PRISMA) guidelines (http://www.prisma-statement.org/).
Systematic Reviews and Meta-Analysis should not exceed 4,000 words, excluding up to 6 tables or figures and up to 100 references.

Imaging and Endoscopy
Manuscript should describe a novel endoscopy or imaging technique and be supported by a video (max. 5 Gb) or high quality images.
The manuscript should include the rationale for the procedure and a detailed description of the procedure including the equipment used.
Manuscript length should be maximum 1,500 words excluding a maximum of 15 references. Videos larger than 15 Mb must be sent to the editorial office (ddi@karger.com) via a large file sharing service.

Consensus Statement and Guidelines
Submitted manuscripts should include a statement intended to guide clinical care as well as the mechanism by which the statement was generated and a review of the evidence for the statement.
Consensus Statement and Guidelines should not exceed 4,000 words, excluding up to 6 tables or figures and up to 100 references.

Editorials
Editorials on special hot topics are primarily invited by the editors.
The maximum length of an Editorial should be 1,500 words excluding a maximum of 15 references.

Letters to the Editor
Letters in reference to a journal article should be received within 2 months after publication of the article. Letters not related to a journal article are also considered.
Letters must not exceed 400 words and have a maximum of five references and one figure or table. They should not be signed by more than three authors.

Conditions

All manuscripts are subject to editorial review. Manuscripts are received with the explicit understanding that they are not under simultaneous consideration by any other publication. Submission of an article for publication implies transfer of the copyright from the author to the publisher upon acceptance. Accepted papers become the permanent property of Digestive Diseases and may not be reproduced by any means, in whole or in part, without the written consent of the publisher. It is the author's responsibility to obtain permission to reproduce illustrations, tables, etc. from other publications.

Peer-Review Policy

Digestive Diseases is a peer-reviewed journal that uses a single-blind peer review. Our aim is to provide authors with fast and constructive feedback regarding their submitted manuscript. The Editor-in-Chief and the Associate Editors ensure a thorough and fair peer review and the highest scientific publishing standards. Submitted manuscripts are checked by the Editorial Office and forwarded to the Editor-in-Chief, who decides whether to accept/reject a manuscript or send it for review to an Associate Editor and at least two reviewers. Reviewers must have a recent publication record in the area of the submission, must not have published with the authors in the previous 3 years, and must not be from the same institution as the authors. The Editor-in-Chief makes a final decision on all papers submitted to the journal and is responsible to maintain high-quality peer review.

Disclosure Statement

Any financial interests (stocks, patents, employment, honoraria, royalties) or nonfinancial relationships (political, personal, professional) that may be interpreted to have influenced the manuscript must be declared in a Conflicts of Interest statement at the end of the main text. If there is no conflict of interest, please state "The authors declare no conflicts of interest".

Ethics Statement

Research must comply with the guidelines for human studies and animal welfare regulations. Copies of these guidelines and policy statements must be available for review by the editors if necessary.

Humans
Manuscripts reporting studies on human subjects should include evidence that the research was conducted ethically in accordance with the World Medical Association Declaration of Helsinki. In particular, authors must provide an Ethics Statement at the end of the main text that all subjects (or their parents or guardians) have given their informed written consent and that the study protocol was approved by an appropriate ethics committee. If no approval was required, this must be stated in this section. All patients should be identified by numbers or aliases, not by their real names. For clinical trials, registration in a public trials registry before or at the time of first patient enrolment is a condition of consideration for publication. The trial registration number must be provided upon submission at the end of the abstract.

Animals
Authors should state that animal experimentation was approved by the appropriate institutional review body. We encourage authors to comply with the Animal Research: Reporting In Vivo Experiments (ARRIVE) guidelines developed by the National Centre for the Replacement, Refinement & Reduction of Animals in Research (NC3Rs).

Plagiarism Policy

Whether intentional or not, plagiarism is a serious violation. We define plagiarism as a case in which a paper reproduces another work with at least 25% similarity and without citation.
If evidence of plagiarism is found before/after acceptance or after publication of the paper, the author will be offered a chance for rebuttal. If the arguments are not found to be satisfactory, the manuscript will be retracted and the author sanctioned from publishing papers for a period to be determined by the responsible Editor(s).

Author Contributions

A short statement detailing the contributions of each person named as an author should be included. Please refer to the ICMJE's criteria for authorship. If an author is removed or added to the manuscript after submission, an explanation and signed statement of agreement for the requested change from all listed authors and from the author to be removed or added is required.

Arrangement

The manuscript should conform to the following order: title page, abstract and key words, body, acknowledgments, references, figure legends, tables and figures. Manuscripts should be written in high-quality English suitable for effective communication to a professional medical audience. For authors whose native language is not English, use of a professional language editing service (http://www.karger.com/Resources/Authors) prior to submission can help to avoid delays with the review process. All pages, including the figure legends, should be numbered in sequence, and the first author's name should appear at the upper right corner of each page. Papers not conforming to the journal style will be returned without review.

Title page: The first page of each paper should indicate a concise title of no more than 150 characters, all authors' names (first name and surname), authors' institutional affiliations, and a short title for use as running head.

Corresponding author: The exact postal address of author(s) to whom correspondence, proofs, and reprint requests should be sent, including the postal code, must be given at the bottom of the title page. Please also supply phone number and e-mail address.

Abstract of Review Articles: Should be divided into the following subsections: Background, Summary and Key Messages. The Background should provide a brief clinical context for the review and is followed by the Summary, which should include a concise description of the main topics covered in the text. The Key Messages encapsulate the main conclusions of the review. Submit

KARGER

E-Mail karger@karger.com
www.karger.com

The Journal Home Page is available at:
www.karger.com/ddi

the abstract on a separate page. The abstract should be less than 300 words.

Key words: Following the abstract, an alphabetical list of five key words that reflect the content of the paper should be given.

Footnotes: Avoid footnotes.

Tables and illustrations: Tables and illustrations (both numbered in sequential Arabic numerals) should be prepared as separate files. Tables require a brief and concise heading. Figures require a legend, prepared as a separate page, after references. Please use scale markers for electron micrographs, and indicate the type of stain used. For the reproduction of illustrations, only good drawings and original photographs can be accepted; negatives or photocopies cannot be used. Due to technical reasons, figures with a screen background should not be submitted. When possible, group several illustrations in one block for reproduction (max. size 180 x 223 mm) or provide crop marks. Electronically submitted b/w half-tone and color illustrations must have a final resolution of 300 dpi after scaling, line drawings one of 800–1,200 dpi.

References: In the text identify references by Arabic numerals [in square brackets]. Material submitted for publication but not yet accepted should be noted as [unpublished data] and not be included in the reference list. The list of references should include only those publications which are cited in the text. Do not alphabetize; number references in the order in which they are first mentioned in the text. The surnames of the authors followed by initials should be given. There should be no punctuation other than a comma to separate the authors. Preferably, please cite all authors. Abbreviate journal names according to the Index Medicus system. Also see International Committee of Medical Journal Editors: Uniform requirements for manuscripts submitted to biomedical journals (www.icmje.org).

Examples
(a) Papers published in periodicals: Chatel JM, Bernard H, Orson FM: Isolation and characterization of two complete Ara h 2 isoforms cDNA. Int Arch Allergy Immunol 2003;131:14–18.
(b) Papers published only with DOI numbers: Theoharides TC, Boucher W, Spear K: Serum interleukin-6 reflects disease severity and osteoporosis in mastocytosis patients. Int Arch Allergy Immunol DOI: 10.1159/000063858.
(c) Monographs: Matthews DE, Farewell VT: Using and Understanding Medical Statistics, ed 4, revised. Basel, Karger, 2007.
(d) Edited books: DuBois RN: Cyclooxygenase-2 and colorectal cancer; in Dannenberg AJ, Dubois RN (eds): COX-2. Prog Exp Tum Res. Basel, Karger, 2003, vol 37, pp 124–137.

Reference Management Software: Use of EndNote® is recommended for easy management and formatting of citations and reference lists.

Page Charges
There is no page charges for papers of 3 or fewer printed pages (including tables, figures, references and acknowledgements). Each additional complete or partial page is charged to the author at CHF 410.00.

Color Illustrations
Online edition: Color illustrations are reproduced free of charge. In the print version, the illustrations are reproduced in black and white. Please avoid referring to the colors in the text and figure legends.
Print edition: Up to 6 color illustrations per page can be integrated within the text at CHF 960.00 per page.

Supplementary Material
Multimedia files and other supplementary files, directly relevant but not essential to the conclusions of a paper, enhance the online version of a publication and increase its visibility on the web. These files will undergo editorial review. The Editors reserve the right to limit the scope and length of the supplementary material. Multimedia and supplementary material should meet production quality standards for publication without the need for any modification or editing. Files should not exceed 10 Mb in size. Figures and tables need to have titles and legends, and all files should be supplied separately and labeled clearly. All supplementary material should be referred to in the main text. A DOI number will be assigned to supplementary material and it will be hosted online at https://karger.figshare.com under a CC BY license. Authors will be charged a processing fee of CHF 250.00 for supplementary material.

Digital Object Identifier (DOI)
S. Karger Publishers supports DOIs as unique identifiers for articles. A DOI number will be printed on the title page of each article. DOIs can be useful in the future for identifying and citing articles published online without volume or issue information. More information can be found at www.doi.org

Self-Archiving/Green Open Access
Karger permits authors to archive their pre-prints (i.e. pre-peer review) or post-prints (i.e. accepted manuscript after peer review but before production) on their personal or their institution's internal website. In addition, authors may post their accepted manuscripts in public Open Access repositories and scientific networks (e.g. ResearchGate or Mendeley) no earlier than 12 months following publication of the final version of their article. For all self-archiving, the posted manuscripts must:

- Be used for noncommercial purposes only
- Be linked to the final version on www.karger.com
- Include the following statement:

"This is the peer-reviewed but unedited manuscript version of the following article: [insert full citation, e.g. Cytogenet Genome Res 2014;142:227–238 (DOI: 10.1159/000361001)]. The final, published version is available at http://www.karger.com/?doi=[insert DOI number]."

It is the author's responsibility to fulfill these requirements.

For papers published online first with a DOI number only, full citation details must be added as soon as the paper is published in its final version. This is important to ensure that citations can be credited to the article.

Manuscripts to be archived in PubMed Central due to funding requirements will be submitted by Karger on the author's behalf [see Funding Organizations (NIH etc.)].

For self-archiving Author's Choice™ (Gold Open Access) articles, see Author's Choice™.

Author's Choice™
Karger's Author's Choice™ service broadens the reach of your article and gives all users worldwide free and full access for reading, downloading and printing at www.karger.com. The option is available for a one-time fee of CHF 3,000.00, which is a permissible cost in grant allocation. More information can be found at www.karger.com/authors_choice.
The final, published version of the article may be posted at any time and in any repository or on other websites, in accordance with the relevant Creative Commons license. Reposted Open Access articles must:

- Follow the terms of the relevant Creative Commons license
- Be linked to the final version on www.karger.com
- Include the following statement:

"The final, published version of this article is available at http://www.karger.com/?doi=[insert DOI number]."

It is the author's responsibility to fulfill these requirements.

For papers published online first with a DOI number only, full citation details must be added as soon as the paper is published in its final version. This is important to ensure that citations can be credited to the article.

Funding Organizations (NIH etc.)
The U.S. National Institutes of Health (NIH) Public Access Policy mandates that accepted, peer-reviewed manuscripts are archived in its digital database, PubMed Central (PMC), within 12 months of the official publication date. As a service to authors, Karger submits NIH-funded articles to PMC on behalf of the authors immediately upon publication. The NIH assigns a PMCID within approximately 1 month and the manuscript will appear in PMC after a 12-month embargo. For authors making their paper Open Access through Author's Choice™, the embargo will be overridden, thereby accelerating the accessibility of the article. Karger also complies with other funders' requirements (including Wellcome Trust and RCUK) for submission to PMC.
Authors should include information on their grant in the Acknowledgements section of their papers.

Proofs
Unless indicated otherwise, proofs are sent to the corresponding author and should be returned with the least possible delay. Alterations other than the correction of printer's errors are charged to the author.

Reprints
Order forms and a price list are sent with the proofs. Orders submitted after the issue is printed are subject to considerably higher prices.

KARGER

E-Mail karger@karger.com
www.karger.com

The Journal Home Page is available at:
www.karger.com/ddi

General Information

Digestive Diseases

ISSN Print Edition: 0257–2753
ISSN Online Edition: 1421–9875

Journal Homepage: www.karger.com/ddi

Publication Data: *Digestive Diseases* is published 6 times a year. Volume 35 with 6 issues appears in 2017.

Subscription Rates: Subscriptions run for a full calendar year. Prices are given per year.

Personal subscription:

Print or Online	**Print+Online combined**
CHF 320.00	CHF 370.00
EUR 288.00	EUR 328.00
USD 348.00	USD 402.00

postage and handling (added to print and print+online)
CHF 48.00 Europe, CHF 69.60 Overseas
EUR 43.20
USD 67.20

Institutional subscription:

Print or Online	**Print+Online combined**
CHF 2864.00	CHF 3294.00
EUR 2580.00	EUR 2967.00
USD 3113.00	USD 3580.00

postage and handling (added to print and print+online)
CHF 60.00 Europe, CHF 87.00 Overseas
EUR 54.00
USD 84.00

Discount subscription prices:
Please enquire about reduced rates for residents.

Back Volumes and Single Issues: Information on availability and prices of single print issues and print or electronic back volumes can be obtained from Customer Service at *service@karger.com.*

Bibliographic Indices: This journal is regularly listed in bibliographic services, including *Current Contents®* and PubMed/MEDLINE.

Subscription Orders:
Orders can be placed at agencies, bookstores, directly with the Publisher

S. Karger AG
Medical and Scientific Publishers
Allschwilerstrasse 10
CH–4009 Basel
Switzerland

t: +41 61 306 11 11
f: +41 61 306 12 34
e: karger@karger.com
w: www.karger.com

(for courier services only:
Allschwilerstrasse 10
CH–4055 Basel)

or further Karger offices or representatives:

Germany
S. Karger GmbH
Postfach
79095 Freiburg
Deutschland
(Hausadresse: Wilhelmstrasse 20A, 79098 Freiburg)
t: +49 761 45 20 70
f: +49 761 45 20 714
e: information@karger.de
w: www.karger.de

Japan
Karger Japan, Inc.
Shiba Daimon Asahi Bldg. 2F
1-2-23 Shiba Daimon
Minato-ku
Tokyo 105-0012
Japan
t: +81 3 6435 6242
f: +81 3 6435 6244
e: publisher@karger.jp
w: www.karger.jp

USA
S. Karger Publishers, Inc.
26 West Avon Road
P.O. Box 529
Unionville, CT 06085
USA
Toll free: +1 800 828 5479
t: +1 860 675 7834
f: +1 860 675 7302
e: kargerusa@karger.com

France
Enter & Read
Albertine Luginbuhl
23, rue du Départ, boite 37
75014 Paris
France
t: +33 (0) 6 81 04 76 85
e: albertineluginbuhl@orange.fr

South East Asia, China and Taiwan
Karger Regional Office (Malaysia)
Level 28-03-03A, PJ Exchange
No. 16A, Persiaran Barat
46050 Petaling Jaya
Selangor Darul Ehsan
Malaysia
t: +60 3 7962 0158
f: +60 3 7962 0001
e: service@karger.cn; r.chew@karger.cn

Karger China
51F Raffles City Centre
268 Xi Zang Middle Road
Huang Pu District
Shanghai 200001
P.R. China
t: +86 21 2312 7673
f: +86 21 2312 7777
e: service@karger.cn
r.chew@karger.cn
w: www.karger.cn

India, Bangladesh, Sri Lanka
Karger India
Plot No. 17, Yusuf Sarai Market
B.L. Glass Building, 2nd Floor
Sri Aurobindo Marg
New Delhi 110 016
India
t: +91 11 46029 633
f: +91 11 46029 634
c: +91 98 91052 128
e: r.kumar@kargerindia.com
w: www.karger.com

Change of Address:
Both old and new address should be sent to the subscription source.

KARGER

E-Mail karger@karger.com
www.karger.com

The Journal Home Page is available at:
www.karger.com/ddi

Digestive Diseases

Clinical Hepatology Practice in 2016: From Science to Therapy

Symposium 204

Official Congress Report
Birmingham, September 2–3, 2016

Editors
G. Hirschfield, Birmingham
D.H. Adams, Birmingham
R. Thimme, Freiburg

16 figures and 13 tables, 2017

KARGER

Basel · Freiburg · Paris · London · New York · Chennai · New Delhi · Bangkok · Beijing · Shanghai · Tokyo · Kuala Lumpur · Singapore · Sydney

S. Karger
Medical and Scientific Publishers
Basel · Freiburg · Paris · London ·
New York · Chennai · New Delhi ·
Bangkok · Beijing · Shanghai · Tokyo ·
Kuala Lumpur · Singapore · Sydney

Disclaimer
The statements, opinions and data contained in this publication are solely those of the individual authors and contributors and not of the publisher and the editor(s). The appearance of advertisements in the journal is not a warranty, endorsement, or approval of the products or services advertised or of their effectiveness, quality or safety. The publisher and the editor(s) disclaim responsibility for any injury to persons or property resulting from any ideas, methods, instructions or products referred to in the content or advertisements.

Drug Dosage
The authors and the publisher have exerted every effort to ensure that drug selection and dosage set forth in this text are in accord with current recommendations and practice at the time of publication. However, in view of ongoing research, changes in government regulations, and the constant flow of information relating to drug therapy and drug reactions, the reader is urged to check the package insert for each drug for any change in indications and dosage and for added warnings and precautions. This is particularly important when the recommended agent is a new and/or infrequently employed drug.

Printed on acid-free and non-aging paper (ISO 9706)
ISBN 978–3–318–05991–5
e-ISBN 978–3–318–05992–2

KARGER

E-Mail karger@karger.com
www.karger.com/ddi

Vol. 35, No. 4, 2017

Digestive Diseases

Contents

KARGER

E-Mail karger@karger.com
www.karger.com/ddi

Digestive Diseases

Dig Dis 2017;35:303
DOI: 10.1159/000457326

Preface

As clinicians face an increasing burden of treating liver diseases in their patient cohorts, opportunities to drive better clinical practice in liver disease continue to emerge. Liver medicine and surgery are at a pivotal moment with rapid advances in basic science underpinning the care of our patients, all of whom seek treatment methods that prevent liver injury, fibrosis and end-stage liver disease complications. Across a spectrum of liver injuries, be they viral, malignant, metabolic, autoimmune or genetic, the key pathways through which a healthy liver traverses to end up in a liver disease are becoming clearer. Where liver disease has specific triggers, it is increasingly the case that directed therapy can be effective, the most dramatic examples being those seen in the cure of viral liver disease; in such cases, substantial investment in specific drug discovery is found to have unquestionable benefits to patients globally. In other liver diseases such as metabolic and autoimmune conditions, progress has been made in terms of gaining mechanistic insights, often uncovering pathways that span apparently unrelated disease, such as the significance of FXR biology to both cholestatic liver disease as well as non-alcoholic fatty liver disease. Such science has driven the generation of an exciting panorama of drugs in clinical trials.

Equally clinical care paradigms have evolved and become more sophisticated and personalised, as a more robust and accessible approach to clinical hepatology practice has emerged. Challenges remain not least with effectively translating science into practice but also in measuring the impact of disease and new interventions against the backdrop of inexorable demands on health care systems internationally. Nonetheless, the practice of hepatology continues to be exciting and dynamic, and our contributors to this collection of articles have captured the essence of the science and clinical practice of hepatology in 2017 elegantly and critically.

Gideon Hirschfield, Birmingham

KARGER

E-Mail karger@karger.com
www.karger.com/ddi

Hepatology 2016 – The Panorama

Digestive Diseases

Dig Dis 2017;35:304–309
DOI: 10.1159/000456580

Lessons from Epidemiology: The Burden of Liver Disease

Ian A. Rowe

University Academic Fellow, Leeds Institute for Data Analytics, University of Leeds, Leeds, UK

Keywords
Alcohol · Cirrhosis · Fibrosis · Non-alcoholic fatty liver · Viral hepatitis

Abstract
Liver cirrhosis is responsible for more than 1 million deaths annually and the majority of these deaths are preventable. There is marked geographical variation in rates of mortality due to cirrhosis, and this variation in liver disease burden exemplifies the links between population risks for liver disease and mortality. The differing geographical distribution of the major risks factors for the development of liver disease including alcohol consumption, hepatitis C virus (HCV) infection, hepatitis B virus infection, and obesity and the metabolic syndrome has the potential to highlight opportunities for intervention, while the evolution of these risk factors provides insights into understanding the future burden of liver disease. This review focuses on the use of population data to identify high-risk areas and populations that would benefit from preventative interventions to reduce the mortality from liver disease. Specific strategies that are effective at the policy and public health levels are discussed to illustrate the impact these can have if widely implemented. The impact of therapies that have the potential to change the natural history of liver disease, including direct acting antivirals for HCV infection is also described. Finally, the challenges of describing the epidemiology of non-alcoholic fatty liver disease are highlighted to illustrate the need to understand the natural history of disease to inform and influence the development of novel therapies.

The profile of liver disease has greatly increased over recent years. The recognition of liver disease and its complications as a major cause of death has been stimulated in part by the continued increase in deaths observed in some parts of the world but also by the development of new treatments, most notably for hepatitis C virus (HCV) infection. The aim of this review was to highlight areas where studies in populations influence practice and research in liver disease.

This review first discusses the global epidemiology of liver disease. I will use examples from each of the 3 most prevalent liver diseases, hepatitis B virus (HBV) infection, HCV infection, and alcohol-related liver diseases (ArLD) to highlight two lessons from the available population data. The first of these is the use of population-based strategies to prevent, or limit, the harm caused by liver disease. The second of these will be to illustrate how the use of currently available treatments for hepatitis C might inform future studies for developing treatments for the increasingly prevalent non-alcoholic fatty liver disease (NAFLD).

The Importance of Liver Disease in Global Mortality Estimates

The investment in global health from the Bill and Melinda Gates Foundation has yielded a number of important contributions. Among these are the reports of the Global Burden of Disease studies. These have variously reported morbidity and mortality assessments for all dis-

KARGER

E-Mail karger@karger.com
www.karger.com/ddi

Ian A. Rowe, MRCP (UK), PhD
University Academic Fellow
Leeds Institute for Data Analytics, University of Leeds
Leeds LS9 7TF (UK)
E-Mail i.a.c.rowe@leeds.ac.uk

eases across the world. The Mortality and Cause of Death Collaborators have made important observations of critical importance to the understanding of liver disease outcomes [1, 2]. First of these is the evolution in causes of death over the last 3 decades. There has been a shift away from mortality and life years lost due to communicable diseases, particularly diarrhoeal disease (that shows a median 62% reduction in life years lost between 1990 and 2013), towards largely non-communicable chronic disease. The consequence of this is that there has been an increase in the number of deaths and life years lost as a result of chronic diseases such as liver disease over the same period. Cirrhosis ranks 13th overall and 4th among chronic diseases in terms of life years after coronary heart disease, cerebrovascular disease and chronic obstructive pulmonary disease. Liver cancer, which is one of the main complications of chronic liver disease and cirrhosis, ranks 21st further highlighting the importance of liver disease as a major cause of premature mortality worldwide. Considering annual mortality from each of these causes, the investigators estimated 1.2 million deaths from cirrhosis and 818,000 deaths from liver cancer, which in total means that complications of chronic liver disease are responsible for more than 2 million deaths every year.

Cause of Cirrhosis in Individuals Dying of Complications of Chronic Liver Disease

Globally, HCV is the leading cause of liver disease–related death accounting for approximately 700,000 deaths annually. HBV infection accounts for in excess of 600,000 deaths and ArLD for almost half a million deaths each year. Other causes of liver disease, including NAFLD, account for 250,000 deaths in total annually. Understanding the geographical distribution of these different diseases provides the potential to observe both opportunities for disease prevention and also patterns of behaviour that are associated with the disease.

Hepatitis B and Prevention of Disease through Vaccination

The global epidemiology of HBV infection identifies the highest disease burden across Asia and in sub-Saharan Africa. In addition to the mortality burden described above, there is a significant morbidity burden in these areas with in excess of 1,000 disability adjusted life years lost per 100,000 persons per year [1, 3]. It is therefore not surprising that it is in Asia where the best evidence supporting the impact of vaccination lies.

Taiwan adopted vaccination of infants from HBV surface antigen positive mothers in 1984 and in 1986 this was extended to all infants [4]. The birth cohort of infants born in the early period of implementation (1984–1986), therefore, contains both vaccinated and unvaccinated individuals. This combined with excellent health records and low population migration has allowed detailed studies of the efficacy of vaccination in preventing hepatocellular carcinoma (HCC). At the latest follow-up point, now almost 30 years after the implementation of the vaccination programme, there is a clear signal that the incidence of HCC is reduced by approximately 60% in vaccinated individuals [5]. This confirmation that disease can be prevented through vaccination is welcome, but the continuing occurrence of HBV-related disease despite vaccination suggests failure of vaccination. These failures are attributed to transmission from highly infectious mothers or due to incomplete vaccination, and these highlight opportunities to further improve the preventative efforts in HBV-related disease.

Prevention of Alcohol-Related Liver Disease

ArLD is the major cause of liver-related mortality in the West with as many as 3 quarters of liver-related deaths being attributed to alcohol consumption [6]. In these individuals, deaths are more frequent due to cirrhosis and liver failure (estimated 383,800 per annum) rather than due to primary liver cancer (92,200 annually) [2]. These epidemiological data support previous reports that the competing risk of liver failure–related mortality reduces the burden of HCC in this group [7] with important implications around screening and surveillance for complications in those patients with ArLD. To put this further into context, it is estimated that 60–80% of liver-related deaths in Europe, mostly from liver failure, are due to excess alcohol consumption [8].

Alcohol consumption at a per capita level is identified as the key driver of high rates of alcohol-attributable fractions of cirrhosis globally, and there is a wealth of observational evidence linking the affordability and availability of alcohol to consumption [8]. Examples of this association come from areas of Europe with high mortality rates from ArLD, Iceland and Russia. In Iceland, there was a population study following the derestriction of beer sales in 1989. Sales of alcohol in Iceland is restricted to a state monopoly and as a consequence, the data on alcohol sales (as a surrogate of consumption) are recorded in detail. Additionally, a national mortality registry incorporating details from death certification allowed detailed mortality data to be examined with data on alcohol sales. The derestriction of beer sales was associated with a steady increase in rates of consumption and also importantly with increased mortality specifically from ArLD [9]. An ecological study of alcohol consumption in the former USSR and later Russia highlights a link between socioeconomic events that correlate with the availability and affordability of alcohol and overall mortality in men [10]. These socioeconomic changes illuminate the potential for policy changes to reduce the overall harms from excess alcohol consumption, including the risks of liver-related mortality.

In several regions, there have been moves towards increasing the cost of alcohol through minimum unit pricing as a mechanism to prevent the harmful effects caused due to excess alcohol consumption. Regions in Canada have had this policy in place for a number of years with an appreciable effect on alcohol-related mortality. For instance, in British Columbia, alcohol-related mortality (the majority from liver disease) fell by 32% within a year of a 10% increase in the minimum unit price of all alcoholic drinks [11, 12]. This rapid reduction in mortality is remarkable and has been reported by other studies as well [13]. This strongly suggests that the introduction of a minimum unit price might have a significant and early effect on liver-related mortality.

In the United Kingdom, where rates of ArLD and consequent mortality have risen over the past 2 decades, there has been enthusiasm among public health physicians and researchers for the introduction of a minimum unit price. The data that support this at a modelling level are strong [14, 15]. For example, at a minimum unit price of 45p there would be an estimated reduction in the number of alcohol-related deaths by 600, and a reduction in the number of alcohol-related hospital admissions by approximately 23,000. It is perhaps surprising therefore that the UK government chose to implement a ban of selling alcohol below its cost price rather than a minimum unit price, particularly when the impact of that strategy when modelled in parallel with that of implementation of minimum unit pricing was negligible both in terms of alcohol-related mortality and alcohol-related hospital admissions [14]. Minimum unit pricing has however been passed into law in Scotland. This has been subject to a legal challenge by the drinks industry and that process is ongoing. Given the rapidity with which changes in alcohol-related mortality are expected once minimum unit pricing is introduced, there should be a clear signal as to its effectiveness early after implementation.

Understanding the Natural History of Disease and the Implications for Therapy

HCV infection is of global importance. The epidemiology shows a more even distribution of mortality across the world with approaching 700,000 deaths attributable to its complications annually [3]. While the greatest burden of disease is in Asia and sub-Saharan Africa, there is also a significant burden across the developed world, including North America. For this reason, there has been an ongoing drive to develop novel direct-acting anti-virals for the treatment of HCV infection. That quest has yielded remarkable results. Following the identification of HCV in 1989 and the development of systems to test antiviral compounds, a number of treatments have been licensed for use in patients with HCV infection. These drugs now offer a very high probability of cure with short-duration treatments and a minimal side-effect burden in contrast to the combination of pegylated interferon and ribavirin used over the last 15 years [16]. These treatment methods have the real prospect of changing the natural history of HCV infection and preventing deaths from liver disease, particularly if treatment is given early in the course of infection before significant liver fibrosis has developed.

The cure of HCV infection is defined by the persistent presence of negative assays for HCV in the blood. This sustained virological response (SVR) has been associated in numerous retrospective studies with improved clinical outcomes most particularly in patients with advanced liver fibrosis or cirrhosis. In this population, there are consistent reports of reduced incidence of both liver failure and HCC subsequent to treatment [17, 18]. SVR has never formally been evaluated in a prospective randomised controlled trial, and for that reason it remains an invalidated surrogate end-point despite all of the clinical evidence supporting the benefits of treatment. As a consequence of the lack of validation, birth cohort screening in the United States that aims to identify individuals with HCV infection for treatment has been questioned [19]. The thrust of the arguments against screening and treatment is twofold. First, there are arguments regarding overdiagnosis and overtreatment. It is clear that not all individuals with HCV in the identified birth cohort – in this case, those born between 1945 and 1965 – will develop end-stage liver disease of HCC as a consequence of their infection. Identification of HCV in that group represents "overdiagnosis" that may have consequences on health-related quality of life and by definition treatment of these individuals is overtreatment since no harm would have resulted from infection and treatment in that circumstance only exposes those individuals to risk. Second, in the interferon era, factors negatively associated with treatment efficacy, for instance age, male gender, advanced fibrosis or cirrhosis, and the presence of type 2 diabetes are also associated with a poor outcome regardless of treatment. It is argued, therefore, that SVR occurs preferentially in patients without those risk factors and the magnitude of the benefit of SVR is therefore exaggerated. There is some truth to these arguments, and while they will never be addressed as part of a large-scale trial comparing treatment with no treatment, the development of highly active agents that cure a vast majority of patients renders much of the debate moot.

The focus on SVR, however, remains of prime importance in trials of antiviral therapy and this remains a barrier to studies of clinical outcomes in individuals with HCV infection, particularly as treatment as prevention type interventions are considered to reduce the global prevalence of HCV. As an example for this, Dore and colleagues recently reported a study of combination therapy to treat HCV in patients receiving opiate substitution therapy [20]. They report high rates of virological cure; in some cases, despite ongoing drug use and while this is a necessary first step, it exemplifies the mindset in study design at present. Targeting treatment to this group where transmission of HCV may be high is rational to reduce the prevalence of HCV and while there is good evidence from modelling studies that this is likely to be effective, it is yet to be tested in a clinical trial [21, 22]. The population that would be evaluated in this scenario has been described in a number of other studies of mortality and it is striking that among these there is substantial competing mortality risk. Particularly, these individuals are at increased risk of death from traumatic injury, suicide, and drug-related deaths [23]. In a study from Norway, mortality rates among persons who inject drugs (PWID) admitted to residential treatment centres were recorded and stratified as either liver or non-liver related [24]. At 30 years after first identification, there was no difference in mortality among HCV-positive and -negative individuals. Additionally, liver-related mortality was not observed until 20 years after first admission when overall mortality in the cohort was approximately 30%. The impact of this competing mortality is not explicitly described in the modelling studies and deserves critical analysis in future clinical studies of antiviral treatment in PWID.

Defining the Natural History of NAFLD

Overdiagnosis, overtreatment, and the importance of competing mortality are potentially relevant to the development of treatments for NAFLD, which is now recognised as the most common liver disease in the developed world [25]. It has recently been estimated that 25% of the global adult population has NAFLD. It is remarkable then that mortality from NAFLD has not yet overtaken that of ArLD or indeed viral hepatitis. There are at least 2 possible explanations for this: either the development of end-stage liver disease from NAFLD has not yet had time to develop in those individuals affected or rather the associated type 2 diabetes and the metabolic syndrome also predispose to the development of cardiovascular disease (and other diseases) that intervene before liver disease becomes advanced.

There is accumulating evidence that there is significant competing mortality in NAFLD that parallels what is seen in PWID with HCV. Large, prospective, long-term follow-up studies of individuals with NAFLD remain scarce as the condition was only recognised relatively recently. As a consequence, the natural history of the disease is poorly defined. It is suggested that NAFLD follows the typical paradigm of all chronic liver diseases. In this case, fatty infiltration of the liver (NAFL) is followed by the development of inflammation (non-alcoholic steatohepatitis [NASH]), and this inflammation results in progressive fibrosis that culminates in cirrhosis [26]. As a consequence of this paradigm, most of the long-term follow-up series have relied on individuals having a liver biopsy at entry to the cohort. This has necessarily biased these cohorts away from containing individuals with the multimorbidity that is typical of this patient group at baseline and inevitably this is likely to exaggerate the risks of liver disease. That said, among the published cohort studies, there are consistent findings. The first finding is that liver disease is an infrequent cause of death among patients with NAFLD at baseline. In one of the most prominent series, less than one in 10 deaths was due to either cirrhosis or HCC and the most frequent cause of death was cardiovascular disease [27]. Non-invasive assessments made as part of the NHANES programme have also suggested similar findings, although the individuals whose data are included in those studies are less thoroughly phenotyped than those in the cohort studies [28]. The other consistent finding was that it is the degree of liver fibrosis, rather than the presence of NASH, that is the most important predictor of outcomes in that group [27, 29, 30]. This is not surprising, but it is a critical observation since the endpoints that have been selected and endorsed in early phase clinical trials for novel therapeutics in NAFLD have been reductions in the degree of inflammation observed with treatment. Investigators have recognised that these are surrogate outcome measures, but the importance of this is underappreciated [31]. As large phase 3 studies get underway for the treatment of NAFLD, it will be fascinating to see to what extent they support the current understanding of the natural history of the disease and whether the proposed surrogate endpoints correlate with clinically meaningful endpoints such as the development of cirrhosis and its complications [32]. Without this understanding, the management of patients with NAFLD will be hampered and the rational targeting of therapies to those patients at greatest risk of progressive liver disease will become critical.

Conclusions

Chronic liver disease and its complications are responsible for more than 2 million deaths annually. The development of effective treatments for viral hepatitis has the potential to change the natural history of these diseases, substantially reducing mortality. The role of antiviral treatment in the prevention of HCV infection remains unproved, but it is an attractive strategy to reduce the incidence of that disease. Lessons from the treatment of HCV and the importance of competing mortality will be relevant as treatments for NAFLD become available in the clinic. The challenge of readily identifying patients with progressive liver disease due to NAFLD who will benefit from treatments is a significant one and without improved information regarding the natural history of disease, this will be a barrier to the implementation of treatment.

Disclosure Statement

There are no relevant disclosures for this work.

References

1 GBD 2013 DALYs and HALE Collaborators, Murray CJ, Barber RM, Foreman KJ, Abbasoglu Ozgoren A, Abd-Allah F, et al: Global, regional, and national disability-adjusted life years (DALYs) for 306 diseases and injuries and healthy life expectancy (HALE) for 188 countries, 1990–2013: quantifying the epidemiological transition. Lancet 2015;386:2145–2191.
2 GBD 2013 Mortality and Causes of Death Collaborators: Global, regional, and national age-sex specific all-cause and cause-specific mortality for 240 causes of death, 1990–2013: a systematic analysis for the Global Burden of Disease Study 2013. Lancet 2015;385:117–171.
3 Stanaway JD, Flaxman AD, Naghavi M, Fitzmaurice C, Vos T, Abubakar I, Abu-Raddad LJ, et al: The global burden of viral hepatitis from 1990 to 2013: findings from the Global Burden of Disease Study 2013. Lancet 2016;388:1081–1088.
4 Chen DS, Hsu NH, Sung JL, Hsu TC, Hsu ST, Kuo YT, Lo KJ, et al: A mass vaccination program in Taiwan against hepatitis B virus infection in infants of hepatitis B surface antigen-carrier mothers. JAMA 1987;257:2597–2603.
5 Chang MH, You SL, Chen CJ, Liu CJ, Lai MW, Wu TC, Wu SF, et al: Long-term effects of hepatitis B immunization of infants in preventing liver cancer. Gastroenterology 2016; 151:472–480.e1.
6 Stein E, Cruz-Lemini M, Altamirano J, Ndugga N, Couper D, Abraldes JG, Bataller R: Heavy daily alcohol intake at the population level predicts the weight of alcohol in cirrhosis burden worldwide. J Hepatol 2016;65:998–1005.
7 Jepsen P, Ott P, Andersen PK, Sorensen HT, Vilstrup H: Risk for hepatocellular carcinoma in patients with alcoholic cirrhosis: a Danish nationwide cohort study. Ann Intern Med 2012;156:841–847, W295.
8 Sheron N: Alcohol and liver disease in Europe – simple measures have the potential to prevent tens of thousands of premature deaths. J Hepatol 2016;64:957–967.
9 Tyrfingsson T, Olafsson S, Bjornsson ES, Rafnsson V. Alcohol consumption and liver cirrhosis mortality after lifting ban on beer sales in country with state alcohol monopoly. Eur J Public Health 2015;25:729–731.
10 Zaridze D, Lewington S, Boroda A, Scelo G, Karpov R, Lazarev A, Konobeevskaya I, et al: Alcohol and mortality in Russia: prospective observational study of 151,000 adults. Lancet 2014;383:1465–1473.
11 Treno AJ, Ponicki WR, Stockwell T, Macdonald S, Gruenewald PJ, Zhao J, Martin G, et al: Alcohol outlet densities and alcohol price: the British Columbia experiment in the partial privatization of alcohol sales off-premise. Alcohol Clin Exp Res 2013;37:854–859.
12 Zhao J, Stockwell T, Martin G, Macdonald S, Vallance K, Treno A, Ponicki WR, et al: The relationship between minimum alcohol prices, outlet densities and alcohol-attributable deaths in British Columbia, 2002–2009. Addiction 2013;108:1059–1069.
13 Nemtsov AV: Alcohol-related human losses in Russia in the 1980s and 1990s. Addiction 2002;97:1413–1425.
14 Brennan A, Meng Y, Holmes J, Hill-McManus D, Meier PS: Potential benefits of minimum unit pricing for alcohol versus a ban on below cost selling in England 2014: modelling study. BMJ 2014;349:g5452.
15 Holmes J, Meng Y, Meier PS, Brennan A, Angus C, Campbell-Burton A, Guo Y, et al: Effects of minimum unit pricing for alcohol on different income and socioeconomic groups: a modelling study. Lancet 2014;383:1655–1664.
16 Pawlotsky JM, Feld JJ, Zeuzem S, Hoofnagle JH: From non-A, non-B hepatitis to hepatitis C virus cure. J Hepatol 2015;62:S87–S99.
17 Bruno S, Stroffolini T, Colombo M, Bollani S, Benvegnu L, Mazzella G, Ascione A, et al: Sustained virological response to interferon-alpha is associated with improved outcome in HCV-related cirrhosis: a retrospective study. Hepatology 2007;45:579–587.
18 van der Meer AJ, Hansen BE, Janssen HL: Sustained virological response to treatment in patients with chronic hepatitis C – reply. JAMA 2013;309:1457.

19 Koretz RL, Lin KW, Ioannidis JP, Lenzer J: Is widespread screening for hepatitis C justified? BMJ 2015;350:g7809.
20 Dore GJ, Altice F, Litwin AH, Dalgard O, Gane EJ, Shibolet O, Luetkemeyer A, et al: Elbasvir-Grazoprevir to treat hepatitis C Virus infection in persons receiving opioid agonist therapy: a randomized trial. Ann Intern Med 2016;165:625–634.
21 Martin NK, Vickerman P, Grebely J, Hellard M, Hutchinson SJ, Lima VD, Foster GR, et al: Hepatitis C virus treatment for prevention among people who inject drugs: modeling treatment scale-up in the age of direct-acting antivirals. Hepatology 2013;58:1598–1609.
22 Martin NK, Vickerman P, Miners A, Foster GR, Hutchinson SJ, Goldberg DJ, Hickman M: Cost-effectiveness of hepatitis C virus antiviral treatment for injection drug user populations. Hepatology 2012;55:49–57.
23 Gibson A, Randall D, Degenhardt L: The increasing mortality burden of liver disease among opioid-dependent people: cohort study. Addiction 2011;106:2186–2192.
24 Kielland KB, Skaug K, Amundsen EJ, Dalgard O: All-cause and liver-related mortality in hepatitis C infected drug users followed for 33 years: a controlled study. J Hepatol 2013;58:31–37.
25 Younossi ZM, Koenig AB, Abdelatif D, Fazel Y, Henry L, Wymer M: Global epidemiology of nonalcoholic fatty liver disease – meta-analytic assessment of prevalence, incidence, and outcomes. Hepatology 2016;64:73–84.
26 Rinella ME, Sanyal AJ: Management of NAFLD: a stage-based approach. Nat Rev Gastroenterol Hepatol 2016;13:196–205.
27 Ekstedt M, Hagstrom H, Nasr P, Fredrikson M, Stal P, Kechagias S, Hultcrantz R: Fibrosis stage is the strongest predictor for disease-specific mortality in NAFLD after up to 33 years of follow-up. Hepatology 2015;61:1547–1554.
28 Kim D, Kim WR, Kim HJ, Therneau TM: Association between noninvasive fibrosis markers and mortality among adults with nonalcoholic fatty liver disease in the United States. Hepatology 2013;57:1357–1365.
29 Angulo P, Kleiner DE, Dam-Larsen S, Adams LA, Bjornsson ES, Charatcharoenwitthaya P, Mills PR, et al: Liver fibrosis, but no other histologic features, is associated with long-term outcomes of patients with nonalcoholic fatty liver disease. Gastroenterology 2015;149:389–397.e10.
30 Angulo P, Bugianesi E, Bjornsson ES, Charatcharoenwitthaya P, Mills PR, Barrera F, Haflidadottir S, et al: Simple noninvasive systems predict long-term outcomes of patients with nonalcoholic fatty liver disease. Gastroenterology 2013;145:782–789.e4.
31 Sanyal AJ; EPA-E Investigators: Reply: to PMID 24818764. Gastroenterology 2015;148:262–263.
32 Sanyal AJ, Neuschwander-Tetri BA, Tonascia J: End points must be clinically meaningful for drug development in nonalcoholic fatty liver disease. Gastroenterology 2016;150:11–13.

Hepatology 2016 – The Panorama

Digestive Diseases

Dig Dis 2017;35:310–313
DOI: 10.1159/000456581

Liver Fibrosis: Understanding the Dynamics of Bidirectional Wound Repair to Inform the Design of Markers and Therapies

John P. Iredale[a] Antonella Pellicoro[b] Jonathan A. Fallowfield[c]

[a]Pro Vice-Chancellor Health, University of Bristol, Senate House, Bristol, [b]Post Doctoral Fellow, and [c]NHS Research Scotland Senior Clinical Fellow, MRC/University of Edinburgh Centre for Inflammation Research, Queen's Medical Research Institute, Edinburgh, UK

Keywords
Fibrosis · Tissue inhibitors of metalloproteinases-1 · Collagen · Relaxin · RXFP1 · Portal hypertension · Fibrosis resolution · Biomarker

Abstract
Background: Liver fibrosis is the final common pathway of iterative or chronic liver damage. When it reaches an advanced stage, cirrhosis develops and this indicates a loss of normal liver architecture, disruption of normal blood flow, the development of nodules of proliferative hepatocytes and consequent functional failure. Cirrhosis is also associated with life-threatening complications. Importantly, this dysregulation of blood flow involves changes resulting from both architectural disruption and a dynamic rise in portal pressure mediated in part by the contraction of myofibroblasts – the major cell mediator of the fibrogenic process – which are derived from hepatic stellate cells (HSC) and termed activated HSC (myofibroblast/activated HSC). ***Key Messages:*** There is now compelling data from both rodent and human models that liver fibrosis is bidirectional. By studying models of progressive and regressing liver fibrosis it has been possible to identify mediators that may be therapeutic targets. Arguably, by identifying the mediators of spontaneous resolution that result in a return of normal architecture, the attributes of a highly effective antifibrotic or pro resolution therapy can be defined. Among these key attributes, understanding the balance of matrix-degrading enzymes and their inhibitors (the metalloproteinases and Tissue inhibitors of metalloproteinases (TIMPs), respectively) led to the identification of both therapeutic targets and the value of TIMP-1 as a serum marker of fibrosis. Furthermore, the action of a potential therapeutic agent, relaxin (RLN) acting through its cognate G-protein coupled receptor (RXFP1) on the surface of activated HSC shows promise. Activation of the RLN-RXFP1-mediated pathway can be detected in vivo by measuring the dynamic contractility of activated HSC and the consequent changes in portal pressure and blood flow as a responsive physical biomarker. ***Conclusion:*** By understanding progressive and resolving liver fibrosis, a series of therapeutic targets have been identified. At the same time, key mediators of fibrosis may have an integral role to play as soluble or physical biomarkers.

Introduction

Liver fibrosis is the final common pathway of iterative or chronic liver damage [1, 2]. When fibrosis reaches an advanced stage, cirrhosis develops – which indicates a

KARGER

E-Mail karger@karger.com
www.karger.com/ddi

John P. Iredale, DM, FRCP, FMedSci, FRSE
Pro Vice-Chancellor Health, University of Bristol
Senate House, Tyndall Avenue
Bristol BS8 1TH (UK)
E-Mail pvc-health@bristol.ac.uk

loss of normal liver architecture, disruption of normal blood flow, the development of nodules of proliferative hepatocytes and consequent functional failure [1, 2]. Cirrhosis is also associated with life-threatening complications, which include the complications of portal hypertension, hepatic failure and the development of hepatocellular cancer. Importantly, the pathological rise in portal pressure associated with fibrosis and cirrhosis results from both the architectural disruption of flow and a dynamic rise in pressure mediated by the contraction of the myofibroblast/activated hepatic stellate cell (HSC) – the major cell mediator of the fibrogenic process (see below) [1–4]. In this review, we describe how we have identified both biomarkers of the fibrotic process and potential antifibrotic approaches by studying cell, molecular, rodent and human models. These have demonstrated that fibrosis is a bidirectional process, demonstrating both progression and regression phases and in some cases spontaneous resolution to a near normal architecture [1, 2]. Further, by using the contractile behaviour of the liver myofibroblast-activated HSC as a bio-readout of receptor targeting on the major fibrogenic cell, we have identified a potential antifibrotic pathway active in vivo, which may also mediate a reduction in portal pressure.

Liver Fibrosis Is Bidirectional

Numerous studies now point to a model of liver fibrogenesis in which resident and incoming innate inflammatory cells, responding to hepatocellular damage, infiltrate the injured liver and through cascades of autocrine and paracrine signalling initiate the fibrogenic response [5, 6]. Prominent among the infiltrating cells is the macrophage. Distinct from the resident tissue macrophage or Kupffer Cell, deletion of recruited inflammatory monocyte-macrophages is associated with a reduction in the resulting fibrotic response, suggesting that these cells orchestrate this initial component [5–7]. Macrophages are important sources of the cytokines-transforming growth factor beta-1 (TGFB-1) and platelet-derived growth factor (PDGF), which regulate the key attributes of the function and phenotype of the HSC [3]. The perisinusoidal HSC are now known to be the key mediators of the fibrogenic process. In response to soluble factors including those released by macrophages, damaged or dead cells and other stimuli, including altered cell-matrix interactions, HSCs undergo a dramatic phenotypic switch, shedding their retinoid droplets, expressing smooth muscle cell contractile filaments (including alpha smooth muscle actin) and adopt a phenotype physically indistinguishable from a myofibroblast [1–4]. In this so-called activated phenotype (myofibroblast/activated HSC), these cells become the liver wound–healing myofibroblast and respond to PDGF and other stimuli by proliferating. Myofibroblast/activated HSC are also the major source of the fibrillar collagens; collagens-I and III, which characterise pathological fibrosis. Indeed myofibroblast/activated HSC are highly responsive to TGFB1 stimulation [3], which by upregulating collagen-I gene expression, functions as the most potent fibrogenic stimulus in the cascades associated with liver injury. Activated HSC also regulate matrix degradation. Inflammatory cells including macrophages and myofibroblast/activated HSC secrete a range of matrix-degrading metalloproteinases (MMPs). In the context of progressive fibrosis, the expression of true interstitial collagenases – the MMPs with activity that results in the initial cleavage of the collagen helix, thereby rendering it susceptible to degradation by more promiscuous enzymes and gelatinases – remains constant or decreases inside the liver [8]. However, in partial response to TGFB1 signalling, myofibroblast/activated HSC have been shown to be a potent source of tissue inhibitors of metalloproteinases (TIMPs) 1 and 2 [1, 2, 8, 9]. Indeed, the activation of HSC is associated with an upregulation of TIMP-1 gene expression that precedes the one seen for collagen-I in the same cell. The presence of these secreted and potent MMP inhibitors holds matrix degradation in check [8, 9]. The result is that progressive fibrosis occurs not only due to a rise in the number of matrix-producing activated HSC expressing fibrillar collagens; but through the expression of TIMPs, the pattern of matrix degradation is altered favouring the net accumulation of scar. In effect, the progression of fibrosis can be considered in part a failure of matrix degradation [8, 9].

Over the last 30 years, this model and its components have proven to be extremely robust and durable. Furthermore, these studies have identified a number of serum markers associated with the process of progressive fibrosis, which have been shown to be more or less useful in various studies of liver fibrosis and its complications and the risks of specific complications. These serum markers include the products of collagen and matrix metabolism associated with its processing as it is laid down (hyaluronic acid, P3NP) and products secreted into the extracellular space that are associated with collagen and other matrix accumulation such as TIMP-1 [10].

Previously considered irreversible, the presence of the matrix-degrading potential in diseased and fibrotic liver suggested that remodelling of existing fibrosis might be possible [1, 2, 8, 9, 11]. We and others have studied this potential using rodent models – work that has been complemented by large-scale therapeutic trials in human models (notably of antivirals deployed in the context of chronic viral hepatitis). Numerous studies now confirm that on withdrawal or suppression of the injurious stimulus, spontaneous resolution of fibrosis with a return or normal or near-normal architecture is possible [1, 2, 8, 9, 11]. Indeed, in advanced cirrhotic models in both humans and rodents, remodelling can be observed. Detailed studies of these models identified that after the withdrawal of the injurious stimulus, the number of myofibroblast/activated HSC decreases significantly and rapidly [1, 2]. This is mediated both through apoptosis [1, 2, 11–14] of these cells and phenotypic reversion to a more quiescent phenotype (although cells that have undergone reversion are primed to respond more avidly to further fibrotic stimuli in comparison to unstimulated quiescent HSC) [15–17]. This net reduction in the number of myofibroblast/activated HSC is associated with a reduction in the expression of collagen but crucially also associated with a reduction in TIMP-1 within the liver. In turn, the net hepatic collagenase activity increases and matrix degradation occurs with consequent remodelling. Interestingly, the recruited inflammatory monocyte-macrophage, crucial to the progression of fibrosis, undergoes a phenotypic switch after cessation of liver injury, which is in part the result of phagocytosis of apoptotic debris. Identifiable by being $LY6C^{hi}$, following cessation of injury the inflammatory monocyte-macrophage downregulates the expression of this marker and expresses collagenase and elastase and mediates matrix degradation [6, 7, 12, 18]. Indeed, cell lineage deletion experiments indicate that loss of this population at the onset of resolution is associated with a critical reduction in hepatic collagenase and a failure of matrix remodelling.

Relaxin as an Antifibrotic/Proresolution Therapy

We and others identified that the mammalian hormone relaxin (RLN) might have value as an antifibrotic (or more accurately proresolution) mediator by virtue of its specific actions [19]. Stimulating a GPCR (RXFP1), RLN appears to act as a paracrine inhibitor of fibrogenesis through the regulation of 3 of the key players in progressive and resolving fibrosis in a manner that would favour net matrix degradation. Specifically, in addition to a series of other effects, RLN downregulates collagen-I and TIMP-1, while upregulating interstitial collagenase (MMP-1 in humans). Furthermore, the activation of HSC is associated with an upregulation of RXFP1. Indeed, RXFP1 expression is upregulated on myofibroblast/activated HSC in fibrotic liver disease in humans and in a variety of experimental fibrotic liver injuries in rats [19]. Early studies using HSC cell culture and experimental fibrosis models demonstrated that RLN would downregulate both collagen-I and TIMP-1 and when administered in the context of ongoing experimental injury was associated with a reduction in fibrosis [19].

RLN and Myofibroblast Contraction – Identifying a Dynamic Physical Biomarker of GPCR Targeting

Because myofibroblast/activated HSC contractility contributes approximately 30% to the increase in intrahepatic vascular resistance seen in fibrosis and cirrhosis, we went on to examine the effect of RLN, mediated via RXFP1, on myofibroblast contraction and portal hypertension. By analysing pathologically distinct models of sinusoidal portal hypertension with simultaneous assessment of gene expression and mediator secretion in response to RLN-RXFP1 signalling, we were able to show that RLN induced a significant reduction in portal pressure with no detrimental effect on systemic arterial pressure [19]. Analysis of liver and serum indicated that RLN stimulation of RXFP1 was associated with the augmentation of intrahepatic NO signaling and a reduction in contractile filament expression in myofibroblasts/activated HSC, but circulating serum levels of NO were unaffected [19]. Recombinant human RLN-2 (serelaxin) is in the process of clinical development for the treatment of acute heart failure and has already been shown to have a favourable pharmacokinetic and safety profile in patients with hepatic impairment (Child–Pugh class A, B, and C) [20]. We are undertaking studies of portal pressure and hepatic and renal blood flow in models of human cirrhosis to further examine the therapeutic effects of RLN (ClinicalTrials.gov identifier: NCT01640964). Thus, we have established that because of common receptor-mediated signalling, the effective targeting of RXFP1 on the myofibroblast/activated HSC can be detected by measuring the portal pressure and blood flow; in effect a physical biomarker. Moreover, the direct effect of RLN on rapid readout parameters during advanced fibrosis and its organ selectivity are useful attributes in clinical trials in cirrhosis patients.

Summary

The last 20 years have seen an explosion in our knowledge regarding the processes and mediators that underlie progressive and resolving fibrosis. The models that have been developed have proven to be durable and highly reproducible and have shown that fibrosis is bidirectional. Furthermore, with our understanding of fibrosis greatly developed, physical and soluble biomarkers have been identified, which may add value to our therapeutic interventions as we approach this major unmet health need.

Disclosure Statement

JPI has advised Novartis on antifibrotic drugs. Remuneration was paid to the Universities of Bristol and Edinburgh.

References

1 Pellicoro A, Ramachandran P, Iredale JP, et al: Liver fibrosis and repair: immune regulation of wound healing in a solid organ. Nat Rev Immunol 2014;14:181–194.
2 Iredale JP: Models of liver fibrosis: exploring the dynamic nature of inflammation and repair in a solid organ. J Clin Invest 2007;117:539–548.
3 Friedman SL: Seminars in medicine of the Beth Israel Hospital, Boston. The cellular basis of hepatic fibrosis. Mechanisms and treatment strategies. N Engl J Med 1993;328:1828–1835.
4 Friedman SL, Roll FJ, Boyles J, et al: Hepatic lipocytes: the principal collagen-producing cells of normal rat liver. Proc Natl Acad Sci U S A 1985;82:8681–8685.
5 Karlmark KR, Weiskirchen R, Zimmermann HW, et al: Hepatic recruitment of the inflammatory Gr1+ monocyte subset upon liver injury promotes hepatic fibrosis. Hepatology 2009;50:261–274.
6 Wynn TA, Barron L: Macrophages: master regulators of inflammation and fibrosis. Semin Liver Dis 2010;30:245–257.
7 Duffield JS, Forbes SJ, Constandinou CM, et al: Selective depletion of macrophages reveals distinct, opposing roles during liver injury and repair. J Clin Invest 2005;115:56–65.
8 Iredale JP: Tissue inhibitors of metalloproteinases in liver fibrosis. Int J Biochem Cell Biol 1997;29:43–54.
9 Yoshiji H, Kuriyama S, Yoshii J, et al: Tissue inhibitor of metalloproteinases-1 attenuates spontaneous liver fibrosis resolution in the transgenic mouse. Hepatology 2002;36(4 pt 1):850–860.
10 Rosenberg WM, Voelker M, thiel R, et al: Serum markers detect the presence of liver fibrosis: a cohort study. Gastroenterology 2004;127:1704–1713.
11 Issa R, Zhou X, Constandinou CM, et al: Spontaneous recovery from micronodular cirrhosis: evidence for incomplete resolution associated with matrix cross-linking. Gastroenterology 2004;126:1795–1808.
12 Ramachandran P, Pellicoro A, Vernon MA, et al: Differential Ly-6C expression identifies the recruited macrophage phenotype, which orchestrates the regression of murine liver fibrosis. Proc Natl Acad Sci U S A 2012;109:E3186–E3195.
13 Preaux AM, D'ortho MP, Bralet MP, et al: Apoptosis of human hepatic myofibroblasts promotes activation of matrix metalloproteinase-2. Hepatology 2002;36:615–622.
14 Wright MC, Issa R, Smart DE, et al: Gliotoxin stimulates the apoptosis of human and rat hepatic stellate cells and enhances the resolution of liver fibrosis in rats. Gastroenterology 2001;121:685–698.
15 Troeger JS, Mederacke I, Gwak GY, et al: Deactivation of hepatic stellate cells during liver fibrosis resolution in mice. Gastroenterology 2012;143:1073–1083.e22.
16 Kisseleva T, Cong M, Paik Y, et al: Myofibroblasts revert to an inactive phenotype during regression of liver fibrosis. Proc Natl Acad Sci U S A 2012;109:9448–9453.
17 Kisseleva T, Brenner DA: Hepatic stellate cells and the reversal of fibrosis. J Gastroenterol Hepatol 2006;21(suppl 3):S84–S87.
18 Pellicoro A, Aucott RL, Ramachandran P, et al: Elastin accumulation is regulated at the level of degradation by macrophage metalloelastase (MMP-12) during experimental liver fibrosis. Hepatology 2012;55:1965–1975.
19 Fallowfield JA, Hayden AL, Snowdon VK, et al: Relaxin modulates human and rat hepatic myofibroblast function and ameliorates portal hypertension in vivo. Hepatology 2014;59:1492–1504.
20 Kobalava Z, Villevalde S, Kotovskaya Y, et al: Pharmacokinetics of serelaxin in patients with hepatic impairment: a single-dose, open-label, parallel group study. Br J Clin Pharmacol 2015;79:937–945.

Digestive Diseases

Hepatology 2016 – The Panorama

Dig Dis 2017;35:314–322
DOI: 10.1159/000456582

Current and Future Magnetic Resonance Technologies for Assessing Liver Disease in Clinical and Experimental Medicine

Stephen J. Bawden R.A. Scott Guruprasad P. Aithal

NIHR Nottingham Digestive Diseases Biomedical Research Unit, Nottingham University Hospitals NHS Trust and University of Nottingham, Nottingham, UK

Keywords
Fibrosis · MRI · Magnetic resonance spectroscopy · Portal hypertension · Steatosis

Abstract

Background: In the past decades, a number of non-invasive methods have emerged for detecting and estimating liver fibrosis; these include both serum-based panels and imaging-based technology. Some of these methods are now being incorporated in clinical practice. However, the limitations of the current techniques include lack of organ specificity, sampling errors and limited ability to reflect the efficacy of interventions. ***Key Messages:*** Novel magnetic resonance (MR)-based techniques provide an opportunity to bring about further changes in the investigations and management of patients with liver diseases. Multimodal quantitative MR techniques enable the estimation of fat, iron accumulation, degree of liver injury/inflammation and fibrosis within the whole liver without the need for administering contrast agents. Architectural changes within the liver can be evaluated concurrently with portal haemodynamic changes allowing non-invasive assessment of portal hypertension and effects of interventions. A combination ultra-high field (7T) provides greater sensitivity with a potential to distinguish inflammation from fibrosis on imaging and determine specific types of fats (saturated vs. unsaturated) present within the liver using MR spectroscopy. ^{13}C MR spectroscopy can estimate glutathione flux and rate of beta oxidation in-vivo providing novel tools for experimental studies that evaluate the efficacy of interventions as well as underlying mechanisms. ***Conclusions:*** Translational research should focus on converting the potentials of these innovative methodologies into clinical applications for the benefit of patients.

Introduction

A number of non-invasive tests have been evaluated over the past decade to assess the degree of structural changes within the liver. These include algorithms derived from a combination of routine tests, panel of biomarkers that directly reflect the pathogenic process involved in liver injury, inflammation and fibrosis as well as imaging modalities, some of which are ready to be used in clinical practice [1]. Magnetic resonance (MR) technologies provide unique methods for imaging the whole liver and abdomen. As a result, several favourable characteristics required to stratify chronic liver diseases are obtained. These methodologies are non-invasive, provide objective measurements, are organ-specific and do not use ionising radiation. They measure multiple parameters in a single scan session and some assess the liver functions through dynamic routines.

KARGER

E-Mail karger@karger.com
www.karger.com/ddi

Prof. Guruprasad Aithal
NIHR Nottingham Digestive Diseases Biomedical Research Unit at the Nottingham University Hospitals NHS Trust and the University of Nottingham, Queens Medical Centre Campus, E Floor, West Block, Derby Road, Nottingham NG7 2UH (UK)
E-Mail guru.aithal@nottingham.ac.uk

More recently, a wider range of MRI measurements have been developed to measure liver disease, including T_1 mapping of liver fibrosis [2], MR elastography [3], R_2* mapping/susceptibility [4] and gradient echo fat-fraction measurements (also referred to as Dixon scanning) [5]. Also, advances in proton and multi-nuclear MR spectroscopy (MRS) have opened up a range of otherwise inaccessible parameters for examination [6, 7]. These tools provide novel opportunities for measuring liver disease, metabolism and oxidative stress in ways that were previously not possible.

This paper reviews some of the new technologies currently being used and developed, leading to exciting possibilities for future hepatic studies in experimental medicine, efficacy and mechanism evaluation.

MRI Measurements

Liver Stiffness

Liver stiffness measurement assessed with ultrasound-based transient elastography (TE) has already found its place in clinical practice as a technique to stratify patients with chronic liver disease with a high negative predictive value for ruling out advanced fibrosis [1]. TE-based controlled attenuation parameter (CAP) measurements provide an opportunity to assess the degree of fat as well as fibrosis at the same time. Accumulation of fat and fibrosis can also be assessed by using MRI-based elastography combined with the estimation of proton density fat fraction (PDFF); MRI techniques have higher diagnostic performance when compared with the technique obtained by combining TE and CAP in the non-invasive assessment of liver fibrosis and steatosis [8]. Interestingly, MRI permits the use of intrinsic internal body motions rather than externally induced vibration waves in elastography. Cardiac-induced [9] or respiratory-induced [10] motion and deformation of the liver can non-invasively assess liver stiffness related to fibrosis using clinically available imaging tools. Liver stiffness assessed with cardiac-induced liver motion and deformation can also stratify between different Child–Pugh grades of cirrhosis [11]. These techniques, however, are constrained by patient factors and assessment is primarily constrained to the left lobe of the liver.

T_1 Measurements of Fibrosis

Two prospective studies have shown that differing measures of liver longitudinal relaxation time (T_1) correlate well to histological fibrosis [12, 13]. For T_1 measures, the acquisition and analysis are highly repeatable in healthy subjects, with a coefficient of variation between visits of 1.8% and low inter- and intra-observer variability with intra-class correlation coefficients of >0.99 [13].

Liver T_1 measurements are influenced by confounding factors, dependent on the MRI technique employed. These include inflammation [13], iron [14–16], fat [17] and oedema [18, 19]. Iron accumulation in liver tissue reduces T2 and T2* relaxation times [15, 16], and an increase in iron will also reduce T_1 in the liver [14]. Iron concentrations can be accurately evaluated with T2* [20], which corrects T_1.

Liver T_1 can be acquired independent of steatosis with fat suppression [13]. Alternative approaches aim to correct T_1 by quantifying hepatic lipid content using localised cardiac-triggered proton spectroscopy in a selected region of interest [12]. However, this approach leaves T_1 vulnerable to hepatic fat interference [21].

The principle unresolved issue with MR measures of liver T_1 is its ability to separate inflammation and fibrosis [13]. MR characteristics of a tissue are exaggerated at higher field strengths. Exploratory work at ultra-high field strength (7T) will hope to identify discriminant hepatic markers to improve diagnostic information at lower field strength scans as they have in other diseases. One such marker could be quantifying the changes in the angio-architecture as cirrhosis progresses. A recent study stratified patients with cirrhosis by evaluating changes in hepatocyte perfusion with ultrasound and injected contrast [22]. MRI may be able to objectively quantify these changes without contrast and overcome the inherent limitations of ultrasound-based techniques.

Portal Pressure

Development of portal hypertension is a major landmark in the natural history of liver cirrhosis, with a majority of clinical manifestations being consequences of portal hypertension. Hepatic venous pressure gradient (HVPG) measurement is the only validated technique to accurately evaluate changes in portal pressure. However, HVPG measurements are invasive and available only in specialised hepatology units, precluding the use of HVPG in routine clinical practice.

MR parameters related to both hepatic architecture and splanchnic circulation have recently been significantly correlated to HVPG [23]. Univariate measures associated with HVPG included liver T_1 relaxation time (Pearson R = 0.835, $p < 0.001$), splenic artery (Pearson R = 0.584, p = 0.003), superior mesenteric artery (Pearson R = 0.534, p = 0.002), and azygous vein (Spearman R = 0.656, $p < 0.001$).

Table 1. A comparison of MRI and MRS methods of measuring the liver-fat fraction

	Fat fraction MR measurement technique	
	MRI	MRS
Terminology used	Dixon, multi-echo, gradient echo, SPGR MRI, IDEAL	^{1}H MRS, MRS, PRESS-MRS, STEAM-MRS, single voxel spectroscopy
Current methodology	6 echoes acquired, complex data fit, 6 peak spectral model	STEAM or PRESS localized (~20 × 20 × 20 mm), acquired at different echo, corrected for T_2 decay
Advantages	Produces fat-fraction maps Visually impressive Many scanners have in-built fitting Easy to interpret	High sensitivity Types of fat can be assessed Fewer assumptions required Less effected by B_0 inhomogeneity
Limitations	Less accurate at low noise Cannot determine types of fat Requires good fitting algorithms Effected by high B_0 inhomogeneity	Acquired in single voxel only May be subject to sampling error Requires more expertise for analysis

A proposed multivariate model combining Liver T_1 and splenic artery velocity accurately correlated with HVPG measurement ($R = 0.90$, $p < 0.001$) uniquely among surrogate markers, including those with clinically significant portal hypertension.

It remains to be established whether these new MRI techniques can stratify changes in HVPG after interventions, for example, to assess beta-blocker therapy for lowering portal pressure (HVPG to <12 mm Hg or reduction of 20% from baseline). Postprandial hyperaemia has long been known to increase the portal pressure [24]. In a pilot study, 10 healthy subjects and 10 patients with compensated cirrhosis were given a liquid meal challenge [25]. Quantitative MRI measures detected significant changes over time in both groups in the portal vein, hepatic artery and azygous vein. The coefficient of variation of these measurements was very small (all <8.5%). This data suggests that newly developed MRI measures are sensitive and accurate in measuring changes as a result of an intervention.

Fat-Water Separation

Many advances have been made in fat-water separation MRI over the last 20 years [26]. The technique has developed over time and as such has been referred to by a number of names as shown in Table 1. The basic principle of all these techniques is the same and relies on a shift in MR frequency between hydrogen nuclei in fat and water. Images are acquired at a number of echo times and the change in signal over time is fitted to a signal model to produce separate fat-only and water-only images, which can then be used to quantify liver fat fraction [27, 28]. This calculated fat fraction is in fact a signal-fat fraction and not a mass-fat fraction as determined through biopsies, and is therefore the ratio of mobile fat molecules to mobile fat and water molecules, and has been termed by some as PDFF [27]. This value can be converted to mass fat fraction by including some assumed tissue properties (which are generally accepted) into the fat fraction calculation [29, 30], but this should be stated in a study's methodology. It is important therefore for clinicians to understand that all MR techniques – both MRI and MRS – provide PDFF, which can be converted to a mass-fat fraction, if required.

There are many publications that have developed and optimized these techniques, focussing on both the acquisition parameters and the fitting algorithms. The most recent methods acquire over a number of echoes and fit for multiple fat peaks, T2* relaxation and field offset [31] providing a quick, non-invasive measurement of liver fat fraction acquired in a single breath-hold. These have been well validated at 1.5T [32] and compared with 3T [33] and uniquely allow for measurements of fat distribution across the liver, whereas biopsies (and MRS) only focus on a small sample. MRI fat-water separation also provides a structural image simultaneously, which can be used for liver volume measurements and blood vessel exclusion, and fitting algorithms also determine T2* relaxation times [34], which are relevant in some conditions such as iron overload [4].

Considering the extensive efforts made to optimize, validate and improve these methods, there are fewer pub-

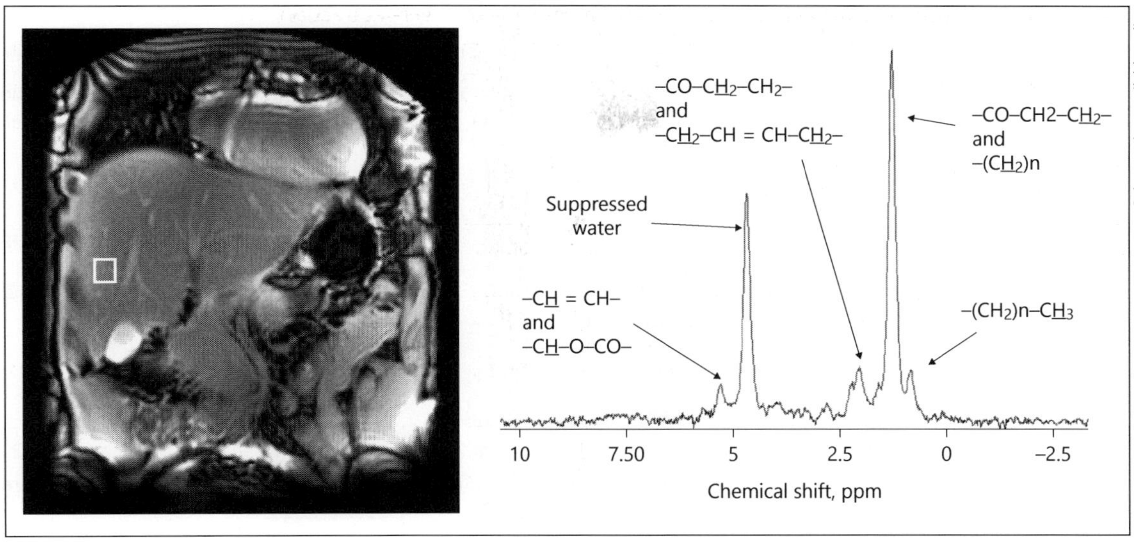

Color version available online

Fig. 1. Magnetic resonance (MR) image of liver showing voxel of interest (left) and example proton MR spectrum, 1H MR spectroscopy, acquired in vivo from the lower right lobe of human liver showing various fatty acid proton peaks.

lications that have used this technique in cross-sectional or interventional studies of fatty liver disease [35] and MRS is still considered the gold standard imaging modality for the estimation of liver fat [36] as discussed at length below. However, the advantages of MRI fat-fraction measurements are increasingly being recognised, and the technique is more readily available on clinical scanners [37] and requires less expertise for analysis.

Proton and Multinuclear MRS

^{1}H MRS Measurements of Liver Fat Fraction

MRI relies on frequency and phase encoding signal from hydrogen nuclei to generate images. By contrast, ^{1}H MRS acquires proton signals from a localised volume to produce a "chemical shift spectrum" with signal peaks corresponding to individual hydrogen nuclei within specific molecules of interest. This provides a powerful tool for quantifying the amount of a specific chemical present within a sample. The dominant signal in biological tissue comes from water (~4.7 ppm), but other substances are also accessible, such as signal from fatty acid chains (main CH_2 peak ~1.3 ppm).

Liver fat fraction can be determined using this technique by taking the fat to water signal ratio. Compared to fat-water MRI techniques described above, which measure fat fractions indirectly through fitting algorithms, MRS is much more sensitive and directly acquires well-resolved signals from hydrogen in the fatty acid chain [38]. As such, MRS also allows for the quantification of specific fatty acid species such as mono- vs. poly- unsaturated and long- vs. short-fatty acid chains as show in Figure 1 [39, 40]. Much work has been done to develop and optimize MRS methodology for in vivo liver fat measurements [41] and current techniques use spin-echo localisation sequences to acquire spectra from a volume of interest (typically 20 × 20 × 20 mm) at a range of echo times used for T_2 correction. This has been validated against absolute fat measurements [29] and histology [42–44] and provides an accurate and repeatable measure of liver fat fraction [30]. A comparison of MRI and MRS fat fraction measurements is presented in Table 1.

^{1}H MRS has been the cornerstone of investigations delineating mechanisms underlying ectopic fat deposition and its response to interventions, which has great clinical significance especially because non-alcoholic fatty liver disease (NAFLD) has become the most common chronic liver disease [45]. In addition, the association of hepatic steatosis with hepatic insulin resistance, which is a key step in the pathogenesis of type 2 diabetes, has resulted in the use of liver fat as an important short-term outcome in the evaluation of dietary and lifestyle interventions in metabolic syndrome.

A previous study, for example, used MRS to investigate the effect of high fat diets and found significant increase in liver fat fraction after only 4 days of intervention

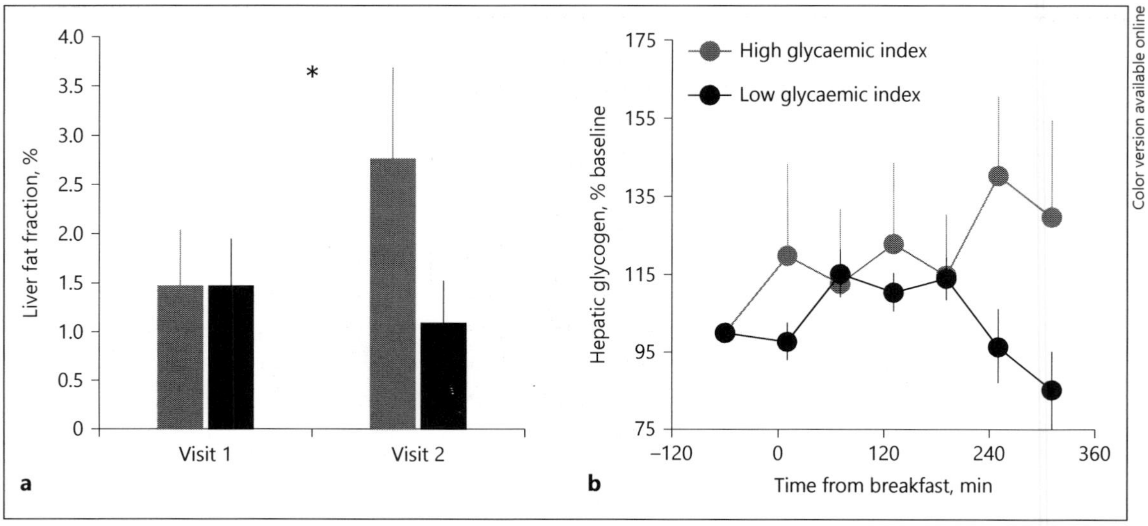

Fig. 2. Liver fat fraction before (visit 1) and after (visit 2) a high versus low glycaemic index diet (**a**); and glycogen response to high versus low glycaemic index test meal (**b**). Reproduced with permission from Bawden et al. [59].

[46] (this effect was actually alleviated when protein was added to the diet). While fat deposition following high fat diets is perhaps expected, less obvious is the impact of carbohydrate intake, which can enter fatty deposition via de novo lipogenesis. Early work suggested that this pathway is not traversed when energy balance (intake versus expenditure) is maintained [47]. However, using high field ^{1}H MRS, a recent study indicated that high carbohydrate diet increased liver fat stores more than high fat diet, and this finding is also supported by other studies [48].

Beyond the amount of carbohydrate consumed, ^{1}H MRS has also enabled the exploration of the effect of different types of carbohydrates, which potentially have different metabolic impacts. For example, previous work had hypothesised that excess fructose intake negatively affected liver health more than glucose [49], whereas a recent randomised controlled trial using ^{1}H MRS to measure liver fat before and after a 2-week excess energy diet of either fructose or glucose showed that increased energy intake caused a significant rise in fat-fraction, but there was not significant difference between glucose and fructose [50]. Similarly, a recent 1-week energy neutral dietary intervention study (no weight loss or gain) found increased liver fat stores following high versus low glycaemic index foods (Fig. 2b) [51], verifying findings from cross-sectional studies [52]. MRS therefore provides a powerful tool to non-invasively test hypotheses in experimental medicine and probe small changes in liver fat fraction induced through lifestyle interventions.

^{13}C MRS Measurements of Liver Glycogen

While many studies have investigated liver lipid deposition, few have explored in vivo control of glycogen stores. Given that glycogen in the liver forms the primary immediate short-term energy store between meals, this provides an important measure to understand metabolic function in the liver and disease pathogenesis. Multinuclear MRS offers a unique method of investigating these stores in real time in vivo and currently provides the only way of monitoring glycogen levels in human subjects without the need for biopsy. As opposed to acquiring the signal from protons, glycogen MRS uses the signal produced from C_1 in the glycogen molecule, which has a chemical shift of 100.5 ppm [53]. There are a number of difficulties that need to be overcome to accurately apply this technique and the measurement is inherently less sensitive than proton MRS. This is largely due to 2 factors – first, only the ^{13}C isotope is MR visible, which has a natural abundance isotopic ratio of ~1% total carbon; and second, the gyromagnetic ratio of ^{13}C is ~25% of hydrogen. Despite this, acquisition routines can be optimized to provide accurate measurements even at low abundance, and in many ways, the liver is an ideal organ for this, as it has a large volume with homogenous tissue type close to the surface of the body. The signal from glycogen can therefore be averaged over a large region of interest using specialized coils positioned over the right upper quadrant. Additionally, the concentration of glycogen is much greater in the liver compared with other tissues in this region of the body so the received signal is dominated by hepatic glycogen stores. From the time that natural abundance ^{13}C MRS measurements of hepatic glycogen levels were first suggested [53], the technique has been validated multiple times [7, 54]. Stephenson et al. [30] also tested measurement repeatability at high field (3T) and reported a single-session coefficient of variation in hepatic ^{13}C MRS measurement of 13% making this a feasible technique for many studies comparing the effects of nutritional intake or exercise [55] and also the differences between healthy volunteers and patients [56]. The low natural abundance of ^{13}C also allows for study designs that specifically track the uptake of consumed or infused ^{13}C labelled substrates. Studies have used this to monitor the incorporation of labelled glucose into glycogen [57] but can potentially trace other hepatic molecular pathways also.

Measurements of fasted hepatic glycogen levels and postprandial response are the most relevant factors that help in understanding liver disease and pathogenesis. While earlier work showed postprandial rises in glycogen stores largely as expected (slow initial rises for around 4 hours, followed by subsequent decline) [7], recent publications have shown a flat response to low energy morning intake [58]. Variations in response to high versus low glycaemic index breakfasts have also been observed (Fig. 2b) [59]. In a recent 1-week dietary intervention crossover study, fasted glycogen stores in the liver were significantly elevated after a high glycaemic index diet when compared with low glycaemic index diet. Other studies have investigated the glycogen response to exercise and recovery and the carbohydrate requirements for glycogen resynthesis [60]. These measurements provide exciting potentials of future research.

^{13}C MRS Measurements of Oxidative Stress

Novel MRI methods have also been developed to investigate measures of oxidative stress, providing a unique and crucial insight into the metabolic pathways that are likely to lead to long-term liver damage. Two such techniques have recently been developed using ^{13}C MRS labelling strategies. Befroy et al. [61] used a labelled ^{13}C acetate infusion to monitor the tricarboxylic acid (TCA) cycle directly by measuring the distinct signal from 2 glutamate peaks. Beta oxidation is a process in which fatty acid molecules are broken down in the mitochondria to generate acetyl-CoA, which is metabolised in the TCA cycle, and therefore the rate of labelled carbon atoms from acetate into glutamate can be used to evaluate the rate of beta oxidation. Similarly, Skamarauskas et al. [62] developed a method to monitor the conversion of glycine to glutathione in an animal model using ^{13}C MRS. Glutathione acts as the primary anti-oxidant for "mopping up" free radicals released during the beta oxidation process, and as such rates of glutathione production indicate the rate of oxidation and the liver's response to stress. In the animal model, there was a significant reduction in glutathione production following a high fat diet, which induced fatty liver. This methodology is now being translated into clinical applications.

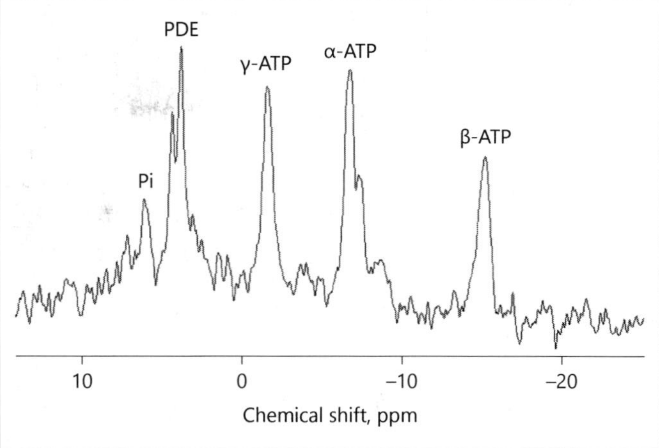

Fig. 3. In vivo 31P MR spectroscopy acquired from the liver showing individual phosphorous groups of adenosine triphosphate (ATP), phosphodiesters and inorganic phosphate. Adenosine diphosphate and monophosphate also sit under ATP peaks.

^{31}P MRS Measurements of Adenosine Triphosphate

NAFLD and its progressive form, NASH, have also been associated with impaired homeostasis of hepatic adenosine triphosphate (ATP) reserves and ^{31}P MRS can be used to provide further insight into healthy and diseased human liver metabolism [63]. Spectra from a localized volume in the liver contain peaks from each phosphate group individually (α-ATP, β-ATP, γ-ATP, inorganic phosphate, and phosphodiesters) as shown in Figure 3. The sensitivity is much greater than ^{13}C MRS due to its high isotopic natural abundance (100%) and can be used to dynamically monitor conversion of ATP to ADP and AMP by directly assessing changes in β-ATP or using saturation-transfer techniques.

Many studies have used this measurement to investigate oxidative production of ATP in liver disease and metabolic disorders. For example, patients with NASH where shown to have a reduced ability to replenish ATP following depletion [64]. It has been suggested that this inability to maintain ATP levels in the liver may lead

Dig Dis 2017;35:314–322
DOI: 10.1159/000456582

prime hepatocytes to become vulnerable to injury by reactive oxygen species and a critical mechanism underlying pathogenesis. In a recent study, an oral fructose challenge was used to deplete liver ATP, and the rate of recovery was monitored in healthy individuals using localized dynamic ^{31}P MRS [65] providing pilot data on a completely non-invasive method to assess liver ATP replenishment. Results also suggested a significant inverse correlation between the rate of ATP replenishment and baseline glycogen levels, providing 2 distinct non-invasive measurements of metabolic function of the liver.

Conclusions

Beyond the current use of MRI in clinical practise that is mainly focused on investigation of focal abnormalities within the liver, technology provides a broad range of methodologies that can be used in experimental medicine and mechanism evaluation. Novel liver T_1 mapping gives an indication of liver fibrosis and combined with measures of splanchnic circulation can produce an alternative measure of portal pressure. Proton MRS provides a non-invasive, operator-independent measure of liver fat-fractions. Development and evaluation of quantitative MRI technology should consider treating MR parameters as continuous variables that reflect the disease process, which lead to the accumulation of fat, inflammation and fibrosis as well as interventions resulting in their resolution [61, 66]. Multinuclear MRS allows for the investigation of underlying metabolism and using these technologies in parallel gives a full picture of the key factor relevant to the cause and progression of metabolic disorders. The next decade is expected to bring in multimodal quantitative MR methodologies that will change the design of experimental medicine studies, end points in clinical trials and eventually clinical algorithms for the management of chronic liver diseases.

Disclosure Statement

This paper presents independent research funded by the National Institute for Health Research (NIHR). The views expressed are those of the authors and not necessarily those of the NHS, the NIHR or the Department of Health. The authors have no conflicts of interest to declare.

References

1 European Association for Study of Liver; Asociacion Latinoamericana para el Estudio del Higado: EASL-ALEH clinical practice guidelines: non-invasive tests for evaluation of liver disease severity and prognosis. J Hepatol 2015;63:237–264.
2 Hoad CL, Palaniyappan N, Kaye P, Chernova Y, James MW, Costigan C, Austin A, Marciani L, Gowland PA, Guha IN, Francis ST, Aithal GP: A study of T_1 relaxation time as a measure of liver fibrosis and the influence of confounding histological factors. NMR Biomed 2015;28:706–714.
3 Singh S, Venkatesh SK, Loomba R, Wang Z, Sirlin C, Chen J, Yin M, Miller FH, Low RN, Hassanein T, Godfrey EM, Asbach P, Murad MH, Lomas DJ, Talwalkar JA, Ehman RL: Magnetic resonance elastography for staging liver fibrosis in non-alcoholic fatty liver disease: a diagnostic accuracy systematic review and individual participant data pooled analysis. Eur Radiol 2016;26:1431–1440.
4 Hernando D, Levin YS, Sirlin CB, Reeder SB: Quantification of liver iron with MRI: state of the art and remaining challenges. J Magn Reson Imaging 2014;40:1003–1021.
5 Liu CY, McKenzie CA, Yu H, Brittain JH, Reeder SB: Fat quantification with IDEAL gradient echo imaging: correction of bias from T(1) and noise. Magn Reson Med 2007;58:354–364.
6 Befroy DE, Perry RJ, Jain N, Dufour S, Cline GW, Trimmer JK, Brosnan J, Rothman DL, Petersen KF, Shulman GI: Direct assessment of hepatic mitochondrial oxidative and anaplerotic fluxes in humans using dynamic 13C magnetic resonance spectroscopy. Nat Med 2014;20:98–102.
7 Taylor R, Magnusson I, Rothman DL, Cline GW, Caumo A, Cobelli C, Shulman GI: Direct assessment of liver glycogen storage by 13C nuclear magnetic resonance spectroscopy and regulation of glucose homeostasis after a mixed meal in normal subjects. J Clin Invest 1996;97:126–132.
8 Imajo K, Kessoku T, Honda Y, Tomeno W, Ogawa Y, Mawatari H, Fujita K, Yoneda M, Taguri M, Hyogo H, Sumida Y, Ono M, Eguchi Y, Inoue T, Yamanaka T, Wada K, Saito S, Nakajima A: Magnetic resonance imaging more accurately classifies steatosis and fibrosis in patients with nonalcoholic fatty liver disease than transient elastography. Gastroenterology 2016;150:626–637.e7.
9 Chung S, Breton E, Mannelli L, Axel L: Liver stiffness assessment by tagged MRI of cardiac-induced liver motion. Magn Reson Med 2011;65:949–955.
10 Watanabe H, Kanematsu M, Kitagawa T, Suzuki Y, Kondo H, Goshima S, Kajita K, Bae KT, Hirose Y, Miotani S, Zhou X, Fujita H: MR elastography of the liver at 3 T with cine-tagging and bending energy analysis: preliminary results. Eur Radiol 2010;20:2381–2389.
11 Chung S, Kim KE, Park MS, Bhagavatula S, Babb J, Axel L: Liver stiffness assessment with tagged MRI of cardiac-induced liver motion in cirrhosis patients. J Magn Reson Imaging 2014;39:1301–1307.
12 Banerjee R, Pavlides M, Tunnicliffe EM, Piechnik SK, Sarania N, Philips R, Collier JD, Booth JC, Schneider JE, Wang LM, Delaney DW, Fleming KA, Robson MD, Barnes E, Neubauer S: Multiparametric magnetic resonance for the non-invasive diagnosis of liver disease. J Hepatol 2014;60:69–77.
13 Hoad CL, Palaniyappan N, Kaye P, Chernova Y, James MW, Costigan C, Austin A, Marciani L, Gowland PA, Guha IN, Francis ST, Aithal GP: A study of T_1 relaxation time as a measure of liver fibrosis and the influence of confounding histological factors. NMR Biomed 2015;28:706–714.
14 Henninger B, Kremser C, Rauch S, Eder R, Zoller H, Finkenstedt A, Michaely HJ, Schocke M: Evaluation of MR imaging with T1 and T2* mapping for the determination of hepatic iron overload. Eur Radiol 2012;22:2478–2486.
15 St Pierre TG, Clark PR, Chua-Anusorn W: Single spin-echo proton transverse relaxometry of iron-loaded liver. NMR Biomed 2004;17:446–458.

16 Wood JC, Enriquez C, Ghugre N, Tyzka JM, Carson S, Nelson MD, Coates TD: MRI R2 and R2* mapping accurately estimates hepatic iron concentration in transfusion-dependent thalassemia and sickle cell disease patients. Blood 2005;106:1460–1465.
17 de Bazelaire CM, Duhamel GD, Rofsky NM, Alsop DC: MR imaging relaxation times of abdominal and pelvic tissues measured in vivo at 3.0 T: preliminary results. Radiology 2004;230:652–659.
18 Zhao F, Wang YX, Yuan J, Deng M, Wong HL, Chu ES, Go MY, Teng GJ, Ahuja AT, Yu J: MR T1ρ as an imaging biomarker for monitoring liver injury progression and regression: an experimental study in rats with carbon tetrachloride intoxication. Eur Radiol 2012;22:1709–1716.
19 Stanisz GJ, Webb S, Munro CA, Pun T, Midha R: MR properties of excised neural tissue following experimentally induced inflammation. Magn Reson Med 2004;51:473–479.
20 Poynard T, Lenaour G, Vaillant JC, Capron F, Munteanu M, Eyraud D, Ngo Y, M'Kada H, Ratziu V, Hannoun L, Charlotte F: Liver biopsy analysis has a low level of performance for diagnosis of intermediate stages of fibrosis. Clin Gastroenterol Hepatol 2012;10:657–663.e7.
21 Mozes FE, Tunnicliffe EM, Pavlides M, Robson MD: Influence of fat on liver T1 measurements using modified look-locker inversion recovery (MOLLI) methods at 3T. J Magn Reson Imaging 2016;44:105–111.
22 Amat-Roldan I, Berzigotti A, Gilabert R, Bosch J: Assessment of hepatic vascular network connectivity with automated graph analysis of dynamic contrast-enhanced US to evaluate portal hypertension in patients with cirrhosis: a pilot study. Radiology 2015;277:268–276.
23 Palaniyappan N, Cox E, Bradley C, Scott R, Austin A, O'Neill R, Ramjas G, Travis S, White H, Singh R, Thurley P, Guha IN, Francis S, Aithal GP: Non-invasive assessment of portal hypertension using quantitative magnetic resonance imaging. J Hepatol 2016;65: 1131–1139.
24 Polio J, Groszmann RJ: Hemodynamic factors involved in the development and rupture of esophageal varices: a pathophysiologic approach to treatment. Semin Liver Dis 1986;6: 318–331.
25 Cox E, Palaniyappan N, Aithal GP, Guha IN, Francis ST: Measuring Dynamic Changes in Liver Perfusion and Blood Flow Following a Meal Challenge: Joint Annual Meeting ISMRM-ESMRMB, Milan, Italy, 2014.
26 Reeder SB, Cruite I, Hamilton G, Sirlin CB: Quantitative assessment of liver fat with magnetic resonance imaging and spectroscopy. J Magn Reson Imaging 2011;34:729–749.
27 Reeder SB, Hu HH, Sirlin CB: Proton density fat-fraction: a standardized MR-based biomarker of tissue fat concentration. J Magn Reson Imaging 2012;36:1011–1014.
28 Reeder SB, Pineda AR, Wen Z, Shimakawa A, Yu H, Brittain JH, Gold GE, Beaulieu CH, Pelc NJ: Iterative decomposition of water and fat with echo asymmetry and least-squares estimation (IDEAL): application with fast spin-echo imaging. Magn Reson Med 2005;54: 636–644.
29 Szczepaniak LS, Babcock EE, Schick F, Dobbins RL, Garg A, Burns DK, McGarry JD, Stein DT: Measurement of intracellular triglyceride stores by H spectroscopy: validation in vivo. Am J Physiol 1999;276(5 pt 1):E977–E989.
30 Stephenson MC, Leverton E, Khoo EY, Poucher SM, Johansson L, Lockton JA, Eriksson JW, Mansell P, Morris PG, Macdonald IA: Variability in fasting lipid and glycogen contents in hepatic and skeletal muscle tissue in subjects with and without type 2 diabetes: a 1H and 13C MRS study. NMR Biomed 2013; 26:1518–1526.
31 Yu H, McKenzie CA, Shimakawa A, Vu AT, Brau AC, Beatty PJ, Pineda AR, Brittain JH, Reeder SB: Multiecho reconstruction for simultaneous water-fat decomposition and T2* estimation. J Magn Reson Imaging 2007;26: 1153–1161.
32 Hines CD, Frydrychowicz A, Hamilton G, Tudorascu DL, Vigen KK, Yu H, McKenzie CA, Sirlin CB, Brittain JH, Reeder SB: T(1) Independent, T(2) (*) corrected chemical shift based fat-water separation with multipeak fat spectral modeling is an accurate and precise measure of hepatic steatosis. J Magn Reson Imaging 2011;33:873–881.
33 Kang GH, Cruite I, Shiehmorteza M, Wolfson T, Gamst AC, Hamilton G, Bydder M, Middleton MS, Sirlin CB: Reproducibility of MRI-determined proton density fat fraction across two different MR scanner platforms. J Magn Reson Imaging 2011;34:928–934.
34 Hernando D, Kellman P, Haldar JP, Liang ZP: Robust water/fat separation in the presence of large field inhomogeneities using a graph cut algorithm. Magn Reson Med 2010;63:79–90.
35 Barchetta I, Del Ben M, Angelico F, Di Martino M, Fraioli A, La Torre G, Saulle R, Perri L, Morini S, Tiberti C, Bertoccini L, Cimini FA, Panimolle F, Catalano C, Baroni MG, Cavallo MG: No effects of oral vitamin D supplementation on non-alcoholic fatty liver disease in patients with type 2 diabetes: a randomized, double-blind, placebo-controlled trial. BMC Med 2016;14:92.
36 Bashir MR, Zhong X, Nickel MD, Fananapazir G, Kannengiesser SA, Kiefer B, Dale BM: Quantification of hepatic steatosis with a multistep adaptive fitting MRI approach: prospective validation against MR spectroscopy. AJR Am J Roentgenol 2015;204:297–306.
37 Vu KN, Gilbert G, Chalut M, Chagnon M, Chartrand G, Tang A: MRI-determined liver proton density fat fraction, with MRS validation: comparison of regions of interest sampling methods in patients with type 2 diabetes. J Magn Reson Imaging 2016;43:1090–1099.
38 Hamilton G, Yokoo T, Bydder M, Cruite I, Schroeder ME, Sirlin CB, Middleton MS: In vivo characterization of the liver fat ^{1}H MR spectrum. NMR Biomed 2011;24:784–790.
39 Yeung DK, Griffith JF, Antonio GE, Lee FK, Woo J, Leung PC: Osteoporosis is associated with increased marrow fat content and decreased marrow fat unsaturation: a proton MR spectroscopy study. J Magn Reson Imaging 2005;22:279–285.
40 Katz-Brull R, Rofsky NM, Morrin MM, Pedrosa I, George DJ, Michaelson MD, Marquis RP, Maril M, Noguera C, Lenkinski RE: Decreases in free cholesterol and fatty acid unsaturation in renal cell carcinoma demonstrated by breath-hold magnetic resonance spectroscopy. Am J Physiol Renal Physiol 2005;288:F637–F641.
41 Hamilton G, Middleton MS, Bydder M, Yokoo T, Schwimmer JB, Kono Y, Patton HM, Lavine JE, Sirlin CB: Effect of PRESS and STEAM sequences on magnetic resonance spectroscopic liver fat quantification. J Magn Reson Imaging 2009;30:145–152.
42 Mcpherson S, Cowin G, O'Rourke P, Volp A, Horsfall L, Burke L, Jonsson J, Clouston A, Fawcett J, Galloway G, Benson M, Powell E: Quantitation of steatosis by magnetic resonance imaging (MRI) and spectroscopy (MRS) in liver disease: effect of hepatic fibrosis. J Hepatol 2009;50:S365–S366.
43 Levene AP, Kudo H, Armstrong MJ, Thursz MR, Gedroyc WM, Anstee QM, Goldin RD: Quantifying hepatic steatosis – more than meets the eye. Histopathology 2012;60:971–981.
44 Runge JH, Bakker PJ, Gaemers IC, Verheij J, Hakvoort TB, Ottenhoff R, Nederveen AJ, Stoker J: Measuring liver triglyceride content in mice: non-invasive magnetic resonance methods as an alternative to histopathology. Magma 2014;27:317–327.
45 Birkenfeld AL, Shulman GI: Nonalcoholic fatty liver disease, hepatic insulin resistance, and type 2 diabetes. Hepatology 2014;59:713–723.
46 Bortolotti M, Kreis R, Debard C, Cariou B, Faeh D, Chetiveaux M, Ith M, Vermathen P, Stefanoni N, Le KA, Schneiter P, Krempf M, Vidal H, Boesch C, Tappy L: High protein intake reduces intrahepatocellular lipid deposition in humans. Am J Clin Nutr 2009;90:1002–1010.
47 Hellerstein MK: De novo lipogenesis in humans: metabolic and regulatory aspects. Eur J Clin Nutr 1999;53(suppl 1):S53–S65.
48 Lagerpusch M, Enderle J, Eggeling B, Braun W, Johannsen M, Pape D, Muller MJ, Bosy-Westphal A: Carbohydrate quality and quantity affect glucose and lipid metabolism during weight regain in healthy men. J Nutr 2013; 143:1593–1601.
49 Lim JS, Mietus-Snyder M, Valente A, Schwarz JM, Lustig RH: The role of fructose in the pathogenesis of NAFLD and the metabolic syndrome. Nat Rev Gastroenterol Hepatol 2010;7:251–264.
50 Johnston RD, Stephenson MC, Crossland H, Cordon SM, Palcidi E, Cox EF, Taylor MA, Aithal GP, Macdonald IA: No difference between high-fructose and high-glucose diets on liver triacylglycerol or biochemistry in healthy overweight men. Gastroenterology 2013;145:1016–1025.e2.

51 Chee C, Mansell P, Stephens F, Cordon S, Kaviani M, Hoad C, Bawden S, Gowland P, Macdonald I: The effects of hyperenergetic carbohydrate vs. fat diets on liver fat content and insulin sensitivity in overweight healthy males. Diabetic Med 2016;33:29.
52 Valtuena S, Pellegrini N, Ardigo D, Del Rio D, Numeroso F, Scazzina F, Monti L, Zavaroni I, Brighenti F: Dietary glycemic index and liver steatosis. Am J Clin Nutr 2006;84:136–142; quiz 268–269.
53 Jue T, Lohman JA, Ordidge RJ, Shulman RG: Natural abundance 13C NMR spectrum of glycogen in humans. Magn Reson Med 1987; 5:377–379.
54 Jue T, Rothman DL, Tavitian BA, Shulman RG: Natural-abundance 13C NMR study of glycogen repletion in human liver and muscle. Proc Natl Acad Sci U S A 1989;86:1439–1442.
55 van der Graaf M, de Haan JH, Smits P, Mulder AH, Heerschap A, Tack CJ: The effect of acute exercise on glycogen synthesis rate in obese subjects studied by 13C MRS. Eur J Appl Physiol 2011;111:275–283.
56 Tomiyasu M, Obata T, Nishi Y, Nakamoto H, Nonaka H, Takayama Y, Autio J, Ikehira H, Kanno I: Monitoring of liver glycogen synthesis in diabetic patients using carbon-13 MR spectroscopy. Eur J Radiol 2010;73:300–304.
57 Jovanovic A, Leverton E, Solanky B, Ravikumar B, Snaar JE, Morris PG, Taylor R: The second-meal phenomenon is associated with enhanced muscle glycogen storage in humans. Clin Sci (Lond) 2009;117:119–127.
58 Bawden SJ, Stephenson MC, Ciampi E, Hunter K, Marciani L, Spiller RC, Aithal GP, Morris PG, Macdonald IA, Gowland PA: A low calorie morning meal prevents the decline of hepatic glycogen stores: a pilot in vivo (13)C magnetic resonance study. Food Funct 2014; 5:2237–2242.
59 Bawden S, Stephenson M, Falcone Y, Lingaya M, Ciampi E, Hunter K, Bligh F, Schirra J, Taylor M, Morris P, Macdonald I, Gowland P, Marciani L, Aithal G: Increased liver fat and glycogen stores following high compared with low glycaemic index food: a randomized cross over study. Diabetes Obes Metab 2016.
60 Casey A, Mann R, Banister K, Fox J, Morris PG, MacDonald IA, Greenhaff PL: Effect of carbohydrate ingestion on glycogen resynthesis in human liver and skeletal muscle, measured by (13)C MRS. Am J Physiol Endocrinol Metab 2000;278:E65–E75.
61 Befroy DE, Perry RJ, Jain N, Dufour S, Cline GW, Trimmer JK, Brosnan J, Rothman DL, Petersen KF, Shulman GI: Direct assessment of hepatic mitochondrial oxidative and anaplerotic fluxes in humans using dynamic 13C magnetic resonance spectroscopy. Nat Med 2014;20:98–102.
62 Skamarauskas JT, Oakley F, Smith FE, Bawn C, Dunn M, Vidler DS, Clemence M, Blain PG, Taylor R, Gamcsik MP, Thelwall PE: Noninvasive in vivo magnetic resonance measures of glutathione synthesis in human and rat liver as an oxidative stress biomarker. Hepatology 2014;59:2321–2330.
63 Oberhaensli RD, Galloway GJ, Taylor DJ, Bore PJ, Radda GK: Assessment of human-liver metabolism by P-31 magnetic-resonance spectroscopy. Brit J Radiol 1986;59:695–699.
64 Cortez-Pinto H, Chatham J, Chacko V, Arnold C, Diehl AM: Impaired liver ATP homeostais in human nonalcoholic steatohepatitis (NASH). Gastroenterology 1999;116:A1116.
65 Bawden SJ, Stephenson MC, Ciampi E, Hunter K, Marciani L, Macdonald IA, Aithal GP, Morris PG, Gowland PA: Investigating the effects of an oral fructose challenge on hepatic ATP reserves in healthy volunteers: a (31)P MRS study. Clin Nutr 2016;35:645–649.
66 Agrawal S, Hoad CL, Francis ST, Guha IN, Kaye P, Aithal GP: Visual morphometry and three non-invasive markers in the evaluation of liver fibrosis in chronic liver disease. Scand J Gastroenterol 2017;52:107–115.

Hepatology 2016 – The Panorama

Digestive Diseases

Dig Dis 2017;35:323–333
DOI: 10.1159/000456583

Genetic Discoveries Highlight Environmental Factors as Key Drivers of Liver Disease

Brian K. Chung[a, b, d] Tom H. Karlsen[b–f]

[a]Centre for Liver Research and National Institute for Health Research (NIHR) Birmingham Liver Biomedical Research Unit, College of Medical and Dental Sciences, Institute of Immunology and Immunotherapy, University of Birmingham, Birmingham, UK; [b]Norwegian PSC Research Center, and [c]Section of Gastroenterology, Department of Transplantation Medicine, Division of Cancer Medicine, Surgery and Transplantation, Oslo University Hospital Rikshospitalet, [d]Institute of Clinical Medicine, Faculty of Medicine, University of Oslo, [e]Research Institute of Internal Medicine, Division of Cancer Medicine, Inflammatory Medicine and Transplantation, Oslo University Hospital, and [f]K.G. Jebsen Inflammation Research Centre, Institute of Clinical Medicine, University of Oslo, Oslo, Norway

Keywords
Phenylketonuria · Tyrosinemia · Cystic fibrosis · Drug-induced liver injury · Autoimmune hepatitis · Primary biliary cholangitis · Primary sclerosing cholangitis

Abstract
Background: Over the last 50 years, genetic studies have uncovered a spectrum of rare and common alleles that confer susceptibility to both Mendelian and complex forms of liver disease. For disorders of Mendelian inheritance, identification of the causal variants has demonstrated that common environmental exposures can elicit severe liver pathogenesis in predisposed individuals. Specific environmental triggers for complex liver disorders are largely unknown; however, large-scale association studies indicate that environmental triggers are the predominant factors in driving liver pathophysiology. ***Key Messages:*** In Mendelian liver disorders, a single rare variant of major effect is often responsible for disease development. Gene-sequencing technologies have greatly facilitated the discovery of causal variants for Mendelian diseases and are increasingly utilized in molecular and clinical genetics for diagnostic and counselling purposes. By contrast, genetic susceptibility for complex liver disorders is heterogeneous, as many different genes acting on multiple distinct pathways influence disease onset and severity. Risk variants for complex liver disorders are relatively common, typically of small effect size and detected by genome-wide association studies (GWAS), which compare the genetic variation of specific loci using thousands of patients and healthy controls. Thus far, GWAS have detected dozens of unique and overlapping risk alleles for complex liver disease, but these account for less than a quarter of the overall disease liability. These observations emphasize that environmental exposures on a background of genetic predisposition are significant drivers of liver pathophysiology. Rare variants of large effect size, undetectable by GWAS, may also affect the development of complex disease on a case-to-case basis but evidence for such a scenario remains to be determined. ***Conclusions:*** Genetic technologies have identified numerous risk genes for Mendelian and complex liver disorders transforming disease recognition. For complex liver disorders, deciphering the interplay between genetic risk and environment determinants remains a significant challenge for unlocking the development of novel and personalized interventions.

Prof. Tom H. Karlsen
Norwegian PSC Research Center, Department of Transplantation Medicine
Division of Cancer Medicine, Surgery and Transplantation, Oslo University Hospital
Rikshospitalet, Pb 4950 Nydalen, NO–0424 Oslo (Norway)
E-Mail t.h.karlsen@medisin.uio.no

Introduction

Advances in genetic technologies have greatly improved the diagnosis and management of rare liver disease. Genetic methodologies, such as positional gene cloning and more recently next-generation sequencing, have uncovered a constellation of novel risk loci that impact the development and behavior of disease. In common liver diseases, genome-wide association studies (GWAS) have identified key molecular pathways and highlighted a major role for environmental insults as risk factors in hepatic pathogenesis. In liver disorders of Mendelian inheritance, a single rare variant can trigger the onset of extreme phenotypes to ubiquitous and otherwise innocuous environmental exposures. Conversely, genetic susceptibility for complex liver disorders is conferred by multiple loci that collectively account for less than 25% of total disease risk (Table 1). These findings highlight the important effect of environment exposures (e.g., diet, medications, toxins or infectious agents) in the pathophysiology of both monogenic and complex liver disease (Fig. 1).

In this study, we discuss genetic risk factors using examples of Mendelian and complex liver disorders and review the utility of these genetic findings for identifying and understanding the role of possible environmental triggers in liver disease development.

Phenylketonuria – Genes or Environment?

Phenylketonuria (PKU) is an autosomal recessive Mendelian disorder caused by mutations to phenylalanine hydroxylase (*PAH*) [1–3]. In patients with PKU, defective expression and function of the liver enzyme PAH lead to the toxic accumulation of phenylalanine in the developing brain [1–4]. For healthy individuals, phenylalanine is a non-toxic amino acid naturally found in dietary protein and metabolized by PAH into tyrosine [5, 6]. When PAH activity is reduced, phenylalanine is converted into phenylpyruvate and detectable in urine [7]. Current management of PKU primarily involves dietary restriction as natural protein sources are replaced with fortified sustenance free of phenylalanine. In roughly 20% of patients, medical intervention with the PAH cofactor tetrahydrobiopterin (THB; BH_4, sapropropterin, Kuvan) restores enzymatic activity and reduces phenylalanine concentrations to physiological levels [8]. With early detection and lifelong dietary compliance, life expectancy of patients is generally normal.

Phenylalanine was discovered as the environmental trigger of PKU in the 1930s and positional cloning of *PAH* in the 1980s significantly advanced the molecular understanding of PKU pathogenesis [1, 2, 9]. Over the last 25 years, more than 950 allelic variations of PAH have been identified, of which 60% are missense mutations, with the remaining consisting of altered splice site and deletion variants (http://www.biopku.org/home/pah/asp) [10]. Growing evidence supports a genotype–phenotype correlation between allelic variants, enzyme activity and responsiveness to THB. In the near future, high-throughput automated sequencing of *PAH* will lead to better disease recognition when applied to confirm and refine a diagnosis [10].

From a conceptual perspective, PKU reflects the complexity of considerations when evaluating what is a "genetic" or "environmental" risk for any disease. In reality, the consumption of a high phenylalanine diet is common and PKU is considered a genetic disease in its entirety. However, if one considers a hypothetical scenario in which everyone carries a *PAH* mutation, phenylalanine would be toxic and PKU would be considered a completely environmental disease [11]. Hence, PKU exemplifies how genetic and environmental risk factors are in fact inseparable and can harbour mechanistic insight for each factor on disease processes.

Tyrosinemia and Cystic Fibrosis – Monogenic Disorders Exhibiting Phenotype Heterogeneity

Tyrosinemia is a group of Mendelian disorders characterized by defects in the metabolism of tyrosine and its catabolic derivatives [12]. Tyrosinemia type 1 is the most severe form and is an autosomal recessive disease associated with fumarylacetoacetate hydrolase (*FAH*) variants. Deficiency of FAH is marked by abnormal elevations of circulating tyrosine, methionine, succinylacetone and alpha-fetoprotein at the time of diagnosis [13–15]. Classically, tyrosinemia type I presents early in life and is a risk factor for hepatocellular carcinoma. Affected infants may demonstrate a failure to thrive, rickets and repeated episodes of diarrhoea, vomiting and epistaxis [16]. Left untreated, affected children develop severe liver and kidney dysfunction and often succumb to the disease before 2 years of age.

Tyrosinemia type 2 (oculocutaneous tyrosinemia, keratosis palmoplantaris with corneal dystrophy and Richner-Hanhart syndrome) features photophobia, scleral inflammation and developmental delay [17, 18]. Patients with tyrosinemia type 2 carry autosomal recessive muta-

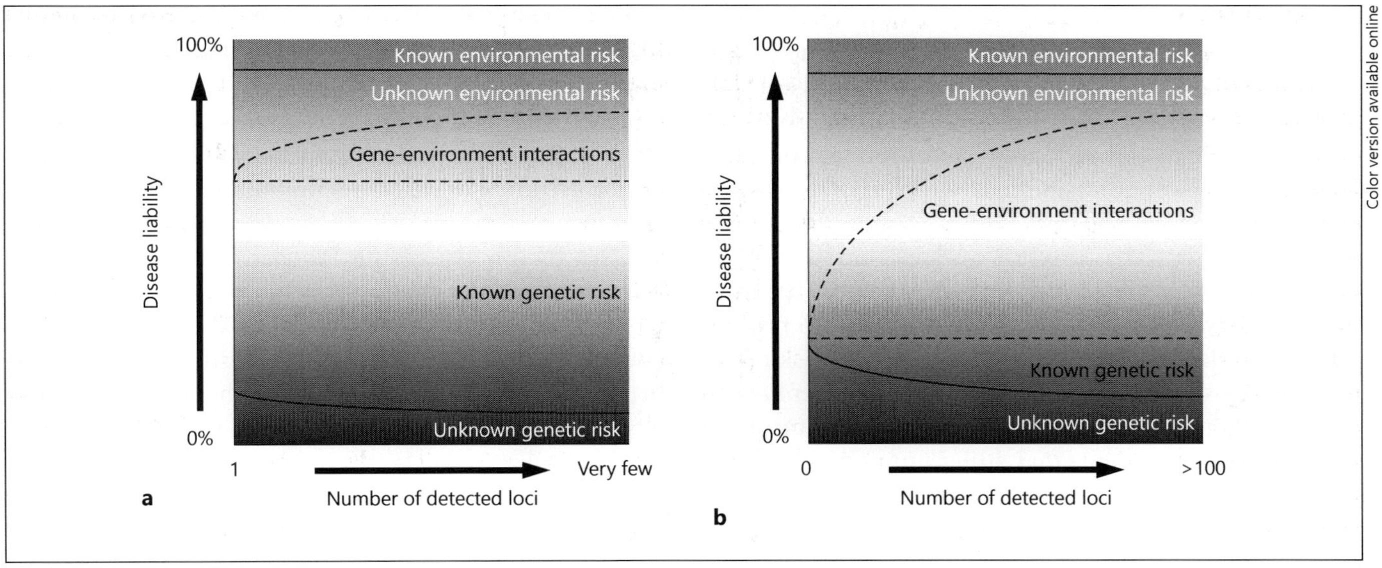

Fig. 1. Mendelian (**a**) and complex (**b**) liver diseases have different genetic contributions. For Mendelian disease, rare variants of large effect size (known genetic risk) significantly contribute to overall disease liability and the number of detected loci (x-axis) responsible for disease is very restricted. In some cases, environmental exposures such as diet, toxins and infections (gene-environment interactions) can unmask underlying genetic conditions and trigger or exacerbate existing phenotypes (dotted lines), thereby increasing the total disease liability of the genetic risk. By contrast, risk variants in complex liver disease identified by genome-wide association studies are common and carry relatively small effect sizes, implying that individuals can carry several risk loci and remain unaffected. The effects of gene-environment interactions in complex liver disease are largely unknown but contribute greatly to total disease liability. Ongoing studies to identify relevant environmental triggers may improve the understanding of gene-environment interactions (dotted lines) and allow for the better understanding of total disease liability for complex liver disorders.

Table 1. Characteristics of Mendelian and complex disease

	Mendelian disease	Complex disease
Disease phenotype	Extreme, early-onset	Mild to severe, adult-onset
Variant frequency	Rare	Common
Number of variants	Monogenic	Polygenic
Penetrance/effect size	Strong/large	Weak/small
Pattern of inheritance	Autosomal dominant, recessive or X-linked	Variable and complex
Effect of environment	Minimal to mild	Significant
Study methodologies	Linkage analysis, exome and whole genome next-generation sequencing	Genome-wide association studies

tions in tyrosine aminotransferase (*TAT*) [19–22]. TAT is primarily produced in the liver and kidneys and TAT deficiencies manifest in patients as high tyrosine concentrations due to the disrupted catabolism of tyrosine into phenylpyruvate [23].

In both forms of tyrosinemia, candidate gene studies confirmed that tyrosine and its metabolites act as environmental triggers in carriers of causal *FAH, TAT* and *HPD* variants. Greater appreciation of the underlying genetic factors has enhanced genetic testing, improved disease recognition and facilitated early implementation of low-protein diets free of phenylalanine and tyrosine for the management of disease. Moreover, genetic and functional confirmation that *FAH* mutations reduce or

Dig Dis 2017;35:323–333
DOI: 10.1159/000456583

abolish FAH activity led to the introduction of 2-(2-nitro-4-trifluoromethylbenzoyl)-1,3-cyclohexanedione (nitisinone) as a highly effective therapy for type 1 disease [12].

To the hepatologist, tyrosinemia type 1 represents another example of complex gene-environment considerations. In essence, tyrosinemia type 1 is liver disease caused by chemical hepatitis. The accumulation of toxic substances leads to tissue injury and development of liver cirrhosis. The metabolites immediately upstream of FAH, fumarylacetoacetate in particular, are also responsible for mutagenesis and drive the excessive risk of hepatocellular carcinoma via DNA injury and enhanced oxidative injury [24]. Although liver injury in most patients is chronic, patients may suffer unpredictable acute liver failure at an early age [25], which demonstrates the variability of circumstantial genetic and environmental factors even in monogenic disorders and underscores that tissue injury and clinical outcome can still differ even in the context of identical genetic risk and environmental exposure.

Cystic fibrosis is another monogenic liver disease that displays phenotypic diversity due to modifying genetic and environmental factors. Cystic fibrosis transmembrane conductance regulator (CFTR) deficiency in cystic fibrosis may lead to sclerosing cholangitis. With regard to genetic modifiers for a cholestatic presentation, it has been shown that individuals who carry deleterious alleles at the *SERPINA1* locus have increased risk of cholestatic liver disease development [26]. As to environmental risk for a cholestatic presentation, it has also been shown in CFTR-knockout murine models that concurrent colonic inflammation enhances the risk of cholestatic liver disease [27]. The local genetic context probably also matters, as exemplified by *ABCB4 (MDR3)*, where the variable severity of mutations can give rise to liver diseases ranging from severe biliary fibrosis in childhood to mild adult phenotypes like gallstone disease and mild cholangiopathy [28]. Hence, although a relatively clear relationship exists between genotype and Mendelian phenotypes, circumstantial genetic (either at the disease locus itself or by other genes) and environment factors modify penetrance and disease presentation such that outcome is never that of a 1:1 relationship.

PNPLA3-Associated Steatohepatitis

Hepatic steatosis or "fatty liver disease" is characterized by a diffuse accumulation of triglycerides within hepatocytes and classified on the basis of alcohol consumption as alcoholic (>20–30 g per day) or non-alcoholic (<20–30 g per day) fatty liver disease (ALD/NAFLD). By imaging and histology, ALD and NAFLD present as overlapping liver pathologies, but each one is clearly defined by distinct etiology and epidemiology considerations [29]. In 10–20% of cases, inflammation and hepatocellular injury are evident (steatohepatitis) and a subset of patients develop advanced steatohepatitis marked by the development of liver cirrhosis and an increased risk of hepatocellular carcinoma [30]. In addition to alcohol, obesity is a common and well-established risk factor for hepatic steatosis. Western diets high in fat and sugar largely contribute to obesity and data from experimental models indicates that western diets rapidly alter the liver transcriptome to promote lipid deposition in the liver [31, 32]. Data also supports an association between liver steatosis and the metabolic syndrome and "metaflammation," encompassing widespread inflammatory processes associated with obesity (central adiposity), alongside insulin resistance, hyperglycemia, dyslipidemia and atherosclerosis [33, 34]. Inflammation and oxidative stress linked to the metabolic syndrome are thought to worsen pre-existing hepatic steatosis and lead to the development of steatohepatitis [35]. Growing evidence implicates the gut microbiome as a major environmental factor in the development of hepatic steatosis and steatohepatitis through poorly understood metabolic and immunological host-microbe interactions [36, 37]. Intriguingly, genetic variability of disease susceptibility genes have been shown to affect the composition of gut microbiota, highlighting a dynamic interaction between the host and environment whereby genetics of the host influence the gut microbiome, which in turn modulates the host immune response [38–43].

In 2008, the first GWAS for NAFLD was published (Table 2), reporting a significant association with the 148M variant (rs738409) of patatin-like phospholipase domain containing 3 protein (*PNPLA3*) [44]. The finding was supported by a second GWAS showing *PNPLA3* associated with elevated plasma levels of alanine aminotransferase [45]. Genetic factors were suspected to influence hepatic steatosis as disease incidence was known to differ between ethnic populations [46]. Subsequent genotyping and meta-data analyses confirmed *PNPLA3* rs738409 as a risk factor for NAFLD [47–49] and several later studies detected prominent *PNPLA3* rs738409 associations with hepatocellular carcinoma [50, 51] and ALD [52, 53] (Table 2) implicating *PNPLA3* rs738409 as an underlying risk determinant for multiple pathologies associated with fatty liver disease.

Table 2. Genome-wide association studies in complex liver disease

Study	Year	Cohort ethnicity	Risk loci ($p < 5 \times 10^{-8}$)
NAFLD			
Romeo et al. [44]	2008	African American, European American, Hispanic	*PDPLA3*
ALD			
Tian et al. [52]	2010	Mixed European, native American	*PDPLA3*
Buch et al. [53]	2015	Mixed European	*PDPLA3*
DILI			
Kindmark et al. [64] (ximelagatran)	2008	Northern European	*HLA*
Daly et al. [68] (flucloxacillin)	2009	Northern European	*HLA*
Singer et al. [69] (lumiracoxib)	2010	Mixed European, Hispanic	*HLA*
Spraggs et al. [70] (lapatinib)	2011	Mixed European, non-European	*HLA*
Lucena et al. [71] (amoxicillin-clavulanate)	2011	Mixed European, European American	*HLA*
Urban et al. [67] (flucloxacillin and amoxicillin-clavulanate)	2012	Mixed European	None
AIH			
de Boer [92]	2014	Northern European	*HLA*
PBC			
Hirschfield et al. [93]	2009	European American	*HLA, IL12A, IL12RB2*
Hirschfield et al. [94]	2010	European American	*IRF5-TNPO3, MMEL1, IKZF3*
Liu et al. [95]	2010	Mixed European	*SPIB, IKZF3, IRF5-TNPO3*
Mells et al. [96]	2011	Mixed American	*DENND1B, STAT4, CD80, NFKB1, IL7R, CXCR5, TNFRSF1A, RAD51L1, CLEC16A, MAP3K7IP1, PLCL2*
Nakamura et al. [97]	2012	Japanese	*RPS6KA4, TNFAIP2, HLA, TNFRSF15*
Cordell et al. [98]	2015	Northern European, mixed European, mixed American	*POU2AF1, IL1R1, CCL20, DGKQ, C5orf30, IL12B, TNFAIP3*
PSC			
Karlsen et al. [99]	2010	Northern European	*HLA*
Melum et al. [100]	2011	Northern European	*HLA, BCL2L11, MST1*
Folseraas et al. [101]	2012	Northern European, mixed European, mixed America European, mixed America	*MMEL1-TNFRSF14*
Srivastava et al. [102]	2012	Northern European	*MST1, IL2RA*
Ellinghaus et al. [103]	2013	Northern European	*GPR35, TCF4*
Liu et al. [104]	2013	Mixed European, mixed American	*HLA, MMEL1-TNFRSF14, CD28, MST1, IL2/IL21, BACH2, IL2RA, SIK2, HDAC7, SH2B3, CD226, FUT2, PSMG1*
Ellinghaus et al. [91]	2016	Pan-European	*ASAP2, NFKB1, RIC8B, LOC107984859*
Ji et al. [105]	2016	Northern European, European American, African, Han Chinese, Japanese	*CCDC88B, CLEC16A, FOXP1, UBASH3A*

Dig Dis 2017;35:323–333
DOI: 10.1159/000456583

The biological relevance of the *PNPLA3* rs738409 association remains under investigation; however, PNPLA3 148M appears to disrupt fat degradation in the liver by accumulating on the surface of lipid droplets [54]. Early studies showed PNPLA3 hydrolyzes and acetylates lipids with PNPLA3 148M demonstrating decreased lipid hydrolysis and increased lipid acetylation compared to the wild-type protein [55–58]. Surprisingly, knockdown or overexpression of endogenous PNPLA3 had no effect on lipid deposition in mice [59, 60], whereas overexpression of PNPLA3 148M triggered liver steatosis in transgenic animals indicating that the expression of PNPLA3 148M is both necessary and sufficient for the development of disease [61]. Indeed, unlike wild-type protein, PNPLA3 148M accumulates at the surface of lipid droplets at very high levels and may promote liver steatosis by inhibiting lipolytic co-factors such as CGI-58/ABHD5 given steatosis was also observed in mice that expressed a catalytically inactive PNPLA3 variant. Importantly, when *PNPLA3* rs738409 expression was controlled physiologically [54], disease appeared only in mice fed with a high-sucrose diet and not a high-fat diet, suggesting that *PNPLA3* rs738409 expression may be driven by insulin and that it serves to highlight how specific environmental factors can modify the impact of the same genetic risk factors carried by different individuals.

Overall, the identification of *PNPLA3* as a significant genetic risk for hepatic steatosis illustrates how multiple environmental risk factors (diet, metabolic syndrome, gut microbiome) may converge and present as a similar phenotype ultimately driven by a common genetic risk factor. Even for a simple and apparently homogeneous histopathological entity like hepatic steatosis, the gene-environmental interactions that underpin disease may be diverse, exemplifying how our normal disease classification (in this case ALD and NAFLD) does not segregate with environmental and genetic risk factors. In the case of hepatic steatosis, discovery of the *PNPLA3* rs738409 association confirmed that diet and alcohol are important environmental risk factors for steatohepatitis as a common denominator for several classical disease definitions. The finding has highlighted a core pathophysiological pathway that may be amendable to medical intervention in all diseases associated with hepatic steatosis.

Idiosyncratic Drug-Induced Liver Injury

Idiosyncratic drug-induced liver injury (DILI) accounts for approximately 10% of acute liver failure and is the second leading cause of failed clinical trials worldwide [62, 63]. In contrast to intrinsic DILI, idiosyncratic DILI is defined as an unanticipated adverse reaction distinct from the known pharmacological mechanism of action and influenced by genetic variability [63]. The first GWAS for idiosyncratic DILI involved the thrombin inhibitor ximelagatran and unexpectedly revealed a profound association between ximelagatran DILI and the human leukocyte antigen (HLA) loci, specifically *HLA-DRB1*07* and *HLA-DQA1*02* [64]. HLA are highly polymorphic proteins that present intra- and extra-cellular peptides and activate T lymphocytes via cognate T-cell receptor (TCR) interactions [65]. Discovery of HLA associations in ximelagatran DILI provided the first evidence that adaptive immune responses contribute to idiosyncratic DILI and rationalized previous reports of lymphocyte sensitization in DILI patients [66]. In addition to ximelagatran DILI, GWAS have also uncovered strong HLA associations for many other models of DILI, thereby supporting a role for adaptive immunity in most idiosyncratic DILI [67] (Table 2). For example, flucloxacillin DILI associated with the treatment of staphylococcal infections strongly correlates with *HLA-B*5701* [68], whereas DILI caused by the treatment of osteoarthritis and acute pain using lumiracoxib strongly associates with *HLA-DRB1*1501* [69]. Furthermore, DILI linked to the breast cancer medication lapatinib is associated with the expression of *HLA-DQA1*0201* [70] and *HLA-A*0201*, and *HLA-DQB1*0602* associations confer increased susceptibility to amoxicillin-clavulanate DILI [71].

While the biological relevance of the HLA associations for idiosyncratic DILI is under investigation [72], lessons from autoimmunity demonstrate how HLA associations can confer disease susceptibility to highly specific environmental factors. In the example of celiac disease, *HLA-DQ2* and *HLA-DQ8* are strongly associated with celiac disease because *HLA-DQ2* and *HLA-DQ8* are structurally capable of presenting gluten antigens, whereas other HLA variants cannot [73]. HLA associations for idiosyncratic DILI likely involve a direct interaction of the drug and DILI-associated HLA variants [74]. In abacavir hypersensitivity syndrome, *HLA-B*57:02* is a strong risk factor because abacavir directly interacts with the peptide-binding cleft of HLA-B*57:01, effectively altering the endogenous peptide repertoire presented by HLA-B*57:01 to T cells [75, 76]. In this scenario, T cells that normally would be unresponsive to self-peptides prior to abacavir treatment recognize the altered peptide repertoire as foreign and are activated to respond. Indirect and direct mechanisms of disease are likely to exist for idiosyncratic DILI, whereby drugs or their metabolites modify antigen exposure and/or antigen immunogenicity [77]. Translating the HLA associations for DILI into discrete mechanisms may provide insights into why HLA associations are so common in disease.

HLA Associations for Immune-Mediated Liver Diseases Point Towards Disease-Specific Antigenic Triggers

Autoimmune hepatitis (AIH), primary biliary cholangitis (PBC), and primary sclerosing cholangitis (PSC) are immune-mediated liver diseases featuring distinct HLA associations of unknown significance. AIH is marked by hypergammaglobulinemia and the production of specific autoantibodies, which define types 1 and 2 AIH subtypes [78]. In type 1 antinuclear antibodies, smooth muscle antibodies and antibodies against soluble liver antigen/liver-pancreas are detected, while patients with type 2 typically generate antibodies to liver/kidney microsomal antigen type-1 and liver cytosol antigen type 1. In most cases, AIH is responsive to immunosuppressants, although adverse effects are common and alternative treatments are lacking [79]. Environmental triggers for AIH are largely unknown but may include drug and toxin exposure, as well as hitherto unidentified viral infections [80].

PBC is a cholestatic liver disease associated with lymphocytic infiltration of the small- to medium-sized interlobular bile ducts [81]. Similar to AIH, PBC typically affects women and presents in adults over the age of 40 years. PBC is considered autoimmune, as autoreactive T-cell and B-cell responses against the mitochondrial E2-domain of pyruvate dehydrogenase complex (PDC-E2) are common with more than 90% of patients producing anti-mitochondrial antibodies to PDC-E2 [82]. The initiation of immune reactivity to PDC-E2 is yet to be determined, but environmental factors, such as smoking, infection and xenobiotics may promote the loss of self-tolerance by means of "molecular mimicry," wherein the exposure to exogenous antigens triggers autoimmunity to endogenous molecules expressing a similar epitope (mimitope) [83]. Treatment for PBC is largely restricted to ursodeoxycholic acid, which delays liver injury successfully for some patients but shows limited efficacy in a significant number of cases [79].

PSC is the most paradoxical of the immune-mediated liver diseases, given that it exhibits classical autoimmune features, such as immune infiltration and HLA associations, but unlike most autoimmune disorders, immunosuppression is ineffective, males are more frequently affected than females (2:1) and so far there is no evidence of disease-specific T cells and/or specific autoantibodies [84]. Recent efforts of characterizing disease-associated antibodies using liver-resident B cells from PSC patients could lead to the identification of relevant autoantibodies, but further work is needed to validate such methodologies [85]. In 30–80% of cases, PSC strongly associates with inflammatory bowel disease (PSC-IBD) suggesting that the gut-liver axis contributes to the pathogenesis of PSC, including lymphocyte migration and the exposure to shared antigens between the gut and liver [86]. Currently, no medical treatment is available for PSC, making it a major indication for liver transplantation in many western countries.

Multiple GWAS conducted for AIH, PBC and PSC (Table 2) have detected an overall genetic architecture characterized by strong HLA associations that closely resemble the situation in prototypical autoimmune disorders, including type 1 diabetes, multiple sclerosis, rheumatoid arthritis and celiac disease [87]. Some of the HLA associations are shared among diseases (e.g., ancestral haplotype 8.1 between PSC and AIH and *HLA-DR4* associations in PBC and AIH), while others are less pleiotropic (e.g., *HLA-DRB1*13:01* in PSC and *HLA-DR8* in PBC) [88].

Importantly, HLA associations AIH, PBC and PSC point towards the involvement of specific environmental co-factors in disease development, similar to what is proposed above for DILI and celiac disease; however, determining the precise relationship between environmental exposures and specific HLA associations remains arduous. Several complementary strategies ranging from HLA elution assays, antibody profiling, high-throughput B cell receptor (BCR) and TCR sequencing and in vitro confirmation of candidate antigens for immune cell reactivity will be necessary, as the source of antigen could be exogenous or endogenous and simultaneously be influenced by diet, drug usage, infection, microbiota and other currently unknown variables (Fig. 2). As demonstrated by the discovery of HLA associations in DILI, antigens may originate from unexpected sources; therefore, a comprehensive approach must be utilized, as relevant candidate triggers may be conventional peptides but could also be derived from small molecules such as drugs or microbial metabolites.

Consideration of HLA associations in such conditions as celiac disease and DILI may aid understanding of the pathophysiology of autoimmune liver diseases, particularly with regard to PSC, where the strong concurrence of IBD suggests that altered gut homeostasis triggers or

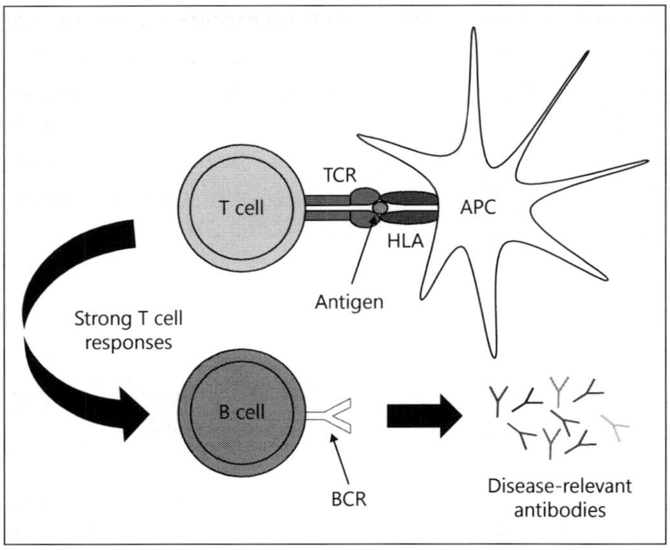

Color version available online

Fig. 2. Human leukocyte antigen (HLA) associations may aid the identification of relevant environmental risk factors in complex liver disease. A majority of complex liver diseases demonstrate strong associations with the HLA complex, which implies the involvement of adaptive immune responses (T and B cells) in disease pathogenesis. HLA on the surface of antigen-presenting cells (APC) display antigens in the context of HLA to cognate T-cell receptors (TCR) expressed by T cells. Antigens that stimulate strong T-cell responses can subsequently activate the production of antibodies from antigen-specific B cells whose specificity reflect the original triggering antigen. Studying B-cell receptor (BCR) clonality using sequencing technologies, and/or antibody reactivity using high-throughput arrays may enable the discovery of disease-relevant environmental exposures that trigger the development of complex liver disorders.

drives disease in the liver. Broadly speaking, a better understanding of the HLA associations in autoimmune liver disease may hold relevance for autoimmunity in general as the increasing incidence of autoimmune liver diseases coincides with the growing epidemic of autoimmune diseases over the last 20–30 years, which cannot be driven by genetic alterations but rather by changes in host-environment interactions. Clearly these will take considerable efforts to reconcile due to their overwhelming complexity; however, they may be guided by the genetic findings made for the HLA-related factors in particular.

In addition to HLA associations, GWAS and targeted genotyping surveys have uncovered several non-HLA loci as risk factors for AIH, PBC and PSC that correspond mainly to immune-related genes and consistently appear as risk factors in other autoimmune conditions (pleiotropy) [89]. This is somewhat reflective of the blurred relationship between classical disease definitions and pathogenic, molecular pathways. It is important to acknowledge that none of these variants are independently capable of establishing disease and likely act as modifiers in a scenario where HLA-antigen interactions are at the centre; however, they themselves possibly also reflect interactions with other environmental factors in the development and/or behaviour of disease [90]. Also, although a majority of the non-HLA loci are pleiotropic, associations nevertheless show disease-specific patterns [91], confirming clinical observations that each disease is a distinct entity, yet also demonstrating that all immune-mediated conditions contain underlying perturbations in common pathways, which appear to promote the onset of self-reactivity in the context of specific environmental drivers. As the field evolves, insights gained from studying other autoimmune diseases with shared genetic susceptibility factors may yield aetiological and mechanistic insights also into AIH, PBC and PSC.

Conclusions

Detailed assessment of genetic risk factors in Mendelian and complex liver disorders has significantly refined concepts of disease pathogenesis in recent years. With such insights, efforts to elucidate the causality between genetic and environmental factors are ongoing and hold promise for understanding the primary contribution of environmental factors in complex disorders and their interaction with the genetic predisposition. Better assessment of genetic risk per se will require larger, well-phenotyped cohorts powered to identify associations of low effect size ("missing heritability") that however may have a minimal impact on total disease liability but represent unexpected pathways targetable by existing or new therapeutic methods. Furthermore, the application of whole exome and genome-sequencing technologies should be considered to identify rare variants of large effect size, as genome-wide surveys are biased towards the detection of common alleles carried by greater than 1–5% of the general population [87]. With the genetic risks for a particular disease in hand, researchers can begin to define the genotypes that truly influence a specific phenotype from those that have a nominal effect on disease outcome but simply associate because of linkage disequilibrium [90]. Whenever feasible, genetic studies should be designed to account for environmental variation, particularly for complex phenotypes where environmental co-factors currently appear to dominate the susceptibility space.

Fundamental challenges remain in translating HLA and non-HLA risk associations into biological understanding particularly for complex disorders such as AIH, PBC and PSC. Interpreting such HLA associations will require several complementary approaches (HLA peptidome analysis, antibody profiling, BCR and TCR sequencing and new technologies under refinement), given that each methodology has inherent limitations, and the source of antigen(s) may be diverse and unanticipated. For non-HLA associations, the effect of specific variants should be mechanistically evaluated in experimental models where their impact on disease-associated biology can be assigned based on the presence or absence of the disease-associated allele and such studies should lead to a greater appreciation of the critical pathways controlling the susceptibility and severity of complex diseases.

In conclusion, the discovery of genetic risk factors in monogenic and complex liver disease provides a strategic path to pursue the identity and impact of specific environmental factors on disease pathophysiology. Although genetic risk accounts for most of the disease liability in Mendelian disorders (Fig. 1), environmental factors influence the phenotypic presentation of carriers of the same disease-associated variant as shown for *ABCB4* and *PNPLA3*-mediated cholangitis. For complex liver disorders, environmental factors largely of unknown origin are thought to trigger and drive the pathology (Fig. 1). Assessments of gene-environment interactions in complex diseases are therefore needed to clearly define the specific environmental factors as such insights may lead to novel treatment paradigms where the elimination of environmental determinants (e.g., gluten in celiac disease) leads to the amelioration of disease.

Acknowledgements

B.K.C. is supported by the European Union Seventh Framework Programme (FP7-PEOPLE-2013-COFUND) under grant agreement #609020 (Scientia Fellows) and received support from the NIHR Birmingham Liver Biomedical Research Unit. This article presents independent research supported by the NIHR Birmingham Liver Biomedical Research Unit based at the University Hospitals Birmingham NHS Foundation Trust and the University of Birmingham. The views expressed in this publication are those of the authors and not necessarily those of the NHS, the NIHR or the Department of Health.

Disclosure Statement

The authors declare no conflict of interest.

References

1 Fölling A: Über ausscheidung von phenylbrenztraubensäure in den harn als stoffwechselanomalie in verbindung mit imbezillität. Hoppe-Seyler's Z Physiol Chem 1934;227:169–181.
2 Penrose LS: Inheritance of phenylpyruvic amentia (phenylketonuria). Lancet 1935;226:192–194.
3 Kenney FT, Reem GH, Kretchmer N: Development of phenylalanine hydroxylase in mammalian liver. Science 1958;127:86.
4 Blau N, van Spronsen FJ, Levy HL: Phenylketonuria. Lancet 2010;376:1417–1427.
5 Jervis GA: Studies on phenylpyruvic oligophrenia; the position of the metabolic error. J Biol Chem 1947;169:651–656.
6 Udenfriend S, Bessman SP: The hydroxylation of phenylalanine and antipyrine in phenylpyruvic oligophrenia. J Biol Chem 1953;203:961–966.
7 Boscott RJ, Bickel H: Detection of some new abnormal metabolites in the urine of phenylketonuria. Scand J Clin Lab Invest 1953;5:380–382.
8 Danks DM, Cotton RG, Schlesinger P: Letter: tetrahydrobiopterin treatment of variant form of phenylketonuria. Lancet 1975;2:1043.
9 Woo SL, Lidsky AS, Güttler F, Chandra T, Robson KJ: Cloned human phenylalanine hydroxylase gene allows prenatal diagnosis and carrier detection of classical phenylketonuria. Nature 1983;306:151–155.
10 Blau N, Shen N, Carducci C: Molecular genetics and diagnosis of phenylketonuria: state of the art. Expert Rev Mol Diagn 2014;14:655–671.
11 Vineis P, Pearce N: Missing heritability in genome-wide association study research. Nat Rev Genet 2010;11:589.
12 Scott CR: The genetic tyrosinemias. Am J Med Genet C Semin Med Genet 2006;142C:121–126.
13 Grenier A, Bélanger L, Laberge C: Alpha1-fetoprotein measurement in blood spotted on paper: discriminating test for hereditary tyrosinemia in neonatal mass screening. Clin Chem 1976;22:1001–1004.
14 Lindblad B, Lindstedt S, Steen G: On the enzymic defects in hereditary tyrosinemia. Proc Natl Acad Sci U S A 1977;74:4641–4645.
15 Tanguay RM, Valet JP, Lescault A, Duband JL, Laberge C, Lettre F, et al: Different molecular basis for fumarylacetoacetate hydrolase deficiency in the two clinical forms of hereditary tyrosinemia (type I). Am J Hum Genet 1990;47:308–316.
16 van Spronsen FJ, Thomasse Y, Smit GP, Leonard JV, Clayton PT, Fidler V, et al: Hereditary tyrosinemia type I: a new clinical classification with difference in prognosis on dietary treatment. Hepatology 1994;20:1187–1191.
17 Macsai MS, Schwartz TL, Hinkle D, Hummel MB, Mulhern MG, Rootman D: Tyrosinemia type II: nine cases of ocular signs and symptoms. Am J Ophthalmol 2001;132:522–527.
18 Rehák A, Selim MM, Yadav G: Richner-hanhart syndrome (tyrosinaemia-II) (report of four cases without ocular involvement). Br J Dermatol 1981;104:469–475.
19 Goldsmith LA, Kang E, Bienfang DC, Jimbow K, Gerald P, Baden HP: Tyrosinemia with plantar and palmar keratosis and keratitis. J Pediatr 1973;83:798–805.
20 Natt E, Kao FT, Rettenmeier R, Scherer G: Assignment of the human tyrosine aminotransferase gene to chromosome 16. Hum Genet 1986;72:225–228.
21 Natt E, Westphal EM, Toth-Fejel SE, Magenis RE, Buist NR, Rettenmeier R, et al: Inherited and de novo deletion of the tyrosine aminotransferase gene locus at 16q22.1-q22.3 in a patient with tyrosinemia type II. Hum Genet 1987;77:352–358.
22 Hühn R, Stoermer H, Klingele B, Bausch E, Fois A, Farnetani M, et al: Novel and recurrent tyrosine aminotransferase gene mutations in tyrosinemia type II. Hum Genet 1998;102:305–313.

23 Canellakis ZN, Cohen PP: Purification studies of tyrosine-alpha-ketoglutaric acid transaminase. J Biol Chem 1956;222:53–62.
24 Bliksrud YT, Ellingsen A, Bjørås M: Fumarylacetoacetate inhibits the initial step of the base excision repair pathway: implication for the pathogenesis of tyrosinemia type I. J Inherit Metab Dis 2013;36:773–778.
25 Durand P, Debray D, Mandel R, Baujard C, Branchereau S, Gauthier F, et al: Acute liver failure in infancy: a 14-year experience of a pediatric liver transplantation center. J Pediatr 2001;139:871–876.
26 Bartlett JR: Genetic modifiers of liver disease in cystic fibrosis. JAMA 2009;302:1076–1083.
27 Blanco PG, Zaman MM, Junaidi O, Sheth S, Yantiss RK, Nasser IA, et al: Gliadin-specific, HLA-DQ(alpha 1*0501,beta 1*0201) restricted T cells isolated from the small intestinal mucosa of celiac disease patients. Am J Physiol Gastrointest Liver Physiol 2004;287:187–196.
28 Trauner M, Fickert P, Wagner M: MDR3 (ABCB4) defects: a paradigm for the genetics of adult cholestatic syndromes. Semin Liver Dis 2007;27:77–98.
29 Scaglioni F, Ciccia S, Marino M, Bedogni G, Bellentani S: ASH and NASH. Dig Dis 2011; 29:202–210.
30 Anstee QM, Targher G, Day CP: Progression of NAFLD to diabetes mellitus, cardiovascular disease or cirrhosis. Nat Rev Gastroenterol Hepatol 2013;10:330–344.
31 Ishimoto T, Lanaspa MA, Rivard CJ, Roncal-Jimenez CA, Orlicky DJ, Cicerchi C, et al: High-fat and high-sucrose (western) diet induces steatohepatitis that is dependent on fructokinase. Hepatology 2013;58:1632–1643.
32 Roberts MD, Mobley CB, Toedebush RG, Heese AJ, Zhu C, Krieger AE, et al: Western diet-induced hepatic steatosis and alterations in the liver transcriptome in adult Brown-Norway rats. BMC Gastroenterol 2015;15: 151.
33 Hotamisligil GS: Inflammation and metabolic disorders. Nature 2006;444:860–867.
34 Rector RS, Thyfault JP, Wei Y, Ibdah JA: Nonalcoholic fatty liver disease and the metabolic syndrome: an update. World J Gastroenterol 2008;14:185–192.
35 Wellen KE, Hotamisligil GS: Inflammation, stress, and diabetes. J Clin Invest 2005;115: 1111–1119.
36 Ferrere G, Wrzosek L, Cailleux F, Turpin W, Puchois V, Spatz M, et al: Fecal microbiota manipulation prevents dysbiosis and alcohol-induced liver injury in mice. J Hepatol 2016; pii:S0168-8278(16)30682-1, doi: 10.1016/j.jhep.2016.11.008 [Epub ahead of print].
37 Tilg H, Cani PD, Mayer EA: Gut microbiome and liver diseases. Gut 2016;65:2035–2044.
38 Blekhman R, Goodrich JK, Huang K, Sun Q, Bukowski R, Bell JT, et al: Host genetic variation impacts microbiome composition across human body sites. Genome Biol 2015; 16:191.
39 Davenport ER, Cusanovich DA, Michelini K, Barreiro LB, Ober C, Gilad Y: Genome-wide association studies of the human gut microbiota. PLoS One 2015;10:e0140301.
40 Turpin W, Espin-Garcia O, Xu W, Silverberg MS, Kevans D, Smith MI, et al: Association of host genome with intestinal microbial composition in a large healthy cohort. Nat Genet 2016;48:1413–1417.
41 Bonder MJ, Kurilshikov A, Tigchelaar EF, Mujagic Z, Imhann F, Vila AV, et al: The effect of host genetics on the gut microbiome. Nat Genet 2016;48:1407–1412.
42 Benson AK: The gut microbiome – an emerging complex trait. Nat Genet 2016;48:1301–1302.
43 Wang J, Thingholm LB, Skieceviciene J, Rausch P, Kummen M, Hov JR, et al: Genome-wide association analysis identifies variation in vitamin D receptor and other host factors influencing the gut microbiota. Nat Genet 2016;48:1396–1406.
44 Romeo S, Kozlitina J, Xing C, Pertsemlidis A, Cox D, Pennacchio LA, et al: Genetic variation in PNPLA3 confers susceptibility to nonalcoholic fatty liver disease. Nat Genet 2008; 40:1461–1465.
45 Yuan X, Waterworth D, Perry JR, Lim N, Song K, Chambers JC, et al: Population-based genome-wide association studies reveal six loci influencing plasma levels of liver enzymes. Am J Hum Genet 2008;83:520–528.
46 Browning JD, Szczepaniak LS, Dobbins R, Nuremberg P, Horton JD, Cohen JC, et al: Prevalence of hepatic steatosis in an urban population in the United States: impact of ethnicity. Hepatology 2004;40:1387–1395.
47 Stickel F, Buch S, Lau K, Meyer zu Schwabedissen H, Berg T, Ridinger M, et al: Genetic variation in the PNPLA3 gene is associated with alcoholic liver injury in caucasians. Hepatology 2011;53:86–95.
48 Corradini SG, Burza MA, Molinaro A, Romeo S: Patatin-like phospholipase domain containing 3 sequence variant and hepatocellular carcinoma. Hepatology 2011;53:1776; author reply 1777.
49 Sookoian S, Pirola CJ: Meta-analysis of the influence of I148M variant of patatin-like phospholipase domain containing 3 gene (PNPLA3) on the susceptibility and histological severity of nonalcoholic fatty liver disease. Hepatology 2011;53:1883–1894.
50 Valenti L, Colombo M, Fargion S: Modulation of the effect of PNPLA3 I148M mutation on steatosis and liver damage by alcohol intake in patients with chronic hepatitis C. J Hepatol 2011;55:1470–1471; author reply 1471–1472.
51 Guyot E, Sutton A, Rufat P, Laguillier C, Mansouri A, Moreau R, et al: PNPLA3 rs738409, hepatocellular carcinoma occurrence and risk model prediction in patients with cirrhosis. J Hepatol 2013;58:312–318.
52 Tian C, Stokowski RP, Kershenobich D, Ballinger DG, Hinds DA: Variant in PNPLA3 is associated with alcoholic liver disease. Nat Genet 2010;42:21–23.
53 Buch S, Stickel F, Trépo E, Way M, Herrmann A, Nischalke HD, et al: A genome-wide association study confirms PNPLA3 and identifies TM6SF2 and MBOAT7 as risk loci for alcohol-related cirrhosis. Nat Genet 2015;47:1443–1448.
54 Smagris E, BasuRay S, Li J, Huang Y, Lai KM, Gromada J, et al: Pnpla3I148M knockin mice accumulate PNPLA3 on lipid droplets and develop hepatic steatosis. Hepatology 2015; 61:108–118.
55 He S, McPhaul C, Li JZ, Garuti R, Kinch L, Grishin NV, et al: A sequence variation (I148M) in PNPLA3 associated with nonalcoholic fatty liver disease disrupts triglyceride hydrolysis. J Biol Chem 2010;285:6706–6715.
56 Huang Y, Cohen JC, Hobbs HH: Expression and characterization of a PNPLA3 protein isoform (I148M) associated with nonalcoholic fatty liver disease. J Biol Chem 2011;286: 37085–37093.
57 Pingitore P, Pirazzi C, Mancina RM, Motta BM, Indiveri C, Pujia A, et al: Recombinant PNPLA3 protein shows triglyceride hydrolase activity and its I148M mutation results in loss of function. Biochim Biophys Acta 2014;1841: 574–580.
58 Kumari M, Schoiswohl G, Chitraju C, Paar M: Adiponutrin functions as a nutritionally regulated lysophosphatidic acid acyltransferase. Cell Metab 2012;15:691–702.
59 Chen W, Chang B, Li L, Chan L: Patatin-like phospholipase domain-containing 3/adiponutrin deficiency in mice is not associated with fatty liver disease. Hepatology 2010;52:1134–1142.
60 Basantani MK, Sitnick MT, Cai L, Brenner DS, Gardner NP, Li JZ, et al: Pnpla3/adiponutrin deficiency in mice does not contribute to fatty liver disease or metabolic syndrome. J Lipid Res 2011;52:318–329.
61 Li JZ, Huang Y, Karaman R, Ivanova PT, Brown HA, Roddy T, et al: Chronic overexpression of PNPLA3I148M in mouse liver causes hepatic steatosis. J Clin Invest 2012; 122:4130–4144.
62 Ostapowicz G, Fontana RJ, Schiødt FV, Larson A, Davern TJ, Han SH, et al: Results of a prospective study of acute liver failure at 17 tertiary care centers in the United States. Ann Intern Med 2002;137:947–954.
63 Leise MD, Poterucha JJ, Talwalkar JA: Drug-induced liver injury. Mayo Clin Proc 2014;89: 95–106.
64 Kindmark A, Jawaid A, Harbron CG, Barratt BJ, Bengtsson OF, Andersson TB, et al: Genome-wide pharmacogenetic investigation of a hepatic adverse event without clinical signs of immunopathology suggests an underlying immune pathogenesis. Pharmacogenomics J 2008;8:186–195.
65 Neefjes J, Jongsma ML, Paul P, Bakke O: Towards a systems understanding of MHC class I and MHC class II antigen presentation. Nat Rev Immunol 2011;11:823–836.
66 Maria VA, Victorino RM: Diagnostic value of specific T cell reactivity to drugs in 95 cases of drug induced liver injury. Gut 1997;41:534–540.

67 Urban TJ, Shen Y, Stolz A, Chalasani N, Fontana RJ, Rochon J, et al: Limited contribution of common genetic variants to risk for liver injury due to a variety of drugs. Pharmacogenet Genomics 2012;22:784–795.
68 Daly AK, Donaldson PT, Bhatnagar P, Shen Y, Pe'er I, Floratos A, et al: HLA-B*5701 genotype is a major determinant of drug-induced liver injury due to flucloxacillin. Nat Genet 2009;41:816–819.
69 Singer JB, Lewitzky S, Leroy E, Yang F, Zhao X, Klickstein L, et al: A genome-wide study identifies HLA alleles associated with lumiracoxib-related liver injury. Nat Genet 2010;42: 711–714.
70 Spraggs CF, Budde LR, Briley LP, Bing N, Cox CJ, King KS, et al: HLA-DQA1*02:01 is a major risk factor for lapatinib-induced hepatotoxicity in women with advanced breast cancer. J Clin Oncol 2011;29:667–673.
71 Lucena MI, Molokhia M, Shen Y, Urban TJ, Aithal GP, Andrade RJ, et al: Susceptibility to amoxicillin-clavulanate-induced liver injury is influenced by multiple HLA class I and II alleles. Gastroenterology 2011;141:338–347.
72 Aithal GP, Grove JI: Genome-wide association studies in drug-induced liver injury: step change in understanding the pathogenesis. Semin Liver Dis 2015;35:421–431.
73 Kim CY, Quarsten H, Bergseng E, Khosla C, Sollid LM: Structural basis for HLA-DQ2-mediated presentation of gluten epitopes in celiac disease. Proc Natl Acad Sci U S A 2004; 101:4175–4179.
74 Pichler WJ, Adam J, Watkins S, Wuillemin N, Yun J, Yerly D: Drug hypersensitivity: how drugs stimulate T cells via pharmacological interaction with immune receptors. Int Arch Allergy Immunol 2015;168:13–24.
75 Illing PT, Vivian JP, Dudek NL, Kostenko L, Chen Z, Bharadwaj M, et al: Immune self-reactivity triggered by drug-modified HLA-peptide repertoire. Nature 2012;486:554–558.
76 Ostrov DA, Grant BJ, Pompeu YA, Sidney J, Harndahl M, Southwood S, et al: Drug hypersensitivity caused by alteration of the MHC-presented self-peptide repertoire. Proc Natl Acad Sci U S A 2012;109:9959–9964.
77 Uetrecht J: Immunoallergic drug-induced liver injury in humans. Semin Liver Dis 2009;29: 383–392.
78 Liberal R, Krawitt EL, Vierling JM, Manns MP, Mieli-Vergani G, Vergani D: Cutting edge issues in autoimmune hepatitis. J Autoimmun 2016;75:6–19.
79 Trivedi PJ, Hirschfield GM: Treatment of autoimmune liver disease: current and future therapeutic options. Ther Adv Chronic Dis 2013;4:119–141.
80 Arndtz K, Hirschfield GM: The pathogenesis of autoimmune liver disease. Dig Dis 2016;34: 327–333.
81 Hirschfield GM, Gershwin ME: The immunobiology and pathophysiology of primary biliary cirrhosis. Annu Rev Pathol 2013;8: 303–330.
82 Bogdanos DP, Invernizzi P, Mackay IR, Vergani D: Autoimmune liver serology: current diagnostic and clinical challenges. World J Gastroenterol 2008;14:3374–3387.
83 Juran BD, Lazaridis KN: Environmental factors in primary biliary cirrhosis. Semin Liver Dis 2014;34:265–272.
84 Hirschfield GM, Karlsen TH, Lindor KD, Adams DH: Primary sclerosing cholangitis. Lancet 2013;382:1587–1599.
85 Chung BK, Guevel BT, Reynolds GM, Gupta Udatha DB, Henriksen EK, Stamataki Z, et al: Phenotyping and auto-antibody production by liver-infiltrating B cells in primary sclerosing cholangitis and primary biliary cholangitis. J Autoimmun 2016;pii :S0896-8411(16)30226-8.
86 Karlsen TH: Primary sclerosing cholangitis: 50 years of a gut-liver relationship and still no love? Gut 2016;65:1579–1581.
87 Karlsen TH, Chung BK: Genetic risk and the development of autoimmune liver disease. Dig Dis 2015;33(suppl 2):13–24.
88 Mells GF, Kaser A, Karlsen TH: Novel insights into autoimmune liver diseases provided by genome-wide association studies. J Autoimmun 2013;46:41–54.
89 Webb GJ, Siminovitch KA, Hirschfield GM: The immunogenetics of primary biliary cirrhosis: a comprehensive review. J Autoimmun 2015;64:42–52.
90 Weiss KM, Terwilliger JD: How many diseases does it take to map a gene with SNPs? Nat Genet 2000;26:151–157.
91 Ellinghaus D, Jostins L, Spain SL, Cortes A, Bethune J, Han B, et al: Analysis of five chronic inflammatory diseases identifies 27 new associations and highlights disease-specific patterns at shared loci. Nat Genet 2016;48:510–518.
92 de Boer YS, van Gerven NM, Zwiers A, Verwer BJ, van Hoek B, van Erpecum KJ, et al: Genome-wide association study identifies variants associated with autoimmune hepatitis type 1. Gastroenterology 2014;147:443–452.e5.
93 Hirschfield GM, Liu X, Xu C, Lu Y, Xie G, Lu Y, et al: Primary biliary cirrhosis associated with HLA, IL12A, and IL12RB2 variants. N Engl J Med 2009;360:2544–2555.
94 Hirschfield GM, Liu X, Han Y, Gorlov IP, Lu Y, Xu C, et al: Variants at IRF5-TNPO3, 17q12-21 and MMEL1 are associated with primary biliary cirrhosis. Nat Genet 2010;42: 655–657.
95 Liu X, Invernizzi P, Lu Y, Kosoy R, Lu Y, Bianchi I, et al: Genome-wide meta-analyses identify three loci associated with primary biliary cirrhosis. Nat Genet 2010;42:658–660.
96 Mells GF, Floyd JA, Morley KI, Cordell HJ, Franklin CS, Shin SY, et al: Genome-wide association study identifies 12 new susceptibility loci for primary biliary cirrhosis. Nat Genet 2011;43:329–332.
97 Nakamura M, Nishida N, Kawashima M, Aiba Y, Tanaka A, Yasunami M, et al: Genome-wide association study identifies TNFSF15 and POU2AF1 as susceptibility loci for primary biliary cirrhosis in the Japanese population. Am J Hum Genet 2012;91:721–728.
98 Cordell HJ, Han Y, Mells GF, Li Y, Hirschfield GM, Greene CS, et al: International genome-wide meta-analysis identifies new primary biliary cirrhosis risk loci and targetable pathogenic pathways. Nat Commun 2015;6: 8019.
99 Karlsen TH, Franke A, Melum E, Kaser A, Hov JR, Balschun T, et al: Genome-wide association analysis in primary sclerosing cholangitis. Gastroenterology 2010;138: 1102–1111.
100 Melum E, Franke A, Schramm C, Weismüller TJ, Gotthardt DN, Offner FA, et al: Genome-wide association analysis in primary sclerosing cholangitis identifies two non-HLA susceptibility loci. Nat Genet 2011;43: 17–19.
101 Folseraas T, Melum E, Rausch P, Juran BD, Ellinghaus E, Shiryaev A, et al: Extended analysis of a genome-wide association study in primary sclerosing cholangitis detects multiple novel risk loci. J Hepatol 2012;57: 366–375.
102 Srivastava B, Mells GF, Cordell HJ, Muriithi A, Brown M, Ellinghaus E, et al: Fine mapping and replication of genetic risk loci in primary sclerosing cholangitis. Scand J Gastroenterol 2012;47:820–826.
103 Ellinghaus D, Folseraas T, Holm K, Ellinghaus E, Melum E, Balschun T, et al: Genome-wide association analysis in primary sclerosing cholangitis and ulcerative colitis identifies risk loci at GPR35 and TCF4. Hepatology 2013;58:1074–1083.
104 Liu JZ, Hov JR, Folseraas T, Ellinghaus E, Rushbrook SM, Doncheva NT, et al: Dense genotyping of immune-related disease regions identifies nine new risk loci for primary sclerosing cholangitis. Nat Genet 2013;45: 670–675.
105 Ji SG, Juran BD, Mucha S, Folseraas T, Jostins L, Melum E, et al: Genome-wide association study of primary sclerosing cholangitis identifies new risk loci and quantifies the genetic relationship with inflammatory bowel disease. Nat Genet 2016, Epub ahead of print.

The Science of Hepatitis

Digestive Diseases

Dig Dis 2017;35:334–338
DOI: 10.1159/000456584

Overcoming CD8+ T-Cell Exhaustion in Viral Hepatitis: Lessons from the Mouse Model and Clinical Perspectives

Dominik Wieland[a–c] Maike Hofmann[a] Robert Thimme[a]

[a]Department of Medicine II, University Hospital Freiburg, [b]Spemann Graduate School of Biology and Medicine, and [c]Faculty of Biology, University of Freiburg, Freiburg, Germany

Keywords

T-cell exhaustion · T-cell restoration · Checkpoint inhibitors

Abstract

About 500 million people all over the world are chronically infected with hepatitis B virus (HBV) or hepatitis C virus (HCV) and are thus at high risk of developing liver fibrosis, cirrhosis or hepatocellular carcinoma. While in adults about 90% of acutely HBV-infected patients clear the virus, only 30% of acute HCV infections clear spontaneously. Several mechanisms contribute to the failure in viral clearance. The main factors responsible for the chronification of HBV and HCV infection are, on the one hand, viral escape mutations leading to lack of recognition by antiviral immune cells and, on the other hand, loss of antiviral effector functions of virus-specific CD8+ T cells, called T-cell exhaustion. This review focuses on the latter highlighting current knowledge about the heterogeneity of exhausted CD8+ T cells and the potential for re-invigoration of exhausted T-cell populations during chronic viral hepatitis. Although direct-acting antivirals successfully clear chronic HCV infection, there is still the need for a prophylactic vaccine to prevent primary infection. Moreover, a therapeutic strategy eliminating HBV infection still does not exist. A better understanding of T-cell exhaustion and the potential for functional recovery will help to develop new immunotherapeutic approaches for chronic viral hepatitis.

CD8+ T-Cell Responses in Hepatitis B Virus and Hepatitis C Virus Infection

Chronic infections with hepatitis B virus (HBV) and hepatitis C virus (HCV) are a global health problem representing a leading cause for hepatic cirrhosis and cancer [1, 2]. Most acutely HBV-infected adults achieve viral clearance (~90%). However, only a minor subgroup of patients can clear acute HCV infection (~30%). Clearance of acute HBV or HCV infection occurs in the presence of strong and broad antiviral CD8+ T-cell responses [3–6]. The key role of virus-specific CD8+ T cells in HBV and HCV clearance has been proven by the depletion of CD8+ T cells in chimpanzees demonstrating prolonged viremia until the reappearance of virus-specific CD8+ T-cell responses in the blood and especially the liver [7, 8]. Patients who establish chronic viral infection

KARGER

E-Mail karger@karger.com
www.karger.com/ddi

Robert Thimme
Department of Medicine II
University Hospital Freiburg
Hugstetter Strasse 55, DE–79106 Freiburg (Germany)
E-Mail robert.thimme@uniklinik-freiburg.de

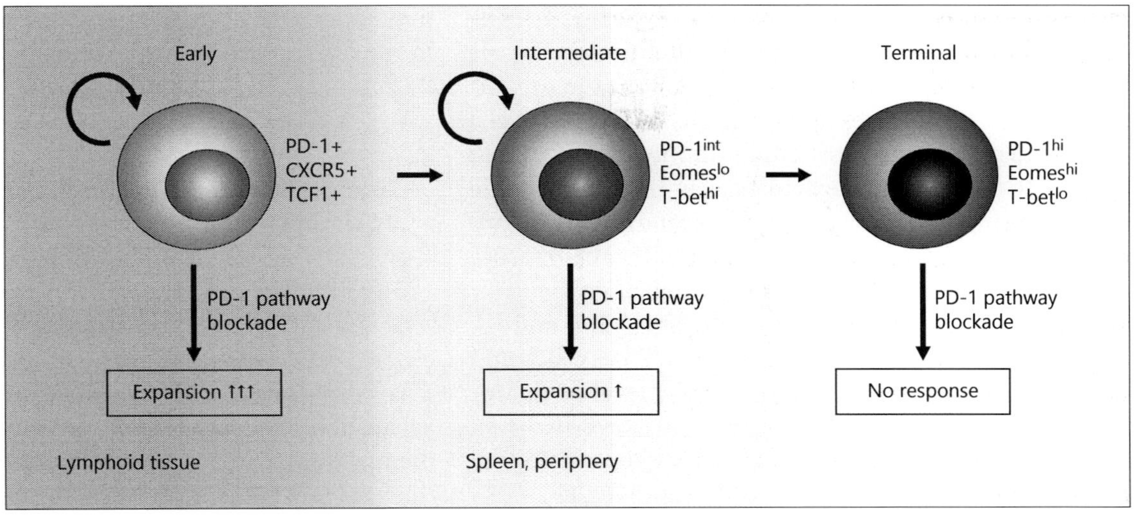

Fig. 1. Major sub-populations of exhausted CD8+ T cells and their responsiveness upon PD-1 pathway blockade. Co-expression of CXCR5, TCF1 and PD-1 defines an early differentiated sub-population of exhausted CD8+ T cells. This sub-population mainly resides in the lymphoid tissue and provides a strong proliferative response upon PD-1 pathway blockade. Further differentiated T-cell populations can be found in the spleen and periphery. Whereas the T-bet^{hi}Eomes^{dim} sub-population still harbors some proliferative potential, the terminally exhausted PD-1^{hi}T-bet^{dim}Eomes^{hi} T-cell sub-population has lost effector functions and is unresponsive to PD-1 pathway blockade.

typically exhibit ineffective CD8+ T-cell responses. One reason for CD8+ T-cell failure is the emergence of viral sequence mutations that can lead to loss of recognition by antiviral CD8+ T cells. In HBV infection, such viral escape seems to play a minor role [9–12]. In contrast, viral escape can be observed in about half the number of HCV-infected patients [9, 13, 14]. A further key determinant for the failure of virus-specific CD8+ T-cell responses is a phenomenon called T-cell exhaustion in which chronic antigen stimulation of virus-specific CD8+ T cells leads to a gradual loss of antiviral effector functions [15–20].

Exhaustion of Virus-Specific CD8+ T Cells

Exhausted virus-specific CD8+ T cells exhibit strongly reduced effector functions upon antigen encounter including low cytokine production, decreased cytotoxicity and impaired proliferative capacity [21]. These functional alterations are accompanied by changes in CD8+ T-cell phenotype like co-expression of multiple inhibitory receptors such as PD-1 or CTLA4, loss of memory markers and an altered transcriptional program [15, 21–27]. Although ongoing antigen triggering seems to be a key driver, the molecular pathways inducing CD8+ T-cell exhaustion are not completely understood and further extrinsic factors like reduced CD4+ T-cell help, increased regulatory T-cell activity or immunoinhibitory cytokines seem to promote T-cell exhaustion [28–33]. The physiological role of T-cell exhaustion is a matter of debate. A common point of view is that T-cell exhaustion limits immunopathology. However, whether CD8+ T-cells functionally adapt to chronic infection by initiating a specific differentiation program or whether CD8+ T-cells passively acquire a state of dysfunction is still controversial [34]. Importantly, recent data reveal that exhausted virus-specific CD8+ T cells targeting one specific viral epitope cannot be considered a homogeneously dysfunctional cell population but instead consist of phenotypically and functionally distinct T-cell sub-populations.

Heterogeneity within Exhausted Virus-Specific CD8+ T-Cell Populations

In human viral hepatitis, in-depth analysis of exhausted T-cell populations is difficult. Low cell numbers that originate from blood or liver isolates limit the possibilities for analyzing HBV- and HCV-specific CD8+ T-cell sub-populations. However, this knowledge is of great demand to establish therapeutic strategies to cure chronic HBV infection [35], or to prevent primary HCV infection or re-infection after clearance with direct acting antivirals (DAA) [36]. Noteworthy, knowledge gathered from mouse models of chronic viral infections gives important novel insights into the organization of single epitope-specific CD8+ T-cell sub-populations. The most common mouse model that is used to study T-cell exhaustion is the lymphocytic choriomeningitis virus (LCMV). Depending on the virus strain that is used, LCMV infection results in acute or chronic viral infection. This model strongly contributed to the understanding of T-cell exhaustion and revealed heterogeneity among exhausted T cells [37, 38]. Early studies focused on the expression level of the inhibitory receptor PD-1 to determine the severity of T-cell exhaustion and demonstrated that terminally exhausted (PD-1^{hi}) as well as less differentiated (PD-1^{int}) T cells exist within a single LCMV-specific CD8+ T-cell population [39]. Further studies investigated the transcriptional program that regulates T-cell exhaustion and revealed that co-expression analysis of the T-box transcription factors T-bet and Eomesodermin (Eomes) can be used to characterize a less differentiated progenitor population of T-$bet^{hi}Eomes^{dim}$ cells and a terminally exhausted T-$bet^{dim}Eomes^{hi}$ population [40]. In contrast to the terminally exhausted subset, the T-$bet^{hi}Eomes^{dim}$ population retained some potential to produce antiviral effector cytokines. Moreover, it has been shown that the 2 sub-populations are in a progenitor/progeny relationship. These data indicated that exhausted T cells not only show phenotypical but also functional heterogeneity. Recently, the transcription factor T-cell factor 1 (TCF1) that is important for the establishment of CD8+ T-cell memory [41] was described to demarcate a circulating sub-population of LCMV-specific CD8+ T cells that sustain the virus-specific CD8+ T-cell pool during chronic viral infection [42]. In addition, a population of TCF1+ LCMV-specific CD8+ T cells expressing the chemokine receptor CXCR5 was found in lymphatic organs that serves as a "stem cell-like" population during chronic viral infection and gives rise to the further differentiated T-cell pool in the periphery [43, 44]. Overall, studies in mice revealed the existence of functionally distinct T-cell sub-populations within exhausted virus-specific CD8+ T cells (Fig. 1). Although currently unknown, the situation in humans might be even more complex. Depending on the setting of human chronic viral hepatitis (e.g., active or inactive chronic HBV infection, viral hepatitis in individuals with or without liver cirrhosis) different T-cell sub-populations might predominate. Thus, studies in HBV and HCV infection are needed to determine T-cell sub-populations in humans and to identify their key roles in the different infection courses before, during and after human chronic viral infection.

The Potential for Reinvigoration of Exhausted CD8+ T Cells in Chronic Viral Infection

Recently, there has been growing interest in blocking interactions of inhibitory receptors with their ligands to recover T-cell functionality [45]. These checkpoint inhibitors have been proven to be highly effective in reversing T-cell exhaustion in cancer [46, 47]. While the success of DAA therapy diminished the need for alternative treatment options in HCV [48], the potential of checkpoint inhibitors in chronic HBV infection is highly appealing. In vitro studies showed that HBV-specific CD8+ T cells respond to the PD-1 pathway blockade by an enhanced proliferative potential and increased cytokine production [22, 49]. Moreover, in vivo studies of chronic hepadnaviral infection in woodchucks showed that a combination therapy of nucleoside analogs, therapeutic DNA vaccination and PD-1 pathway blockade recovered the functionality of virus-specific CD8+ T cells and resulted in an improved sustained viral control and even complete viral clearance in some animals [50]. Great effort has been made to understand the mechanisms of checkpoint inhibitors. Interestingly, data from the LCMV mouse model showed that not all exhausted virus-specific CD8+ T cells respond upon checkpoint blockade. Early reports by Blackburn et al. [39] have shown that the terminally exhausted fraction of LCMV-specific T cells (PD-1^{hi}) was unresponsive to the PD-1 pathway blockade and prone to cell death by apoptosis. It was the less differentiated PD-1^{int} LCMV-specific CD8+ T-cells (later identified as T-$bet^{hi}Eomes^{dim}$) that could be rescued by PD-1 pathway blockade resulting in reduced apoptosis while enhancing T-cell expansion and protective immunity [40]. Most recent results then assigned the major proliferative responsiveness upon PD-1 pathway blockade to the CXCR5+TCF1+ progenitor population of LCMV-specific CD8+ T cells that resides in the lymphoid tissue [43, 44] (Fig. 1). These insights into the mechanisms of therapeutic PD-1 pathway blockade demonstrate that it is necessary to understand the heterogeneity of virus-specific CD8+ T-cell populations in human chronic hepatitis to predict the responsiveness upon checkpoint blockade. Although the success of the inhibitory receptor pathway blockade in cancer therapy is promising, recent work in the LCMV mouse model revealed that PD-1 pathway blockade only temporarily improves T-cell functionality and cannot re-program exhausted T cells to acquire the epigenetic signature of effector or memory T cells [51]. These results suggest that T-cell exhaustion is heavily imprinted and that inhibition of the PD-1 pathway is not able to ultimately overcome T-cell exhaustion in chronic viral infection. Of note, in this study, it might be possible that ongoing T-cell stimulation during chronic viral infection precluded T-cell recovery. However, work in the clinically relevant model of HCV-infected chimpanzees showed that virus-specific CD8+ T-cell responses could not prevent HCV re-infection even 1 year after DAA-mediated HCV clearance [52]. This suggests that the imprinting of T-cell exhaustion is maintained even after cessation of chronic antigen stimulation. In contrast, however, Martin et al. [53] could show that at least the proliferative capacity of exhausted HCV-specific CD8+ T cells improves during DAA-mediated HCV clearance. Further studies in patients receiving DAA therapy need to address this critical question in more detail and describe the fate of exhausted CD8+ T cells after cessation of chronic antigen stimulation in humans. Whether long-term antigen clearance eventually licenses exhausted CD8+ T cells to regain antiviral effector functions remains to be clarified. Overall, as latest work in T-cell exhaustion indicates that the potential for functional restoration differs between T-cell sub-populations, characterization of the diverse sub-populations is necessary to uncover new molecular pathways beside inhibitory receptor pathway blockade that can be targeted by immunomodulation.

Conclusion and Future Perspectives

Checkpoint inhibitors like PD-1 pathway blockade already demonstrate great therapeutic potential in cancer studies. However, manipulating physiological mechanisms of T-cell inhibition come with safety concerns that require careful evaluation. In addition, the approach of checkpoint inhibition does not seem to overwrite the genetic program of T-cell exhaustion and thus long-term success for reinvigoration of exhausted T-cells still is controversial. Of note, current research has shown that exhausted virus-specific CD8+ T cells consist of diverse sub-populations with different functional responsiveness. This knowledge allows the development of immunotherapeutic approaches that target a specific T-cell sub-population and the respective molecular pathways to balance beneficial and detrimental effects. However, as most data is obtained from mouse models of chronic viral infection, studies in the human setting are greatly needed. Future work in human chronic viral infection will have to determine the relevance of data from the mouse model for the human system and thus highlight the most promising sub-populations and pathways of human exhausted T cells for immunotherapeutic approaches.

Disclosure Statement

Nothing to disclose.

References

1 Schweitzer A, et al: Estimations of worldwide prevalence of chronic hepatitis B virus infection: a systematic review of data published between 1965 and 2013. Lancet 2015;386:1546–1555.
2 Messina JP, et al: Global distribution and prevalence of hepatitis C virus genotypes. Hepatology 2015;61:77–87.
3 Cooper S, et al: Analysis of a successful immune response against hepatitis C virus. Immunity 1999;10:439–449.
4 Lechner F, et al: Analysis of successful immune responses in persons infected with hepatitis C virus. J Exp Med 2000;191:1499–1512.
5 Rehermann B, et al: The cytotoxic T lymphocyte response to multiple hepatitis B virus polymerase epitopes during and after acute viral hepatitis. J Exp Med 1995;181:1047–1058.
6 Thimme R, et al: Viral and immunological determinants of hepatitis C virus clearance, persistence, and disease. Proc Natl Acad Sci U S A 2002;99:15661–15668.
7 Shoukry NH, et al: Memory CD8+ T cells are required for protection from persistent hepatitis C virus infection. J Exp Med 2003;197:1645–1655.
8 Thimme R, et al: CD8(+) T cells mediate viral clearance and disease pathogenesis during acute hepatitis B virus infection. J Virol 2003;77:68–76.
9 Nitschke K, et al: CD8+ T-cell responses in hepatitis B and C: the (HLA-) A, B, and C of Hepatitis B and C. Dig Dis 2016;34:396–409.
10 Rehermann B, et al: Hepatitis B virus (HBV) sequence variation of cytotoxic T lymphocyte epitopes is not common in patients with chronic HBV infection. J Clin Invest 1995;96:1527–1534.
11 Desmond CP, et al: Viral adaptation to host immune responses occurs in chronic hepatitis B virus (HBV) infection, and adaptation is greatest in HBV e antigen-negative disease. J Virol 2012;86:1181–1192.
12 Kefalakes H, et al: Adaptation of the hepatitis B virus core protein to CD8(+) T-cell selection pressure. Hepatology 2015;62:47–56.
13 Neumann-Haefelin C, et al: Virological and immunological determinants of intrahepatic virus-specific CD8+ T-Cell failure in chronic hepatitis C virus infection. Hepatology 2008;47:1824–1836.
14 Cox AL, et al: Cellular immune selection with hepatitis C virus persistence in humans. J Exp Med 2005;201:1741–1752.
15 Boni C, et al: Characterization of hepatitis B virus (HBV)-specific T-cell dysfunction in chronic HBV infection. J Virol 2007;81:4215–4225.
16 Gruener NH, et al: Sustained dysfunction of antiviral CD8+ T lymphocytes after infection with hepatitis C virus. J Virol 2001;75:5550–5558.
17 Lechner F, et al: Analysis of successful immune responses in persons infected with hepatitis C virus. J Exp Med 2000;191:1499–1512.
18 Gallimore A, et al: Induction and exhaustion of lymphocytic choriomeningitis virus-specific cytotoxic T lymphocytes visualized using soluble tetrameric major histocompatibility complex class I-peptide complexes. J Exp Med 1998;187:1383–1393.

19 Zajac AJ, et al: Viral immune evasion due to persistence of activated T cells without effector function. J Exp Med 1998;188:2205–2213.
20 Angelosanto JM, et al: Progressive loss of memory T cell potential and commitment to exhaustion during chronic viral infection. J Virol 2012;86:8161–8170.
21 Wherry EJ: T cell exhaustion. Nat Immunol 2011;12:492–499.
22 Bengsch B, et al: Coexpression of PD-1, 2B4, CD160 and KLRG1 on exhausted HCV-specific CD8+ T cells is linked to antigen recognition and T cell differentiation. PLoS Pathog 2010;6:e1000947.
23 Schurich A, et al: Role of the coinhibitory receptor cytotoxic T lymphocyte antigen-4 on apoptosis-prone CD8 T cells in persistent hepatitis B virus infection. Hepatology 2011; 53:1494–1503.
24 Owusu Sekyere S, et al: A heterogeneous hierarchy of co-regulatory receptors regulates exhaustion of HCV-specific CD8 T cells in patients with chronic hepatitis C. J Hepatol 2015;62:31–40.
25 Wherry EJ, et al: Molecular signature of CD8+ T cell exhaustion during chronic viral infection. Immunity 2007;27:670–684.
26 Blackburn SD, et al: Coregulation of CD8+ T cell exhaustion by multiple inhibitory receptors during chronic viral infection. Nat Immunol 2009;10:29–37.
27 Buggert M, et al: T-bet and Eomes are differentially linked to the exhausted phenotype of CD8+ T cells in HIV infection. PLoS Pathog 2014;10:e1004251.
28 Knolle PA, Thimme R: Hepatic immune regulation and its involvement in viral hepatitis infection. Gastroenterology 2014;146:1193–1207.
29 Battegay M, et al: Enhanced establishment of a virus carrier state in adult Cd4+ T-cell-deficient mice. J Virol 1994;68:4700–4704.
30 Ng CT, Oldstone MB: IL-10: achieving balance during persistent viral infection. Curr Top Microbiol Immunol 2014;380:129–144.
31 Boettler T, et al: T cells with a CD4+CD25+ regulatory phenotype suppress in vitro proliferation of virus-specific CD8+ T cells during chronic hepatitis C virus infection. J Virol 2005;79:7860–7867.
32 Cabrera R, et al: An immunomodulatory role for CD4(+)CD25(+) regulatory T lymphocytes in hepatitis C virus infection. Hepatology 2004;40:1062–1071.
33 Stoop JN, et al: Regulatory T cells contribute to the impaired immune response in patients with chronic hepatitis B virus infection. Hepatology 2005;41:771–778.
34 Speiser DE, et al: T cell differentiation in chronic infection and cancer: functional adaptation or exhaustion? Nat Rev Immunol 2014;14:768–774.
35 Liang TJ, et al: Present and future therapies of hepatitis B: from discovery to cure. Hepatology 2015;62:1893–1908.
36 Baumert TF, et al: A prophylactic hepatitis C virus vaccine: a distant peak still worth climbing. J Hepatol 2014;61(1 suppl):S34–S44.
37 Moskophidis D, et al: Virus persistence in acutely infected immunocompetent mice by exhaustion of antiviral cytotoxic effector T cells. Nature 1993;362:758–761.
38 Zhou X, et al: Role of lymphocytic choriomeningitis virus (LCMV) in understanding viral immunology: past, present and future. Viruses 2012;4:2650–2669.
39 Blackburn SD, et al: Selective expansion of a subset of exhausted CD8 T cells by alphaPD-L1 blockade. Proc Natl Acad Sci U S A 2008;105: 15016–15021.
40 Paley MA, et al: Progenitor and terminal subsets of CD8+ T cells cooperate to contain chronic viral infection. Science 2012;338: 1220–1225.
41 Zhou X, et al: Differentiation and persistence of memory CD8(+) T cells depend on T cell factor 1. Immunity 2010;33:229–240.
42 Utzschneider DT, et al: T cell factor 1-expressing memory-like CD8(+) T cells sustain the immune response to chronic viral infections. Immunity 2016;45:415–427.
43 Im SJ, et al: Defining CD8+ T cells that provide the proliferative burst after PD-1 therapy. Nature 2016;537:417–421.
44 He R, et al: Follicular CXCR5-expressing CD8+ T cells curtail chronic viral infection. Nature 2016;537:412–428.
45 Pauken KE, Wherry EJ: Overcoming T cell exhaustion in infection and cancer. Trends Immunol 2015;36:265–276.
46 Barber DL, et al: Restoring function in exhausted CD8 T cells during chronic viral infection. Nature 2006;439:682–687.
47 Brahmer JR, et al: Safety and activity of anti-PD-L1 antibody in patients with advanced cancer. N Engl J Med 2012;366:2455–2465.
48 Webster DP, Klenerman P, Dusheiko GM: Hepatitis C. Lancet 2015;385:1124–1135.
49 Fisicaro P, et al: Antiviral intrahepatic T-cell responses can be restored by blocking programmed death-1 pathway in chronic hepatitis B. Gastroenterology 2010;138:682–693, 693.e1–e4.
50 Liu J, et al: Enhancing virus-specific immunity in vivo by combining therapeutic vaccination and PD-L1 blockade in chronic hepadnaviral infection. PLoS Pathog 2014;10: e1003856.
51 Pauken KE, et al: Epigenetic stability of exhausted T cells limits durability of reinvigoration by PD-1 blockade. Science 2016;354: 1160–1165.
52 Callendret B, et al: T-cell immunity and hepatitis C virus reinfection after cure of chronic hepatitis C with an interferon-free antiviral regimen in a chimpanzee. Hepatology 2014; 60:1531–1540.
53 Martin B, et al: Restoration of HCV-specific CD8+ T cell function by interferon-free therapy. J Hepatol 2014;61:538–543.

Hepatitis Treatment: The Challenges

Digestive Diseases

Dig Dis 2017;35:339–346
DOI: 10.1159/000456585

Treating Hepatitis C in Patients with Renal Failure

Sabela Lens[a] Sergio Rodriguez-Tajes[a] Laura-Patricia Llovet[a]
Francisco Maduell[b] Maria-Carlota Londoño[a]

[a]Liver Unit, CIBERehd, and [b]Nephrology Department, Hospital Clínic Barcelona, IDIBAPS, Barcelona, Spain

Keywords
End-stage renal disease · Hepatitis C · Direct-acting antivirals

Abstract

Background: There is a strong relationship between hepatitis C virus (HCV) infection and the kidney. Approximately 10–16% of the patients with HCV infection develop renal disease, and the prevalence of HCV infection in patients with renal dysfunction is higher than that of the general population (9.5 vs. 1.6%). Moreover, HCV-positive patients on hemodialysis (HD) have higher mortality rates as compared to HCV-negative patients also on HD, not only due to liver-related complications but also owing to cardiovascular disease. ***Key Messages:*** In the interferon era, the treatment of HCV infection in patients on HD was hampered due to a significant number of treatment-related adverse events (predominately anemia and infectious complications). The development of direct-acting antivirals (DAAs) has revolutionized the field allowing viral eradication in these very sick patients. Two recently published clinical trials assessed the efficacy and safety of DAAs in patients with end-stage renal disease (ESRD). The combination of grazoprevir and elbasvir has been studied in the C-SURFER trial with 94% of the patients achieving sustained virological response (SVR). Adverse events were mild and only a small number of patients discontinued therapy early due to adverse events. The 3D regimen was evaluated in the RUBY-I trial. Here, a 90% SVR rate was achieved in 20 patients with ESRD, most of them on HD. Although sofosbuvir is eliminated by the kidney and its use in patients with glomerular filtration rate <30 mL/min is not recommended, real-life data have shown good results for this drug in terms of efficacy and safety. ***Conclusions:*** The use of DAAs has safely permitted the treatment of patients with renal dysfunction with excellent efficacy results.

Introduction

It has been estimated that approximately 170 million people around the world are living with hepatitis C virus (HCV) infection and 500,000 people died because of HCV-related liver disease in 2010. Hepatitis C is tightly bound to the kidney function. Thus, the prevalence of hepatitis C in patients on hemodialysis (HD) is higher than that found among the general population. A study published in 2013 by Dialysis Outcomes and Practice Pattern Study with data from more than 49,000 patients from different countries around the world showed that the prevalence of HCV infection in patients on HD was 9.5%, ranging between 3.3 and 16.8% [1]. Moreover, HCV infection confers a higher morbidity and mortality risk to patients on HD. Hence, a meta-analysis of 14 observational studies confirmed that the presence of anti-HCV antibodies was an independent risk factor for death in patients on maintenance HD with a relative risk (RR) of 1.35 (95% CI 1.25–1.47). Interestingly, the increased risk of death in these patients was not only due to liver-related

KARGER

E-Mail karger@karger.com
www.karger.com/ddi

Maria-Carlota Londoño, MD
Liver Unit
Hospital Clínic Barcelona
Calle Villarroel 170, ES–08036 Barcelona (Spain)
E-Mail MLONDONO@clinic.ub.es

mortality (RR 3.82; 95% CI 1.92–7.61), but it was also related to cardiovascular disease with an RR of 1.26 (95% CI 1.10–1.45) despite adjusting for confounding factors such as age, gender, time on HD and diabetes. These data suggest a potential atherogenic role of the HCV, which is probably produced through the aggravation of the individual components of the metabolic syndrome [2].

On the other hand, the HCV impairs the kidney. The most common cause of renal dysfunction in HCV-positive patients is the presence of mixed cryoglobulinemia, which is characterized by an immune complex-mediated vasculitis affecting small vessels, as a result of a non-malignant clonal stimulation of B lymphocytes generating cryoglobulins [3]. Other glomerular diseases have been rarely reported. In a large study conducted among US veterans, there was a significantly higher proportion of membranoproliferative glomerulonephritis among the HCV-positive patients included in the cohort as compared to those without the HCV infection [4]. In addition, several studies have observed an impact of HCV infection in the risk of developing/progressing kidney damage. Tsui et al. [5] analyzing data from more than 15,000 patients from NHANES III evidenced an age-dependent significant association between HCV seropositivity and the presence of albuminuria. Moreover, a very large study including data from 474,369 veterans showed that HCV-positive patients had a higher risk of developing end-stage renal disease (ESRD) as compared to their negative counterparts (4.26 vs. 3.05 per 1,000 person-years, respectively) [6]. More recently, Chen et al. [7], with data from the Taiwan National Health Insurance Research Database found that after a mean follow-up of 7.12 years, the incidence of chronic kidney disease (CKD) was 1.66-fold higher in the HCV-positive cohort as compared to HCV-negative patients. Finally, a recent meta-analysis from 14 observational studies evaluated the risk of CKD in 336,227 individuals infected with hepatitis C and compared it with the risk in 2,665,631 uninfected patients. The study showed that HCV-positive patients have a 26% greater risk of developing or having progression of CKD [8]. Altogether these data support the relevance of the interaction between HCV and the kidney.

Evaluation of Renal Function in Patients with Hepatitis C

Given the important association between HCV and renal impairment, all patients with HCV infection should be evaluated for the presence of albuminuria/proteinuria, hematuria, decreased glomerular filtration rate (GFR) and hypertension. According to Kidney Disease: Improving Global Outcomes (KDIGO) guidelines, a random urine sample must be collected to determine the presence of hematuria and the albumin-to-creatinine ratio (ACR; or protein-to-creatinine ratio), together with the estimation of GFR (eGFR) annually in patients with HCV infection. The presence of an ACR >30 mg/g or an eGFR <60 mL/min that persist for more than 3 months leads to the diagnosis of CKD [9]. Patients with impaired renal function, hematuria or proteinuria should complete the study by undergoing testing for cryoglobulins, complement levels and rheumatoid factor. A kidney biopsy should also be considered in order to establish the cause of renal dysfunction.

Evaluation of Liver Disease in Patients with Renal Failure

EASL guidelines recommend the assessment of liver fibrosis before starting antiviral therapy in patients with HCV infection. Detecting patients with advanced fibrosis or cirrhosis in order to determine the prognosis and the need for surveillance of hepatocellular carcinoma is especially important [10]. Non-invasive tests including liver stiffness measurements or blood biomarkers have been widely validated in the assessment of liver fibrosis and therefore liver biopsy can be reserved to cases of uncertainty or those in which other etiologies are suspected. Moreover, the presence of hemostatic disorders in patients with ESRD on HD could increase the risk of hemorrhagic complications of the liver biopsy hampering its applicability [11].

In patients on HD, the non-invasive evaluation of liver fibrosis has been less studied. Liu et al. [12], compared the performance of transient elastography (TE) and APRI score (AST-to-platelets ratio) with liver biopsy in 284 patients with chronic hepatitis C on HD. The authors found that TE was good and superior to APRI score in the assessment of the severity of liver fibrosis with areas under the receiver operating characteristic (AUROC) curve >0.9 for fibrosis stages ≥F2, ≥F3, or F4. The main concern with the use of TE in patients on HD is whether volume overload overestimates liver fibrosis. A recent study conducted in 36 patients on HD showed no significant changes in liver stiffness determined by TE before and after an HD session with a mean volume withdrawal of 2.55 L. However, in patients in whom the net volume withdrawal was greater than 2.55 L, the authors observed a statistically significant decrease in liver stiffness after the HD session. Although for obvious reasons the study lacked liver biopsies, it suggests that volume overload at pre-HD could yield a falsely elevated determination of liver stiffness [13]. Non-invasive biomarkers of fibrosis have also been scarcely studied in patients on HD. Varaut et al. [14] determined the diagnostic accuracy of Fibrotest® in the evaluation of liver fibrosis in patients on HD and in kidney transplant (KT) recipients. There were no significant differences between KT recipients and patients on HD. However, the AUROC curve for the diagnosis of significant fibrosis was poor for patients on HD (0.47 vs. 0.71 in KT recipients). These results are not unexpected since most of the components of Fibrotest® are affected by renal dysfunction: levels of α2 macroglobulin increase in dialysis patients due to chronic inflammation, apolipoprotein A1 levels are low, hemolysis in the context of HD increases bilirubin and decreases haptoglobin, and finally gamma-glutamil transferase levels are lower in HD patients. Although AST levels and platelet counts could be affected by dialysis (lower transaminase levels and heparin-induced low platelet counts), a study showed that the APRI score with adjusted cut-off points has an AUROC curve of 0.81 in the prediction of significant fibrosis [11].

In summary, and in spite of the scarcity of information, TE seems to be able to correctly evaluate fibrosis in patients on HD, especially when this technique is performed in the absence of fluid overload. The use of blood biomarkers of fibrosis could not be recommended due to the variations in the score components in patients on HD.

Treatment

Whom to Treat?

The KDIGO guidelines recommend that all patients with CKD should be screened for the presence of HCV infection. The decision to treat should be individualized but must take into consideration the potential risks and benefits of antiviral therapy. Traditionally, and according to KDIGO recommendations, all HCV-positive patients with CKD (dialysis dependent or not) on the waiting list for a KT were candidates who were to receive antiviral therapy. The benefits of viral eradication in these patients were the slowing of liver fibrosis progression and the avoidance of the extra-hepatic complications of HCV after KT (including de novo glomerulonephritis, post-transplant diabetes mellitus, humoral rejection, or chronic allograft nephropathy [15]). From a theoretical point and because HCV has been linked with an accelerated atherogenesis [16], it is possible that an additional benefit of viral eradication would be a decrease in cardiovascular morbidity and mortality. However, there are no data on the long-term effects of viral eradication.

Despite the benefits of viral eradication, in the interferon (IFN) era, the use of antiviral treatment in patients on HD was hampered by the high number of adverse events related to therapy, especially anemia and infections. In fact, data from the DOPS showed that only 1% of 4,589 HCV-positive patients on HD received an IFN-based therapy [1]. The development of direct-acting antivirals (DAAs) has completely changed the scenario enabling the treatment of more difficult patients including those with ESRD. The advantages of DAAs in patients with ESRD are (1) the increase in the efficacy results, (2) the improvement in safety, and (3) the possibility to treat the patients after KT (the use of IFN after KT was not recommended due to the high risk of allograft rejection). The later is a very important issue because it opens a discussion regarding the appropriate time to indicate the antiviral therapy to KT candidates. The scarcity of organ donors and the significant number of patients awaiting KT have led to the acceptance of HCV-positive organs for transplantation in order to decrease waiting times. Data on the use of an HCV-positive donor in an HCV-positive KT recipient are controversial. Some studies have shown an increase in the risk of dead, graft loss and severe liver disease [17–19] but a prospective, multicenter study from Spain showed that the use of HCV-positive donors in HCV-positive KT recipients (n = 162) was not an independent risk factor for liver disease severity, and graft and patient survival [20].

Despite the potential concerns on the use of HCV-positive donors raised in the previously mentioned studies, there are some issues that favor the use of these donors: (1) the minimization of dialysis time is a priority because HCV-positive patients who receive a KT live longer than HCV-positive patients on HD [21] (the exception for this statement would be the presence of significant fibrosis or cirrhosis that increases the risk of disease progression or clinical decompensations), (2) current data with the use of new DAAs are excellent in terms of efficacy and safety after KT [22–25] even in patients who had received an HCV-positive donor [26]. With all these factors in mind and where the use of HCV-positive donors is acceptable, some authors suggest the postponement of antiviral therapy until the post-transplant period in patients with mild to moderate liver fibrosis in order to decrease waiting times. The main concern with this strategy is the possibility of infecting a patient with a difficult-to-treat genotype,

Dig Dis 2017;35:339–346
DOI: 10.1159/000456585

Table 1. Pharmacokinetics of direct-acting antivirals in patients with end-stage renal disease

DAA	Elimination	GFR 50–80 mL/min	GFR 30–50 mL/min	GFR <30 mL/min
Sofosbuvir [38]	Renal 80%	GS-331007 AUC↑ 56%	GS-331007 AUC↑ 90%	GS-331007 AUC↑ 456%
Dasabuvir [39]	GI 90% Renal <2%	AUC↑ 21%	AUC↑ 37%	AUC↑ 50%
Daclatasvir [40]	GI 88% Renal 6%	No change	No change	No change
Ledipasvir [41]	GI 86% Renal 1%	No change	No change	No change
Ombitasvir [39]	GI 90% Renal <2%	No change	No change	No change
Elbasvir [42]	Renal <1%	No change	No change	No change
Velpatasvir [43]	GI 77%	No data	No data	No change
Simeprevir [44]	GI 91% Renal <0.4%	No change	No change	No change
Paritaprevir/ritonavir [39]	GI 90% Renal <2%	AUC↑ 19%/ AUC↑ 42%	AUC↑ 33%/ AUC↑ 80%*	AUC↑ 45%/ AUC↑ 114%*
Grazoprevir [42]	Renal <1%	No change	No change	No change

* Lower exposure as compared to higher doses of ritonavir use in HIV treatments. DAA, direct-acting antiviral; GFR, glomerular filtration rate; GI, gastrointestinal; AUC, area under the curve.

such as genotype 3 for which current DAA treatments are less effective [27–29] and the data in KT recipients are very limited. On the contrary, in patients with advanced liver disease or in those with a living donor available, viral eradication should be attempted before KT in order to achieve sustained virological response (SVR) and to avoid the potential risk of disease transmission or liver disease progression [30, 31].

More data are needed to evaluate the results of the previous strategy and to determine the best moment to start the antiviral therapy in patients with ESRD who are candidates for a KT.

DAAs and the Kidney

The pharmacokinetics of the different DAAs in patients with ESRD is shown in Table 1. Most of the currently approved DAAs are metabolized by the liver with minimal renal clearance. However, sofosbuvir (SOF), the backbone of a majority of antiviral regimens, is a pro-drug that is phosphorylated into an active metabolite (GS461203) and subsequently dephosphorylated into its inactive metabolite (GS331007) [32]. SOF and the GS331007 metabolite are eliminated by the kidney and therefore they accumulate in patients with a GFR <30 mL/min. Given the lack of clinical trials evaluating the safety and efficacy of SOF in patients with ESRD, the label does not recommend its use in these patients. However, a recent study by Desnoyer et al. [33], compared the plasma concentrations of SOF and its inactive metabolite (GS331007) in patients receiving a SOF-based therapy with a standard dose of SOF (400 mg/day, n = 7) or SOF administered 3 times per week (n = 5). The authors found that neither SOF nor its metabolite GS331007 accumulates between HD sessions or during the period of the study. In addition, the GS331007 extraction rate was 52%, which was similar to historical data. There were no side effects related to the treatment. More information is needed to confirm these results, but it seems plausible to allow the use of SOF-based therapies in patients with ESRD and no other treatment options with very careful monitoring.

On the other hand, it is important to remember that patients with ESRD, especially those on HD are poly-medicated and there is a potential for drug–drug interactions (DDI) between concomitant medication and antiviral drugs.

Table 2. Summary of clinical trial and real-life cohorts evaluating antiviral therapy in patients with end-stage renal disease

Author	Type of study	Number	Regimen	Dialysis	Efficacy, %	AEs
Roth et al. [45]	Clinical trial	224	GZV + EBV	76%	94	SAEs in 16%
Pockros et al. [46]	Clinical trial	20	OMV/PTV/r/DSV ± RBV	65%	90	Mild (anemia in the 13 patients with RBV)
Gane et al. [47]	Clinical trial	10	SOF (200) + RBV	No	40	Mild (5 had anemia)
Martin et al. [48]	Clinical trial	10	SOF (400) + RBV	No	60	
Perumpail et al. [49]	Clinical case	1	SOF (200) + SMV	$n = 1$	100	None
Bhamidimarri et al. [34]	Case series	15	SOF (200) + SMV	$n = 12$ (1 with PD)	87	Mild (fatigue [20%], pruritus [13%], diarrea [7%], anemia [13%])
Hundemer et al. [50]	Case series	6	SOF (400) + SMV ($n = 3$) SOF (400) + RBV ($n = 2$) SOF (400) + PR ($n = 1$)	$n = 2$	67	Anemia in the 3 patients with RBV, worsening renal function in 1 patient
Nazario et al. [35]	Case series	17	SOF (400) + SMV	$n = 15$	100	Mild (insomnia, worsening anemia, headache, nausea)
Beinhardt et al. [37]	Case series	10	SOF (400) + PR ($n = 1$) SOF (400) + SMV ($n = 2$) SOF (400) + DCV ($n = 4$) SOF (400) + RBV ($n = 1$) UK ($n = 2$)	$n = 10$ (2 with PD)	90	5 of 6 patients with AEs had SAEs
Gane et al. [51]	Clinical trial	18	OMV/PTV/r/DSV	$n = 12$	100%	4 patients had SAEs. No patients had grade 3 anemia
Gane et al. [52]	Clinical trial	104	GLE + PIB	82%	100%	SAEs in 25%
Dumortier et al. [53]*	Case series	50	SOF + PR ($n = 2$) SOF + SMV ± RBV ($n = 11$) SOF + DCV ± RBV ($n = 30$) SOF + RBV ($n = 7$)	$n = 35$	86	3 patients receiving RBV presented severe anemia

GZV, grazoprevir; EBV, elbasvir; OMV, ombitasvir; PTV/r, paritaprevir/ritonavir; DSV, dasabuvir; RBV, ribavirin; SOF, sofosbuvir; SMV, simeprevir; PR, pegylated interferon + ribavirin; DCV, daclatasvir; GLE, glecaprevir, PIB, pibrentasvir; UK, unknown; AEs, adverse events; SAEs, serious adverse events.

* All patients in HD received SOF at reduced dose.

Therefore, it is mandatory to check for DDI before starting antiviral treatment [10]. In addition, the presence of cardiovascular disease ideally warrants for a ribavirin (RBV)-free regimen to avoid the risk of developing or worsening anemia that complicates the tolerance to therapy.

Efficacy and Safety of DAAs in Patients with Renal Failure

Two studies have been specifically designed to determine the safety and the efficacy of different combinations of DAAs in patients with ESRD (Table 2). The RUBY-1 trial evaluated the combination of ombitasvir (NS5A inhibitor), paritaprevir/r (ritonavir-boosted protease inhibitor) and dasabuvir (non-nucleoside NS5B inhibitor) with or without RBV in 20 genotype 1-infected patients with CKD stages 4 and 5. Thirteen patients were infected with genotype 1a and received the 3D antiviral combination with RBV. The remaining 7 patients infected with genotype 1b received the 3D combination alone. Most of the patients were male and had stage 5 CKD (14 of them on HD). All 20 patients achieved end-of-treatment response, but 90% (18 out of the 20 patients) of them finally achieved SVR12 (in the intention to treat analysis). One of the patients who did not achieved SVR died 14 days after discontinuing antiviral therapy (unrelated to therapy) and one other remaining patient presented a relapse at post-treatment week 4. This was a genotype 1a infected patient with advanced fibrosis and a relatively low dose adherence reported who had discontinued RBV during therapy due to anemia. In addition, resistance-associated substitutions were detected in this patient at the time of failure in NS5A. Regarding safety, most of the patients presented adverse events, although mild or moderate in severity, and in fact, none of the patients discontinued therapy due to adverse events. Anemia was the most common adverse event and was developed only in genotype 1a patients in whom RBV was administered per protocol. It is important to note that all the patients receiving RBV interrupted the drug at some point during antiviral therapy. Four patients also required erythropoietin and none of them was transfused. RBV could be reassumed in 3 patients.

On the other hand, in the C-SURFER study, 224 genotype 1 infected patients with CKD stages 4 and 5 were randomly assigned to receive the combination of grazoprevir (second generation protease inhibitor) and elbasvir (NS5A inhibitor; $n = 111$) once daily for 12 weeks or placebo ($n = 113$). Patients in the placebo arm also received active treatment in a deferred manner. Eleven patients participated in an intensive pharmacokinetic study and were included in the immediate treatment arm. Most of the patients were naïve (80%) and infected with genotype 1a (52%). Six percent of the patients had cirrhosis and 76% were on HD. In the full set analysis, 94 and 95% of patients in the immediate and the deferred treatment groups, respectively, achieved SVR12. Three patients experienced a relapse and 9 patients discontinued therapy early due to adverse events not considered to be related to antiviral therapy. Among the relapse patients, 2 were infected with genotype 1a and 1 patient with genotype 1b; all of them were non-cirrhotics and had baseline resistant-associated substitutions in NS5A at baseline and at the time of failure. As compared to placebo, the percentage of serious adverse events (SAEs) or early treatment discontinuations due to adverse events was lesser in the immediate treatment group (19 vs. 16% and 5 vs. 0% respectively).

As mentioned above, according to the label, the use of SOF in patients with GFR <30 mL/min is not recommended. However, some real-life data have shown that an SOF-based therapy is efficacious and well tolerated in patients with ESRD (Table 2). Bhamidimarri et al. [34] evaluated half a dose of SOF (200 mg/day or 400 mg 3 times per week) in combination with Simeprevir (SMV) in 15 patients with ESRD (12 on dialysis). Eighty-seven percent of the patients achieved SVR and there were no major adverse events. Nazario et al. [35] reported the results of 17 patients with ESRD (15 of them on HD) treated with standard doses of SOF (400 mg/day) and SMV for 12 weeks. Most of the patients were found to be with an advanced fibrosis stage (F3-F4, $n = 12$) and were infected with genotype 1a ($n = 13$). All 17 patients completed the course of therapy and achieved SVR. There were only 4 mild adverse events (insomnia, headache, nausea and worsening anemia). Saxena et al. [36], with data from the HCV-TARGET cohort, compared the results in terms of efficacy and safety in patients with a GFR ≤45 mL/min ($n = 82$, 5 of them on HD) or >45 mL/min ($n = 1,811$) receiving a SOF-based therapy. The authors found similar results in terms of efficacy (SVR of 83 vs. 82%, respectively) but a significantly higher number of adverse events, especially anemia (22 vs. 6%, $p < 0.001$) and worsening renal function (15 vs. 1%, $p < 0.001$) in the group of patients with a GFR ≤45 mL/min. However, there are no follow-up data to evaluate whether renal function is restored after treatment discontinuation. More recently, Beinhardt et al. [37] reported their experience with SOF-based therapies in 25 patients treated in the pre- or post-KT setting. Ten of the patients had ESRD on HD and all of them received a standard dose of SOF (400 mg/day). Nine of the 10 patients achieved SVR and 6 presented adverse events that were considered SAEs in 5 patients. None of the SAEs were related to therapy although in one case it led to the reduction of SOF dose. Despite these very promising results, the current information available comes from a small series of cases with different doses of SOF and treatment durations. A clinical trial evaluating an SOF-based therapy would be useful to determine the appropriate dose and the best treatment regimen for patients on HD. Meanwhile, patients with ESRD with an urgent need of therapy and no other available treatment options (genotype 2 or 3) would benefit from SOF. A very close monitoring of these patients is necessary in order to rapidly detect any adverse event.

Conclusions

The development of DAAs was an outstanding achievement in the treatment of hepatitis C. These new drugs have safely allowed the treatment of hard-to-treat populations in whom previous therapies were associated with low rates of SVR and a high number of adverse events. Patients with ESRD are comprised among this group of patients. Different combinations of antiviral drugs have proved to be safe and efficacious in patients even in patients on HD. Although more data and longer follow-up are needed, it is probable that these therapies will improve survival and quality of life before and after KT.

Disclosure Statement

S.L. received advisory fees from Gilead and Janssen. M.-C.L. received advisory fees from Gilead, Janssen, BMS and MSD. The other authors declare no conflict of interest.

References

1 Goodkin DA, Bieber B, Gillespie B, Robinson BM, Jadoul M: Hepatitis C infection is very rarely treated among hemodialysis patients. Am J Nephrol 2013;38:405–412.

2 Fabrizi F, Dixit V, Messa P: Impact of hepatitis C on survival in dialysis patients: a link with cardiovascular mortality? J Viral Hepat 2012;19:601–607.

3 Dammacco F, Sansonno D: Therapy for hepatitis C virus-related cryoglobulinemic vasculitis. N Engl J Med 2013;369:1035–1045.

4 El-Serag HB, Hampel H, Yeh C, Rabeneck L: Extrahepatic manifestations of hepatitis C among United States male veterans. Hepatology 2002;36:1439–1445.

5 Tsui JI, Vittinghoff E, Shlipak MG, O'Hare AM: Relationship between hepatitis C and chronic kidney disease: results from the third national health and nutrition examination survey. J Am Soc Nephrol 2006;17:1168–1174.

6 Tsui JI, Vittinghoff E, Shlipak MG, Bertenthal D, Inadomi J, Rodriguez RA, O'Hare AM: Association of hepatitis C seropositivity with increased risk for developing end-stage renal disease. Arch Intern Med 2007;167:1271–1276.

7 Chen YC, Lin HY, Li CY, Lee MS, Su YC: A nationwide cohort study suggests that hepatitis C virus infection is associated with increased risk of chronic kidney disease. Kidney Int 2014;85:1200–1207.

8 Park H, Adeyemi A, Henry L, Stepanova M, Younossi Z: A meta-analytic assessment of the risk of chronic kidney disease in patients with chronic hepatitis C virus infection. J Viral Hepat 2015;22:897–905.

9 KDIGO clinical practice guidelines for the prevention, diagnosis, evaluation, and treatment of hepatitis C in chronic kidney disease. Kidney Int Suppl 2013;3:1–149.

10 European Association for Study of Liver: EASL recommendations on treatment of hepatitis C 2015. J Hepatol 2015;63:199–236.

11 Schiavon LL, Schiavon JL, Filho RJ, Sampaio JP, Lanzoni VP, Silva AE, Ferraz ML: Simple blood tests as noninvasive markers of liver fibrosis in hemodialysis patients with chronic hepatitis C virus infection. Hepatology 2007;46:307–314.

12 Liu CH, Liang CC, Huang KW, Liu CJ, Chen SI, Lin JW, Hung PH, Tsai HB, Lai MY, Chen PJ, Chen JH, Chen DS, Kao JH: Transient elastography to assess hepatic fibrosis in hemodialysis chronic hepatitis C patients. Clin J Am Soc Nephrol 2011;6:1057–1065.

13 Khunpakdee N, Jayanama K, Kaewdoung P, Promson K, Rattanasiri S, Warodomwichit D, Kantachuvesiri S, Sobhonslidsuk A: Transient elastography in end-stage renal disease patients on hemodialysis: the effect of net fluid withdrawal. Blood Purif 2015;40:256–259.

14 Varaut A, Fontaine H, Serpaggi J, Verkarre V, Vallet-Pichard A, Nalpas B, Imbertbismuth F, Lebray P, Pol S: Diagnostic accuracy of the fibrotest in hemodialysis and renal transplant patients with chronic hepatitis C virus. Transplantation 2005;80:1550–1555.

15 Fabrizi F, Aghemo A, Messa P: Hepatitis C treatment in patients with kidney disease. Kidney Int 2013;84:874–879.

16 Fabrizi F, Verdesca S, Messa P, Martin P: Hepatitis C virus infection increases the risk of developing chronic kidney disease: a systematic review and meta-analysis. Dig Dis Sci 2015;60:3801–3813.

17 Bucci JR, Lentine KL, Agodoa LY, Peters TG, Schnitzler MA, Abbott KC: Outcomes associated with recipient and donor hepatitis C serology status after kidney transplantation in the united states: analysis of the USRDS/UNOS database. Clin Transpl 2004:51–61.

18 Abbott KC, Lentine KL, Bucci JR, Agodoa LY, Peters TG, Schnitzler MA: The impact of transplantation with deceased donor hepatitis c-positive kidneys on survival in wait-listed long-term dialysis patients. Am J Transplant 2004;4:2032–2037.

19 Bucci JR, Matsumoto CS, Swanson SJ, Agodoa LY, Holtzmuller KC, Peters TG, Abbott KC: Donor hepatitis C seropositivity: clinical correlates and effect on early graft and patient survival in adult cadaveric kidney transplantation. J Am Soc Nephrol 2002;13:2974–2982.

20 Morales JM, Campistol JM, Dominguez-Gil B, Andres A, Esforzado N, Oppenheimer F, Castellano G, Fuertes A, Bruguera M, Praga M: Long-term experience with kidney transplantation from hepatitis C-positive donors into hepatitis c-positive recipients. Am J Transplant 2010;10:2453–2462.

21 Bloom RD, Sayer G, Fa K, Constantinescu S, Abt P, Reddy KR: Outcome of hepatitis C virus-infected kidney transplant candidates who remain on the waiting list. Am J Transplant 2005;5:139–144.

22 Kamar N, Marion O, Rostaing L, Cointault O, Ribes D, Lavayssiere L, Esposito L, Del Bello A, Metivier S, Barange K, Izopet J, Alric L: Efficacy and safety of sofosbuvir-based antiviral therapy to treat hepatitis C virus infection after kidney transplantation. Am J Transplant 2016;16:1474–1479.

23 Sawinski D, Kaur N, Ajeti A, Trofe-Clark J, Lim M, Bleicher M, Goral S, Forde KA, Bloom RD: Successful treatment of hepatitis C in renal transplant recipients with direct-acting antiviral agents. Am J Transplant 2016;16:1588–1595.

24 Lin MV, Sise ME, Pavlakis M, Amundsen BM, Chute D, Rutherford AE, Chung RT, Curry MP, Hanifi JM, Gabardi S, Chandraker A, Heher EC, Elias N, Riella LV: Efficacy and safety of direct acting antivirals in kidney transplant recipients with chronic hepatitis C virus infection. PLoS One 2016;11:e0158431.

25 Colombo M, Aghemo A, Liu L, Hyland R, Yun C, Brainard D, McHutchinson J, Bourliere M, Peck-Radosavljevic M, Manns M, Pol S: Ledipasvir/sofosbuvir for 12 or 24 weeks is safe and effective in kidney transplant recipients with chronic genotype 1 or 4 HCV infection. J Hepatol 2016;64:S183.

26 Sawinski D, Lee DH, Doyle AM, Blumberg EA: Successful posttransplant treatment of hepatitis C with ledipasvir-sofosbuvir in HIV+ kidney transplant recipients. Transplantation 2016, Epub ahead of print.

27 Zeuzem S, Dusheiko GM, Salupere R, Mangia A, Flisiak R, Hyland RH, Illeperuma A, Svarovskaia E, Brainard DM, Symonds WT, Subramanian GM, McHutchison JG, Weiland O, Reesink HW, Ferenci P, Hezode C, Esteban R: Sofosbuvir and ribavirin in HCV genotypes 2 and 3. N Engl J Med 2014;370:1993–2001.

28 Nelson DR, Cooper JN, Lalezari JP, Lawitz E, Pockros PJ, Gitlin N, Freilich BF, Younes ZH, Harlan W, Ghalib R, Oguchi G, Thuluvath PJ, Ortiz-Lasanta G, Rabinovitz M, Bernstein D, Bennett M, Hawkins T, Ravendhran N, Sheikh AM, Varunok P, Kowdley KV, Hennicken D, McPhee F, Rana K, Hughes EA: All-oral 12-week treatment with daclatasvir plus sofosbuvir in patients with hepatitis C virus genotype 3 infection: ALLY-3 phase III study. Hepatology 2015;61:1127–1135.

29 Leroy V, Angus P, Bronowicki JP, Dore GJ, Hezode C, Pianko S, Pol S, Stuart K, Tse E, McPhee F, Bhore R, Jimenez-Exposito MJ, Thompson AJ: Daclatasvir, sofosbuvir, and ribavirin for hepatitis C virus genotype 3 and advanced liver disease: a randomized phase III study (ALLY-3+). Hepatology 2016;63:1430–1441.

30 Ladino M, Pedraza F, Roth D: Hepatitis c virus infection in chronic kidney disease. J Am Soc Nephrol 2016;27:2238–2246.
31 Sawinski D, Bloom RD: Novel hepatitis C treatment and the impact on kidney transplantation. Transplantation 2015;99:2458–2466.
32 Kirby BJ, Symonds WT, Kearney BP, Mathias AA: Pharmacokinetic, pharmacodynamic, and drug-interaction profile of the hepatitis C virus NS5B polymerase inhibitor sofosbuvir. Clin Pharmacokinet 2015;54:677–690.
33 Desnoyer A, Pospai D, Le MP, Gervais A, Heurgue-Berlot A, Laradi A, Harent S, Pinto A, Salmon D, Hillaire S, Fontaine H, Zucman D, Simonpoli AM, Muret P, Larrouy L, Bernard Chabert B, Descamps D, Yazdanpanah Y, Peytavin G: Pharmacokinetics, safety and efficacy of a full dose sofosbuvir-based regimen given daily in hemodialysis patients with chronic hepatitis C. J Hepatol 2016;65: 40–47.
34 Bhamidimarri KR, Czul F, Peyton A, Levy C, Hernandez M, Jeffers L, Roth D, Schiff E, O'Brien C, Martin P: Safety, efficacy and tolerability of half-dose sofosbuvir plus simeprevir in treatment of hepatitis C in patients with end stage renal disease. J Hepatol 2015;63: 763–765.
35 Nazario HE, Ndungu M, Modi AA: Sofosbuvir and simeprevir in hepatitis c genotype 1-patients with end-stage renal disease on haemodialysis or GFR <30 ml/min. Liver Int 2016;36:798–801.
36 Saxena V, Koraishy FM, Sise ME, Lim JK, Schmidt M, Chung RT, Liapakis A, Nelson DR, Fried MW, Terrault NA: Safety and efficacy of sofosbuvir-containing regimens in hepatitis C-infected patients with impaired renal function. Liver Int 2016;36:807–816.
37 Beinhardt S, Al Zoairy R, Ferenci P, Kozbial K, Freissmuth C, Stern R, Stattermayer AF, Stauber R, Strasser M, Zoller H, Watschinger B, Schmidt A, Trauner M, Hofer H, Maieron A: Daa-based antiviral treatment of patients with chronic hepatitis C in the pre- and post-kidney transplantation setting. Transpl Int 2016;29:999–1007.
38 Cornpropst M, Denning J, Clemons D, et al: The effect of renal impairment and end stage renal disease on the single-dose pharmacokinetics of PSI-7977. J Hepatol 2012; 56:S433.
39 Khatri A, Dutta S, Marbury TC, Preston RA, Rodrigues L Jr, Wang H, Awni WM, Menon RM: Pharmacokinetics and tolerability of anti-hepatitis C virus treatment with ombitasvir, paritaprevir, ritonavir, with or without dasabuvir, in subjects with renal impairment. Clin Pharmacokinet 2017;56:153–163.
40 Garimella T, Wang R, Luo WL, Hwang C, Sherman D, Kandoussi H, Marbury TC, Alcorn H, Bertz R, Bifano M: Single-dose pharmacokinetics and safety of daclatasvir in subjects with renal function impairment. Antivir Ther 2015;20:535–543.
41 Mogalian E, Mathias AA, Yang JC, Pang PS, Moorehead L, Hernandez M, Lasseter KC, Ries D, Robson RA, Klein G: The pharmacokinetics of ledipasvir, an HCV specific NS5A inhibitor, in HCV-uninfected subjects with severe renal impairment. Hepatology 2014; 60.
42 Yeh WW, Caro L, Guo Z, Pung Feng H, Davis HU, Kozisek M, Stypinski D, Feng C, Mitchell C, Gillespie A, Ichhpurani N, Marshall WL, Lasseter KC, Marbury TC, Butterton JR: Pharmacokinetics of co-administered HCV protease inhibitor mk-5172 and NS5A inhibitor mk-8742 in volunteers with end-stage renal disease on hemodialysis or severe renal impairment not on hemodialysis. Hepatology 2014;60:1137A.
43 Gilead Sciences, Inc.: Epclusa. Product monograph 2016. https://www.gilead.com/~/media/files/pdfs/medicines/liver-disease/epclusa/epclusa_pi.pdf?la=en.
44 Ouwerkerk-Mahadevan S, Beumont-Mauviel M, Mortier S, Peeters M, Verloes R, Truyers C, Mannens G, Wynant I, Simion A: Evaluation of the pharmacokinetics and renal excretion of simeprevir in subjects with renal impairment. Drugs R D 2015;15:261–270.
45 Roth D, Nelson DR, Bruchfeld A, Liapakis A, Silva M, Monsour H Jr, Martin P, Pol S, Londono MC, Hassanein T, Zamor PJ, Zuckerman E, Wan S, Jackson B, Nguyen BY, Robertson M, Barr E, Wahl J, Greaves W: Grazoprevir plus elbasvir in treatment-naive and treatment-experienced patients with hepatitis C virus genotype 1 infection and stage 4–5 chronic kidney disease (the C-SURFER study): a combination phase 3 study. Lancet 2015;386:1537–1545.
46 Pockros PJ, Reddy KR, Mantry PS, Cohen E, Bennett M, Sulkowski MS, Bernstein DE, Cohen DE, Shulman NS, Wang D, Khatri A, Abunimeh M, Podsadecki T, Lawitz E: Efficacy of direct-acting antiviral combination for patients with hepatitis c virus genotype 1 infection and severe renal impairment or end-stage renal disease. Gastroenterology 2016; 150:1590–1598.
47 Gane E, Robson R, Bonacini M, Maliakkal B, Kirby B, Liu L, Sajwani K, Stamm L, Brainard D, McHutchison J, Stedman C, Lawitz E: Safety, antiviral efficacy, and pharmacokinetics of sofosbuvir in patients with severe renal impairment. Hepatology 2014;60:667A.
48 Martin P, Gane E, Ortiz-Lasanta G, Liu L, Sajwani K, Kirby B, Stamm L, Brainard D, McHutchison J, Lawitz E, Gordon E, Robson R: Safety and efficacy of treatment with daily sofosbuvir 400 mg + ribavirin 200 mg for 24 weeks in genotype 1 or 3 HCV-infected patients with severe renal impairment. Hepatology 2015;62:765A.
49 Perumpail RB, Wong RJ, Ha LD, Pham EA, Wang U, Luong H, Kumari R, Daugherty TJ, Higgins JP, Younossi ZM, Kim WR, Glenn JS, Ahmed A: Sofosbuvir and simeprevir combination therapy in the setting of liver transplantation and hemodialysis. Transpl Infect Dis 2015;17:275–278.
50 Hundemer GL, Sise ME, Wisocky J, Ufere N, Friedman LS, Corey KE, Chung RT: Use of sofosbuvir-based direct-acting antiviral therapy for hepatitis c viral infection in patients with severe renal insufficiency. Infect Dis (Lond) 2015;47:924–929.
51 Gane E, Sola R, Cohen E, Roberts SK, George J, Skoien R, Riordan S, Mobashery N, Abunimeh M, Cohen D, Agarwal K: RUBY-II: Efficacy and Safety of a Ribavirin-Free Ombitasvir/Paritaprevir/Ritonavir ± Dasabuvir Regimen in Patients With Severe Renal Impairment or End-Stage Renal Disease and HCV Genotype 1a or 4 Infection. Hepatology 2016;64(suppl 1):470A.
52 Gane E, Lawitz E, Pugatch D, Papatheodoridis G, Bräu N, Brown A, Pol S, Leroy V, Persico M, Moreno C, Colombo M, Yoshida E, Nelson D, Lei Y, Kosloski M, Mensa F: EXPEDITION-4: Efficacy and Safety of Glecaprevir/Pibrentasvir (ABT-493/ABT-530) in Patients With Renal Impairment and Chronic Hepatitis C Virus Genotype 1–6 Infection. Hepatology 2016;64(suppl 1):1125A.
53 Dumortier J, Bailly F, Pageaux GP, Vallet-Pichard A, Radenne S, Habersetzer F, Gagnieu MC, Grangé JD, Minello A, Guillaud O, Kamar N, Alric L, Leroy V: Sofosbuvir-based antiviral therapy in hepatitis C virus patients with severe renal failure. Nephrol Dial Transplant 2016;pii:gfw348 [Epub ahead of print].

Hepatitis Treatment: The Challenges

Digestive Diseases

Dig Dis 2017;35:347–350
DOI: 10.1159/000456586

Pre- and Post-Transplant Treatment of Viral Hepatitis C

David Mutimer

Birmingham University and NIHR Liver Biomedical Research Unit, Birmingham, UK

Keywords

Hepatitis C virus · Antiviral treatment · Direct-acting antivirals · Liver failure · Liver transplantation

Abstract

Background: Hepatitis C (HCV) is a common cause of liver failure and liver cancer, and is a frequent indication for liver transplantation (LT). Until recently, a majority of transplanted patients were viraemic at the time of transplantation and they inevitably underwent recurrent infection of the graft. Prior to the availability of specific direct-acting antiviral (DAA) drugs, HCV infection was seldom successfully treated before or after transplantation. ***Key Messages:*** During the past 2 years, the use of interferon-free DAA therapy has transformed the management of patients post-LT and of patients on the transplant waiting list. DAA treatment post-LT can eradicate infection and normalize liver function tests in a majority of treated patients. An improvement in long-term graft and patient outcome can be anticipated. DAA treatment of patients with liver failure awaiting LT eliminates infection and is associated with an improvement in the liver function for a majority of treated patients. The majority still require transplantation, though some may improve sufficiently and quickly enough to be removed from the LT waiting list. ***Conclusions:*** Eventually, as greater numbers of patients with compensated cirrhosis are successfully treated with DAAs, HCV-associated liver failure may become an uncommon indication for LT.

Introduction

Liver failure and/or liver cancer complicating hepatitis C (HCV) infection are the predominant indications for liver transplantation (LT) in many western countries, including the United Kingdom (UK). In the financial year 2014–2015, 170 UK patients underwent LT for these indications, comprising 15–20% of adult liver transplants performed in that year. In many countries, the proportion is significantly greater.

Until recently, with the advent of potent and well-tolerated antiviral therapy, a majority of patients were viraemic at the time of LT. Recurrent infection of the graft was inevitable and chronic hepatitis was established. Recurrent infection is associated with accelerated liver damage (in comparison to chronic hepatitis of the native liver) [1]. Median time from transplantation to the development of graft cirrhosis is less than 10 years (compared with 30 years in the immunocompetent); only 60% survive 3 years after the development of cirrhosis (compared with 90% 5-year survival in the immunocompetent), and only 50% survive at least one year after the development of liver failure (50% 5-year survival is seen in the immunocompetent) [2]. In addition to the accelerated progression to cirrhosis and liver failure, aggressive fibrosing cholestatic hepatitis (FCH) may cause acute or subacute graft failure in HCV-infected graft recipients.

KARGER

E-Mail karger@karger.com
www.karger.com/ddi

David Mutimer
Professor of Clinical Hepatology
Birmingham University and NIHR Liver Biomedical Research Unit
Birmingham (UK)
E-Mail david.mutimer@uhb.nhs.uk

Antiviral Treatment Post-LT

Until recently, the results of antiviral treatment post-LT were disappointing. A small proportion of transplanted patients were suitable for treatment with interferon (IFN) and ribavirin. Published series were consistent in demonstrating low rates of sustained virological response (SVR) in the LT setting [3]. In addition, IFN treatment could cause significant graft dysfunction including a risk for graft rejection. Many post-LT patients have renal dysfunction, and ribavirin dose reduction is frequently required. HCV genotype is an important determinant of successful treatment of LT patients with IFN and ribavirin. Indeed, in our experience, high rates of SVR could be achieved with carefully selected genotype 3 (G3) patients. Since 2003 and prior to the recent availability of direct-acting antivirals (DAAs) for G3-infected LT recipients, we achieved an SVR rate of 84% (21/25 patients). These patients were treated prior to the development of graft cirrhosis. Many had failed the same combination of IFN and ribavirin before LT, highlighting the importance of fibrosis stage in determining treatment outcome in G3 patients in both pre- and post-LT settings. Results of treatment of G1-infected patients were disappointing with a majority of published series reporting SVR rates between 20 and 30%. The development of first-generation HCV-specific protease inhibitors (PIs) offered an improvement in the treatment of G1-infected patients [4] but with additional side-effects. In particular, PI use was associated with significant drug–drug interactions. Specifically, both telaprevir and boceprevir are potent inhibitors of the cytochrome p450 3A4 isoenzyme, the main enzyme that metabolises both tacrolimus and cyclosporin. Thus, during antiviral treatment with these drugs, significant reduction of tacrolimus and cyclosporin doses and careful therapeutic drug monitoring are required. The rapid pace of antiviral drug development and licensing, with availability of more potent and less toxic drug regimens, has made the first generation of PIs obsolete after a brief period of clinical use. Though the interaction could be managed, it is preferable to avoid antivirals with significant p450 3A4 inhibition if possible.

All-Oral Antiviral Treatment Post-LT

The outstanding results of all-oral DAA regimens in treatment of non-immunosuppressed chronic HCV patients have been rapidly translated to the post-LT setting. The Gilead-sponsored studies, SOLAR-1 and SOLAR-2, evaluated the combination of ledipasvir (an HCV NS5A protein inhibitor) with sofosbuvir (a nucleotide HCV polymerase inhibitor), given with ribavirin for 12 or 24 weeks to patients with liver failure or post-LT [5, 6]. Patients infected with either G1 or G4 HCV were eligible for this treatment. The combined post-LT population included 463 patients, 426 with G1 and 37 with G4. The treated post-LT population included patients with any fibrosis stage, including cirrhotic patients with graft failure. Also, a population of 11 patients with FCH was treated. The results of the treatment were remarkable, and SVR was achieved for 194 out of 200 (97%) patients with fibrosis stages 0–3, for 105 out of 108 (97%) patients with cirrhosis (Child–Pugh grade A), for 84 out of 91 (92%) cirrhotic patients with CP class B, and for 11 out of 16 (69%) of patients with CP class C. Virological failure was rare, and much of the treatment failure was due to patient death, reflecting the advanced stage of graft failure in many patients before commencement of treatment. The cure rate for G4 patients was 31/37 (84%). The response to treatment of the 11 patients with FCH was also remarkable. All were cured, and prompt resolution of severe liver dysfunction was observed.

The AbbVie 3 drug regimen has also been evaluated in G1-infected post-LT patients [7]. It comprises a ritonavir-boosted PI (paritaprevir), an NS5A inhibitor (ombitasvir) and a non-nucleoside polymerase inhibitor (dasabuvir). Thirty-four patients with graft fibrosis stage of 2 or less were treated and 33 were cured. In that study, treatment appeared safe so long as careful reduction of tacrolimus was made in reaction to the potent cytochrome p450 inhibition by ritonavir. A single case of virological relapse (in a G1a-infected patient) was observed.

In addition to these pivotal studies, a growing number of case series have been published. The majority have treated predominantly G1-infected LT patients with combinations of sofosbuvir, simeprevir (a PI inhibitor) and daclatasvir (NS5A inhibitor), with or without ribavirin. It is clear that SVR rates greater than 90% are readily achieved. A much smaller experience with G3-infected patients has been included in these reports, though the response to a combination of sofosbuvir and daclatasvir appears quite potent for this genotype.

Our own experience in Birmingham is consistent with these published reports, with SVR rates of 52/53 (98%) observed for treatment of G1 infection with either the Gilead or the AbbVie regimens, and 10/12 (83%) for G3 patients receiving combination sofosbuvir with daclatasvir and ribavirin.

Thus, the majority of HCV-infected LT patients can be cured by all-oral DAA treatment. These regimens have been available only for a couple of years, but a majority of patients in many transplant units have already been cured of infection. It is too early for published data to demonstrate the impact of successful treatment on graft and patient survival, but a significant positive impact seems very likely.

Antiviral Treatment before LT

The aims of antiviral treatment in the pre-transplant patient with HCV-associated liver failure include the eradication of HCV infection and consequent improvement of liver function that may permit the removal of the patient from the LT waiting list. In addition, SVR, documented before LT, avoids HCV recurrence and post-LT graft damage. The aim of treating the waiting list patient with well-compensated cirrhosis complicated by liver cancer is less clear. HCV eradication will not affect the indication for LT, so successful treatment simply prevents post-LT HCV recurrence. Based on the excellent results achieved by antiviral treatment post-LT (discussed above), there is an option to use antivirals either before or after LT for this subset of HCV patients.

Curry et al. [8] were the first to demonstrate the potential of DAA treatment, given to waiting list patients, to achieve HCV clearance and to prevent post-transplant HCV recurrence. They showed that serum HCV negativity could be achieved by the use of sofosbuvir with ribavirin given to waitlisted patients until the time of LT. Post-LT HCV recurrence was seldom observed in patients who had serum HCV RNA negativity for at least 4 weeks before LT. In comparison, those patients with serum negativity for less than 4 weeks before LT were very likely to experience HCV relapse post-LT. With the availability of combination DAA regimens, however, the treatment paradigm has already shifted away from suppressive regimens, given the indefinite waiting time until LT, to a paradigm that aims to cure waiting list patients (and other patients with advanced liver disease) with combination treatment of finite, short duration. The cure rate of combination treatment and the impact of treatment on the liver function are now well defined.

Gilead-sponsored studies, SOLAR-1 and SOLAR-2, treated patients with advanced liver disease (Child–Pugh class B or C) with the combination of ledipasvir and sofosbuvir with ribavirin for 12 or 24 weeks [5, 6]. There was no significant difference between the efficacies of the 2 treatment durations. Virological cure rate for patients with CP-B at baseline was 96/115 (83%), and for patients with CP-C was 75/91 (82%). Treatment failure was due to virological failure ($n = 15$) or patient death ($n = 13$). Comparison of MELD scores at baseline with those calculated 12 weeks after conclusion of treatment demonstrated an improvement in liver function (i.e., a reduction in MELD score) for the majority of treated patients. Thus, these studies showed that virological cure can be achieved for most patients and that virological response is mirrored by clinical improvement. An impact on the need for transplantation would be predicted, but this is harder to demonstrate. For instance, SOLAR 2 was an international multicenter study, and patient selection for transplantation, waiting times on the transplant waiting list and protocols for allocation of organs to waitlisted patients will likely vary from centre to centre and between countries. In particular, time on waiting list may vary significantly. An analysis of liver failure patients treated with DAAs at our Birmingham Liver Unit shows that improvement of liver function continues for many patients for up to 6 months after the completion of DAA treatment. However, in real-world practice, a significant number of DAA-treated patients will be transplanted before treatment is completed and before 6 months follow-up post-treatment has elapsed. For those patients, the observation period after treatment commencement and before LT may be too short to permit clinical improvement to occur to its maximum potential. In our own initial experience with DAA treatment of 89 consecutive HCV patients with liver failure or a history of hepatic decompensation, 13 of those were on the waiting list at time of commencement of treatment. Of these, 1 patient died awaiting LT, 2 patients were delisted (1 with non-adherence to management, 1 with newly diagnosed oral cancer), and the remaining 10 underwent transplantation (5 during antiviral treatment and an additional 4 within 6 months of treatment completion). Also, an additional 8 of the 89 patients were added to the waiting list during or after the antiviral treatment, and all of these underwent LT. Thus, though we can demonstrate antiviral efficacy (SVR for 80%) and clinical improvement (an improvement in MELD score for the majority), we cannot clearly identify an impact on the need for LT. If waiting times for LT had been much longer, then an impact on the need for LT may have been observed. Recently, in a multicenter European study of 103 waitlisted patients with HCV-associated liver failure, Belli and colleagues observed the impact of DAA treatment on the need for LT. In that cohort, clinically significant improvement was observed for 34 patients, and 21 of those patients were de-listed [9]. Predictably perhaps, clinically significant improvement was more likely to be observed in those patients with lower baseline MELD (i.e., before DAA treatment) and greater MELD reduction between baseline and follow-up week 24. Indeed, a majority of de-listed patients had a baseline MELD <15, and all improved by at least 1 MELD point.

Dig Dis 2017;35:347–350
DOI: 10.1159/000456586

Thus, DAA treatment of patients with advanced HCV cirrhosis will achieve viral eradication in approximately 80%, a majority of treated patients will demonstrate measurable clinical improvement during short-term follow-up, and a minority of waitlisted patients may improve to an extent that permits removal from the waiting list.

Management of Patients Who Are Transplanted before Completion of Antiviral Treatment

A liver donation may become available during antiviral treatment. The study of Curry et al. [8], giving antiviral therapy to waitlisted patients until the time of LT suggests that explantation after at least 4 weeks of on-treatment serum HCV RNA negativity is associated with a low risk of recurrent HCV post-LT. This would be a reasonable, though unproven, approach to the post-transplant management of patients who had not completed a course of DAA treatment by the time of LT. An alternative approach to this group of partially treated patients, and a recommended approach for the management of patients who had serum RNA negativity for less than 4 weeks at the time of LT, is to continue antiviral treatment after LT. There are few data to describe the impact of hepatectomy during antiviral treatment. Our own experience of 4 patients treated for a total duration of 12 weeks spread across the pre- and post-LT periods has been encouraging. All 4 achieved SVR without recurrence following LT.

Conclusion

In summary, DAA therapy of HCV has transformed the management of patients with advanced liver disease and patients after LT. Intention-to-treat analysis of DAA treatment of liver failure patients shows a high rate of SVR (80% at least), and a majority of patients demonstrate measurable clinical improvement (perhaps 70–80% at 12 weeks post-treatment), and some listed patients (perhaps 20%) improve to the point where they can be removed from the LT waiting list. Liver failure patients represent only the tip of the cirrhosis iceberg. At present, patients with cirrhosis are being identified and targeted for DAA therapy. The antiviral cure rate for well-compensated cirrhosis is better than 90%. HCV elimination at this stage dramatically affects the risk of future decompensation for these patients. A more substantial reduction in need for LT should be observed during long-term follow-up of these patients. As was observed for patients with HBV cirrhosis receiving long-term suppressive antiviral treatment, the phenotype of the HCV patient in need of LT will almost certainly change. The majority will have well-compensated cirrhosis after successful antiviral therapy, but they would have developed primary liver cancer as an indication for LT.

DAA treatment has transformed the outcome for post-LT patients. DAA treatment is substantially safer than IFN-based treatment, and a majority of patients are expected to be successfully treated. Reflecting the success of antivirals that are administered pre-LT, HCV recurrence post-LT will become uncommon and will be easily cured. We have probably already reached the stage where we can say that graft and patient survival are no longer affected by recurrent HCV infection of the graft.

In addition, the predictable efficacy of DAA treatment opens the door to the use of HCV-positive donors for all recipients regardless of the recipient HCV status.

Disclosure Statement

David Mutimer has received honoraria for participation in advisory boards and/or speaker's fees from Gilead Sciences, AbbVie, MSD and BMS.

References

1 Gane EJ: The natural history of recurrent hepatitis C and what influences this. Liver Transpl 2008;14(suppl 2):S36–S44.

2 Firpi RJ, Clark V, Soldevila-Pico C, et al: The natural history of hepatitis C cirrhosis after liver transplantation. Liver Transpl 2009;15:1063–1071.

3 Berenguer M: Systematic review of the treatment of established recurrent hepatitis C with pegylated interferon in combination with ribavirin. J Hepatol 2008;49:274–287.

4 Forns X, Didier S, Mutimer D, et al: Efficacy of telaprevir-based therapy in stable liver transplant patients with chronic genotype 1 hepatitis C. Ann Hepatol 2016;15:512–523.

5 Manns M, Samuel D, Gane EJ, et al: Ledipasvir and sofosbuvir plus ribavirin in patients with genotype 1 or 4 hepatitis C virus infection and advanced liver disease: a multicentre, open-label, randomised, phase 2 trial. Lancet Infect Dis 2016;16:685–697.

6 Charlton M, Everson GT, Flamm SL, et al: Ledipasvir and sofosbuvir plus ribavirin for treatment of HCV infection in patients with advanced liver disease. Gastroenterology 2015;149:649–659.

7 Kwo PY, Mantry PS, Coakley E, et al: An interferon-free antiviral regimen for HCV after liver transplantation. N Engl J Med 2014;371:2375–2382.

8 Curry MP, Forns X, Chung RT, et al: Sofosbuvir and ribavirin prevent recurrence of HCV infection after liver transplantation: an open-label study. Gastroenterology 2015;148:100–107.e1.

9 Belli L, Berenguer M, Cortesi PA, et al: Delisting of liver transplant candidates with chronic hepatitis C after viral eradication: a European study. J Hepatol 2016;65:524–531.

Digestive Diseases

Dig Dis 2017;35:351–358
DOI: 10.1159/000456587

Hepatitis B Reactivation: The Controversies Continue

Jordan J. Feld

Toronto Centre for Liver Disease, Toronto General Hospital, University Health Network, Sandra Rotman Centre for Global Health, University of Toronto, Toronto, ON, Canada

Keywords
Hepatitis B reactivation · Chemotherapy · Immunosuppressive therapy · Rituximab

Abstract
Hepatitis B virus (HBV) reactivation is a serious but largely avoidable complication of immunosuppressive therapy. The consequences of reactivation range from subclinical increases in HBV DNA to fulminant liver failure, which can be prevented with the appropriate use of prophylactic antiviral therapy. However, which patients need to be screened and whether all patients who test positive for any serological test require antiviral therapy are issues that still remain unclear. Additional issues such as the choice of antiviral and the duration of treatment also need clarification. Some of the confusion comes from the use of varying definitions in the literature to define outcomes. In this review, areas of controversy from definitions of reactivation to management of patients who are hepatitis B surface antigen and lone anti-core antibody positive in different clinical settings are discussed. The recently recognized issue of reactivation in the setting of hepatitis C antiviral therapy is also addressed as well as some recommendations for areas of future research to help clarify best practices.

Introduction

The natural history of chronic hepatitis B virus (HBV) infection is highly dependent on the immune response of the infected individual. Classically, the course of chronic infection is described as progressing from a period of immune tolerance, characterized by high levels of viremia with no associated liver inflammation, through an immune active phase with flares of hepatitis and ultimately reaching the final immune control stage of infection in which HBV DNA levels are suppressed and liver inflammation resolves [1].

Although some have questioned the accuracy of the names for these phases recently, the fact that liver injury is caused by the immune response to the virus rather than a direct cytopathic effect of viral replication is useful for conceptualizing the natural history of the disease. The importance of the immune response is highlighted by the fact that immune suppression significantly impacts the course of the infection and the degree of liver injury. Specifically, loss of immune control through systemic immunosuppressive therapy may result in increases in viral replication followed by hepatitis at the time of immune reconstitution [2]. HBV reactivation refers to an increase of HBV DNA replication in the setting of immunosup-

KARGER

E-Mail karger@karger.com
www.karger.com/ddi

Jordan J. Feld
Toronto Centre for Liver Disease
200 Elizabeth Street 9EB-240
Toronto, ON M5G 2C4 (Canada)
E-Mail Jordan.feld@Uhn.ca

Table 1. Controversies in hepatitis B reactivation

Category	Controversy	Proposed solution
Definitions	Definitions of HBV reactivation and its complications?	Use standardized definitions to take into account virological, hepatic and immunosuppressive aspects of HBV reactivation (Table 2)
HBsAg+	Preferred agent? Duration of therapy?	Entecavir superior to lamivudine Uncertain optimal duration making it necessary to watch carefully for withdrawal flares
HBsAg–/anti-HBc+	When to screen?	Most guidelines recommend screening all patients. Screening in low-risk situations like solid-tumor chemotherapy is of questionable benefit
	When to treat?	Prophylactic antiviral therapy or close monitoring indicated for: Anti-CD20 therapy or stem cell transplant Anti-TNF + 2nd agent Not required for standard solid tumor chemotherapy or similar degrees of immunosuppression
During HCV treatment	Whom to screen with what? Management of HBsAg+? Management of HBsAg–/anti-HBc+?	Screen HBsAg and anti-HBc Treat with HBV antiviral or monitor closely Risk very low – no treatment necessary Consider measurement of HBV DNA if ALT rises or fails to normalize on therapy

pressive therapy. Although first described in patients with inactive chronic HBV infection who remained hepatitis B surface antigen (HBsAg) positive, subsequent reports documented the reappearance of HBsAg even in those with so-called resolved HBV who were HBsAg-negative with anti-hepatitis B core antibodies (anti-HBc) as the only markers of HBV exposure [2]. The reappearance of HBsAg in the serum is referred to as "reverse seroconversion" and provides the best evidence that the term "resolved infection" is a really a misnomer because most, if not all, patients with this serological profile (HBsAg–/HBc+) have replication competent HBV DNA in hepatocytes, which is quiescent due to potent HBV-specific immunity [3]. With loss of this immune control, HBV replication and its potential consequences may return.

Although HBV reactivation in the setting of immunosuppression has been recognized for decades and progress has been made in both its understanding and management, controversy still exists in a number of aspects of this clinical entity. This review focuses on areas of specific controversy in the management of patients with HBV infection undergoing immunosuppressive therapy, highlighting research gaps and offering suggestions for clinical management in areas with continued uncertainty. The areas of focus include issues in the management of HBsAg+ patients, the role of screening and treatment in HBsAg–/HBc+ patients, particularly in the context of potent immunosuppression and finally a discussion of reactivation with newer immunosuppressive regimens, including antiviral therapy for chronic hepatitis C virus (HCV) infection (Table 1).

Definitions

A source of considerable confusion in the "HBV reactivation" literature relates to the definitions used by different authors to describe related but non-identical clinical entities. HBV reactivation itself is usually defined by either a 1-log (10 fold) increase in HBV DNA in the serum or a return of HBV DNA viremia in a patient with undetectable HBV DNA at baseline. Some authors also include reverse seroconversion (return of HBsAg in a HBsAg-negative individual) under the term "HBV reactivation"; however, given the extent of immune suppression required to trigger reverse seroconversion, this entity should be considered separately [4]. In addition to considering the serological profile and levels of viremia, it is critical to consider the degree of liver injury. While an asymptomatic rise in HBV DNA may still be of some relevance, it is of much less consequence than a case of severe or even fatal hepatitis. Studies should report the rates of HBV-associated hepatitis, which requires HBV reactivation plus an associ-

Table 2. Proposed grading system for HBV reactivation [4]

Virological		Hepatic		Immunosuppression	
V_1	HBV DNA increase by >1 log IU/mL (or from undetectable to detectable)	H_0	No hepatitis: ALT remains <2 ULN, no change in bilirubin or INR	I_0	No consequence
V_2	Reverse seroconversion: reappearance of HBsAg with or without associated rise in HBV DNA (as in A)	H_1	Hepatitis: ALT 2–10 × ULN with no associated change in bilirubin or INR	I_1	No interruption but increased frequency of HBV DNA and ALT monitoring
		H_2	Severe hepatitis: ALT>10 × ULN and/or elevation of bilirubin (>2 ULN) or INR (>1.3)	I_2	Interruption of immunosuppressive therapy with re-initiation of same drug after hepatitis flare resolved
		H_3	Fulminant hepatitis: criteria for 2 with development of encephalopathy or ascites	I_3	Interruption of immunosuppressive regimen with re-initiation of 2nd line, suboptimal, therapy
		H_4	Death: due to liver failure	I_4	Discontinuation of immunosuppression

ated elevation of alanine aminotransferase (ALT). The most relevant threshold of ALT elevation is not clear but most studies where it has been defined have used 3× the upper limit of normal or 100 U/L. In addition to the degree of hepatic inflammation, changes in hepatic function should be documented, specifically the presence of icterus, coagulopathy, encephalopathy and ascites. Liver-related death (and liver transplant) should also be reported. Beyond liver-related issues, it is also important to document consequences to the underlying condition for which the immunosuppressive therapy is being given. With most literature coming from the oncology field, rates of chemotherapy interruption/discontinuation and cancer-related outcomes including all-cause mortality should be reported. Unfortunately, many studies do not clearly define outcomes using standardized approaches, making it difficult to compare results across studies. A scoring system that documents virological, hepatic and oncologic consequences has been proposed, which would allow for greater uniformity in reporting across studies (Table 2) [4]. The challenges with definitions and incomplete reporting have complicated attempts at meta-analysis and systematic review, hampering efforts to generate precise risk estimates. Hopefully journals will start insisting on adopting more standardized outcome definitions to improve the overall quality of the literature in this field.

HBsAg-Positive Patients

The rates and consequences of HBV reactivation have been best studied in patients with inactive chronic HBV infection (HBsAg+) undergoing cancer chemotherapy. A recent meta-analysis of HBV reactivation in patients receiving treatment for solid tumors found significant variability across studies, making it difficult to report precise tumor-specific or regimen-specific reactivation rates [5]. However, despite the heterogeneity, they found the risk of HBV reactivation to be highest among patients with breast cancer, particularly in those receiving anthracycline-based chemotherapy (median 29%), followed by those receiving platinum-based regimens for lung, head and neck cancers (median 25%), with a slightly lower risk seen in those receiving anti-metabolite therapy for gastrointestinal cancers (median 20%). Pooling data across studies, they were able to estimate the benefit of antiviral prophylaxis to prevent secondary complications of HBV reactivation, showing significant reductions in HBV-associated hepatitis (OR 0.18, 0.10–0.32) and chemotherapy interruption (OR 0.10, 0.04–0.27) and non-significant trends in acute liver failure (OR 0.31, 0.09–1.02) and death (OR 0.43, 0.15–1.20). Apart from the type of cancer and chemotherapy, other risk factors for reactivation include male gender, younger age and hepatitis B e antigen and/or HBV DNA positivity at baseline [5].

The risks of HBV reactivation are highest in patients with hematological malignancies. Studies have reported rates of reactivation approaching 60% with the highest rates reported in patients receiving anthracyclines, high-dose glucocorticoids and anti-CD20 agents like rituximab. To determine the optimal strategy to prevent HBV reactivation, landmark studies evaluated the effect of prophylactic antiviral therapy started before chemotherapy compared to “on-demand” therapy, which is given at the time of either a rise in HBV DNA or ALT [6]. All studies have shown lower rates of HBV reactivation and its com-

Dig Dis 2017;35:351–358
DOI: 10.1159/000456587

plications with prophylactic antiviral therapy, making this a preferred strategy [7, 8]. More recently, 2 studies have evaluated whether the antiviral agent used impacts on the rates and consequences of HBV reactivation. Both studies randomized patients to receive lamivudine or entecavir as prophylactic therapy and both reported lower rates of HBV reactivation and complications with entecavir [9, 10]. The benefit of entecavir was most pronounced in patients with HBV DNA levels above 2,000 IU/mL at baseline. In patients with HBV DNA levels below this threshold, lamivudine was highly effective, leading the American Association for the Study of Liver Disease (AASLD) to recommend any agent for those with low level viremia (<2,000 IU/mL) but only entecavir or tenofovir in patients with higher level viremia at baseline [11]. Notably the cause for reactivation in a number of patients with high DNA levels randomized to lamivudine was the emergence of lamivudine-resistant HBV, highlighting the importance of ongoing monitoring during antiviral therapy [9].

In addition to the preferred agent, there is some lack of clarity as to the optimal duration of antiviral therapy. Most studies have evaluated an additional 3–6 months of antiviral therapy following the completion of immunosuppressive therapy, but no direct comparisons have been made, thereby limiting the ability to make strong recommendations. Late reactivations have been reported, particularly in patients receiving rituximab-based therapy [12]. Importantly, reactivation, including fatal episodes, has been reported after the completion of antiviral therapy, highlighting the importance of following patients closely for evidence of a withdrawal flare at the time of cessation of antiviral prophylaxis [7]. The optimal monitoring strategy is not clear, but frequent HBV DNA and ALT measurements are likely necessary in the first few months after stopping the antiviral.

HBsAg-Negative/HBc-Positive Patients

Unlike the way it is for HBsAg-positive patients, the management of patients who have cleared HBsAg and remain anti-HBc-positive with or without anti-HBs antibodies remains very controversial. There are 2 major considerations: the relatively low rate of reactivation (compared to those who are HBsAg+) and the frequency of this serological profile (HBsAg–/cAb+). In HBV-endemic countries, 20–50% of the population may have been exposed to HBV [13]. With a high prevalence and a low risk of HBV reactivation, a strategy of screening and treating all individuals will result in a large number of people being treated unnecessarily with significant associated costs.

In patients receiving standard immunosuppressive regimens, such as solid tumor chemotherapy, the risk of HBV reactivation is very low, with the largest studies reporting rates well below 1% [5]. With such low rates of reactivation, it is unlikely that prophylactic therapy would be the preferred strategy, particularly from a cost-effectiveness standpoint. Alternatively, other approaches would include more frequent monitoring with either HBV DNA and/or HBsAg with plans to introduce therapy if either becomes positive or simply to forego testing altogether given the low risk of any consequence. There is no consensus on the optimal strategy with different clinical practice guidelines offering differing and sometimes conflicting recommendations.

With the more potent immunosuppression used for hematological malignancies, the risk of HBV reactivation even in those who have cleared HBsAg is significant. The highest risk of HBV reactivation has been reported with anti-CD20 agents, particularly rituximab. In the first prospective study, Yeo et al. [14] followed patients with diffuse large B-cell lymphoma receiving either CHOP or CHOP plus rituximab. In those on CHOP alone, no patients experienced HBV reactivation; however, in the group receiving rituximab, 24% became HBsAg positive and there was a 5% mortality rate. A more recent study from Hong Kong reported even higher rates of HBV reactivation. Seto et al. [15] measured HBV DNA monthly during and following rituximab-based chemotherapy for lymphoma and found that 42% of patients experienced an HBV reactivation during follow-up. However, this study highlights some of the issues with interpreting the literature. The authors concluded that HBV reactivation was extremely frequent with rituximab and recommended that patients should be considered for prophylactic antiviral therapy. However, the conditions under which HBV reactivation was defined were very stringent, with all patients requiring only an HBV DNA titre of 10 IU/mL. As soon as patients had detectable HBV DNA, they were promptly started on open-label entecavir therapy. Notably, there were no clinical consequences of HBV reactivation with no cases of severe HBV-associated hepatitis, chemotherapy interruption, liver failure or liver-related death. As such, one could equally interpret the results to support a strategy of instituting antiviral therapy upon appearance of HBV DNA. In reality, with such a low level of HBV DNA, it is not even clear if all patients required therapy. While this strategy certainly proved safe, whether monthly HBV DNA testing is feasible or cost-effective in standard clinical practice is very questionable.

Another study randomized HBsAg–/cAb+ patients receiving rituximab-based therapy to prophylactic entecavir or "on-demand" therapy upon evidence of HBV reactivation, defined in this study as an HBV DNA of 2,000 IU/mL or appearance of HBsAg (reverse seroconversion). Using this strategy, they found that only 4% of patients randomized to prophylactic entecavir experienced HBV reactivation and none had a reverse seroconvesion, whereas those without pre-treatment had a rate of 26% reactivation and 10.3% reverse seroconversion [16]. Although the authors' conclusion that prophylactic therapy was more effective at preventing HBV reactivation and should therefore be adopted seems logical, similar to the Seto study, there were no consequences to HBV reactivation or reverse seroconversion in the patients in the "on-demand" therapy arm. There were no cases of HBV-associated hepatitis or any more serious complications. The results could thus alternatively be interpreted to support the "on-demand" approach. Furthermore, the fact that there were no consequences even in patients with an HBV DNA above 2,000 IU/mL suggests that the very low threshold used by Seto et al. [15] (10 IU/mL) was probably stricter than necessary. In fact, based on these results, one might question whether HBV DNA testing is required at all or if it could be replaced by HBsAg monitoring, a much cheaper strategy. To date, HBsAg monitoring alone has not been studied but may be a reasonable strategy with a plan to promptly initiate therapy in those who become HBsAg positive. Collectively these studies highlight why the optimal strategy for monitoring and treating HBsAg-negative patients receiving even rituximab-based therapy remains unclear.

To help clarify who might need prophylactic therapy, Seto et al. [15] looked for risk factors for HBV reactivation in their study. They found that the presence of anti-HBs antibodies was a strong predictor of reactivation. The cumulative incidence of HBV reactivation at 2 years was 68% among patients with no anti-HBs antibodies compared to 34% in those positive for anti-HBs titres. Based on their findings, the authors recommended that patients negative for anti-HBs at baseline should receive prophylactic antiviral therapy and other patients should be followed closely and treated upon appearance of HBV DNA. While this is an interesting approach that certainly merits further study, 2 systematic reviews (including the Seto study) have not found a statistically significant benefit to the presence of anti-HBs antibodies in reducing the risk of HBV reactivation [17].

Screening Guidelines

HBV reactivation is a potentially serious but also a largely preventable complication of systemic immunosuppressive therapy. Because patients with inactive or even "resolved" HBV infection are usually asymptomatic, most are unaware of their infection and its associated risk. With a simple screening test and relatively straightforward and effective intervention, HBV reactivation seems like an ideal condition for which screening would be helpful. Screening recommendations have been put forward by multiple societies; however, there are significant variations in terms of which tests are recommended for which populations and even on how to manage positive results.

In 2008, the Centers for Disease Control and Prevention changed their approach from recommending risk-based screening to advocating for testing all individuals for HBsAg, anti-HBc and anti-HBs prior to immunosuppressive therapy [18]. While the AASLD and the European Association for the Study of the Liver promoted a similar screening approach, the American Society of Clinical Oncology (ASCO) strongly opposed widespread screening [19–21]. In a Provisional Clinical Opinion, they argued that the evidence was insufficient to determine the net benefits and harms of routine screening for chronic HBV infection [19]. They stated that physicians may consider screening in patients with known risk factors for HBV or those receiving highly immunosuppressive regimens with a consideration to use antiviral therapy in those who tested HBsAg positive. They raised concerns that the studies supporting screening were small and of relatively poor quality, that there was insufficient data on the costs of screening, and there was concern that screening may lead to delays in chemotherapy and/or treatment may interfere with chemotherapy by either causing drug–drug interactions or adverse events from antiviral therapy.

To address some of the data gaps identified by ASCO, cost-effectiveness studies were undertaken. Zurawska et al. [22] found that screening for HBsAg in patients scheduled to receive R-CHOP chemotherapy for high-grade lymphoma was not only cost-effective but actually cost-saving. Similarly, Day et al. [23] found that screening for HBsAg alone, but not HBsAg plus anti-HBc, was also cost-effective prior to breast cancer therapy. With increasing reports of HBV reactivation, including fatal cases, with the use of rituximab, the Federal Drug Administration (FDA) added a "black box" warning to the rituximab label highlighting the risk of HBV reactivation and recommending screening for HBV in all patients prior to starting rituximab with either close monitoring or antiviral therapy in those found to be positive. With accumulating data and the FDA recommendation, the ASCO panel elected to review and revise their Provisional Clinical Opinion in 2015 [24].

After re-reviewing the evidence, the ASCO panel came to the conclusion that screening may be useful in certain populations of patients. They advocated for a "risk-adapted" screening approach with a recommendation to screen patients at high risk of HBV or patients receiving highly immunosuppressive therapy for HBV. They advised testing for both HBsAg and anti-HBc with a plan to institute antiviral therapy in patients found to be HBsAg+ and either close monitoring or prophylactic antiviral therapy in those found to be HBsAg– but anti-HBc+ [24]. Notably, a minority opinion was put forward by 2 members of the panel. They argued that screening should be based on the risk of reactivation and the presence of a clear strategy for intervention rather than the risk of HBV exposure in the individual patient. Given the very low risk of reactivation in HBsAg/cAb+ patients receiving standard low-risk immunosuppressive therapy (e.g., solid tumor chemotherapy), identifying the presence of anti-HBc is unlikely to be helpful. This raises the issue of the harms of screening. Identifying patients who are anti-HBc+ but do not need prophylactic antivirals may lead to unnecessary treatment, additional visits for the patient for unnecessary monitoring as well as potentially confusion and even stigma on the part of the patient. In HBV-endemic regions, this approach would be particularly unhelpful, given the high prevalence of lone anti-HBc positivity [13]. As such, the minority opinion recommended testing all patients for HBsAg but reserving anti-HBc for those receiving highly immunosuppressive regimens such as anti-CD20 depleting agents or an allogeneic stem-cell or bone marrow transplant. This strategy ensures that all patients are screened for the low prevalence but high-risk HBsAg, and only those at risk with lone anti-HBc have this test performed. Additionally, this approach does not require oncologists or other practitioners to be familiar with risk factors for HBV, which multiple studies have shown is an important reason for risk-based screening to have been ineffective in the past [25]. Clearly additional studies are required to show the benefits of each approach to help guide ASCO and other societies in formulating guidelines.

Novel Immunosuppressant Agents

Beyond cancer chemotherapy, immunosuppressive regimens are increasingly being used in other areas of medicine. Reports of HBV reactivation have been published in the rheumatology, dermatology and gastroenterology literature in patients receiving biologics for autoimmune disease. Unfortunately, the published literature to date is of poor quality, consisting of case reports and small case series with very few prospective cohort studies. Without robust data, it is very difficult to assess the risk of HBV reactivation, making it very hard to offer recommendations on clinical management.

To date, the most extensive data exist for anti-tumor necrosis factor (anti-TNF) agents used for rheumatologic conditions and inflammatory bowel disease. Although individual cases of reactivation have been reported in HBsAg–/cAb+ patients, the risk is clearly much higher in patients who are HBsAg+. In fact, all cases of reactivation reported in HBsAg–/cAb+ patients occurred in patients receiving combination therapy with an anti-TNF agent and another immunomodulator, whereas reactivation has been reported with anti-TNF monotherapy in HBsAg+ individuals [26]. Based on the limited data available, the risk seems to be somewhat higher in patients receiving infliximab compared to other anti-TNF agents; however, the studies are small, limiting high-quality comparisons. Based on the available data, Perillo proposed an algorithm in which patients scheduled to receive anti-TNF monotherapy are screened for HBsAg only and put on antiviral prophylaxis if found positive. On the other hand, those who are scheduled to receive combination therapy are screened for both HBsAg and anti-HBc with a plan to treat HBsAg+ individuals and monitor those positive only for anti-HBc with ALT every 2–3 months, adding HBV DNA in those in whom the ALT rises [27]. While not validated, this approach seems like a good strategy that could be applied to other agents for which the risk of reactivation is poorly documented.

More recently, cases of HBV reactivation have been reported in patients treated for HCV infection with oral direct-acting antivirals (DAAs) in the absence of any overt immunosuppression. It is well known that HCV may inhibit HBV replication either through direct competition in the hepatocyte or possibly by stimulating a non-specific immune response in the liver. Because of this competition, it is relatively uncommon to have detectable viremia for both viruses simultaneously. In the era of interferon-based therapy for HCV, reports of HBV reactivation were cited. However, they were quite rare, possibly owing to the fact that HBV is also inhibited by interferon. Recently, 2 cases of HBV reactivation were reported in patients treated with sofosbuvir and simeprevir [28]. In the first case, the patient was HBsAg+ with detectable HBV DNA and cirrhosis. By week 8 of DAA therapy, the ALT was noted to rise and HBV DNA was found to be markedly increased. HCV therapy was stopped and tenofovir/emtricitabine was instituted. Fortunately, HBV was suppressed and the patient made a full recovery, including achieving a sustained virological response for the HCV infection. The second case involved a patient who was HBsAg– but anti-HBc+. In this case, the HBV DNA was monitored and it increased within 4 weeks of DAA therapy leading to the institution of tenofovir with prompt control of HBV without complication. These reports raised concerns that HBV reactivation may be a greater concern with DAA therapy.

Since these initial reports, 3 studies have examined this issue. In a study from Hong Kong, 3 of 10 patients who were HBsAg positive at the time of starting DAA therapy experienced HBV reactivation including a case of icteric hepatitis and a case of liver failure [29]. In another small study in New Zealand, Gane et al. [30] found that of 8 patients who were HBsAg+, 7 had a rise in HBV DNA during treatment, but fortunately there were no associated consequences. The HBV DNA did not rise above 20,000 IU/mL in any patient and no hepatitis was noted during sofosbuvir/ledipasvir therapy. Collectively these studies suggest that there is likely at least a modest risk of HBV reactivation in HBsAg positive patients and these patients should therefore be monitored carefully or preemptively treated with antiviral therapy. There is very limited global experience to date because HBsAg+ patients were excluded from all trials and are still not eligible for therapy in some jurisdictions. As more data accumulate, particularly from Asia, the magnitude of the risk will hopefully be better quantified.

In patients who are HBsAg–/cAb+, the risk appears to be very low. Despite the one case report, in 2 other relatively large series, no cases of HBV reactivation have been reported in patients during DAA therapy. In a review of patients treated in phase II studies of sofosbuvir/ledipasvir in Korea and Taiwan, of 103 patients who were anti-HBc+, none reactivated during treatment [31]. Similarly, no reactivations were seen in 124 HBsAg–/cAb+ patients treated with DAAs in Hong Kong [29]. Overall, these data suggest that the risk of HBV reactivation in those who are HBsAg– is very low and antiviral therapy is not indicated. Whether any specific monitoring beyond routine ALT assessment should be required in these patients is not clear but is quite relevant, given the large number of HCV-infected patients who are also anti-HBc+ in both HBV-endemic regions and in those who acquired HCV through injection drug use.

Summary

HBV reactivation is a potentially serious and largely preventable complication of immunosuppressive therapy. Fortunately, increasing the awareness of HBV reactivation has led to the evolution of more studies to generate the evidence to guide optimal management. For patients with chronic HBV infection (HBsAg+) receiving immunosuppressive therapy, the risk of reactivation is high and prophylactic antiviral therapy is highly effective, leaving the only controversy as the optimal duration of antiviral therapy after completion of immunosuppression. This is unlikely to be answered by a clinical trial and thus clinicians must remain vigilant and monitor for withdrawal flares. For those who are HBsAg–/HBc+, strategies for screening and treatment remain less clear. The risk of reactivation is very low with all but the most immunosuppressive regimens and thus an argument could be made to limit screening and intervention to only those receiving anti-CD20 therapy or stem-cell transplantation. Even among such patients, whether prophylactic therapy is required or monitoring with on-demand therapy would be adequate is still unclear, resulting in differing recommendations from different clinical practice guidelines. Hopefully as the data gaps are filled, there will be greater consensus to guide therapy. Similarly as new agents appear, high-quality prospective data will have to be collected using appropriate definitions to help quantify the risk of HBV reactivation and thus the appropriate interventions. While progress has been made, at least for now, some controversies remain.

Disclosure Statement

J.J.F. received consulting and/or research support from Abbvie, Abbott, Gilead, Janssen and Merck.

References

1 Gish RG, et al: Chronic hepatitis B: virology, natural history, current management and a glimpse at future opportunities. Antiviral Res 2015;121:47–58.
2 Hoofnagle JH: Reactivation of hepatitis B. Hepatology 2009;49(5 suppl):S156–S165.
3 Feitelson MA, Lee J: Hepatitis B virus integration, fragile sites, and hepatocarcinogenesis. Cancer Lett 2007;252:157–170.
4 Visram A, Feld JJ: Defining and grading HBV reactivation. Clin Liver Dis 2015;5:35–38.
5 Paul S, et al: Hepatitis B virus reactivation and prophylaxis during solid tumor chemotherapy: a systematic review and meta-analysis. Ann Intern Med 2016;164:30–40.

6 Lau GK, et al: Early is superior to deferred preemptive lamivudine therapy for hepatitis B patients undergoing chemotherapy. Gastroenterology 2003;125:1742–1749.
7 Hsu C, et al: A revisit of prophylactic lamivudine for chemotherapy-associated hepatitis B reactivation in non-Hodgkin's lymphoma: a randomized trial. Hepatology 2008;47:844–853.
8 Loomba R, et al: Systematic review: the effect of preventive lamivudine on hepatitis B reactivation during chemotherapy. Ann Intern Med 2008;148:519–528.
9 Huang H, et al: Entecavir vs lamivudine for prevention of hepatitis B virus reactivation among patients with untreated diffuse large B-cell lymphoma receiving R-CHOP chemotherapy: a randomized clinical trial. JAMA 2014;312:2521–2530.
10 Chen WC, et al: A comparison of entecavir and lamivudine for the prophylaxis of hepatitis B virus reactivation in solid tumor patients undergoing systemic cytotoxic chemotherapy. PLoS One 2015;10:e0131545.
11 Terrault NA, et al: AASLD guidelines for treatment of chronic hepatitis B. Hepatology 2016;63:261–283.
12 Niitsu N, et al: Prospective analysis of hepatitis B virus reactivation in patients with diffuse large B-cell lymphoma after rituximab combination chemotherapy. J Clin Oncol 2010;28: 5097–5100.
13 Te HS, Jensen DM: Epidemiology of hepatitis B and C viruses: a global overview. Clin Liver Dis 2010;14:1–21, vii.
14 Yeo W, et al: Hepatitis B virus reactivation in lymphoma patients with prior resolved hepatitis B undergoing anticancer therapy with or without rituximab. J Clin Oncol 2009;27:605–611.
15 Seto WK, et al: Hepatitis B reactivation in patients with previous hepatitis B virus exposure undergoing rituximab-containing chemotherapy for lymphoma: a prospective study. J Clin Oncol 2014;32:3736–3743.
16 Huang YH, et al: Randomized controlled trial of entecavir prophylaxis for rituximab-associated hepatitis B virus reactivation in patients with lymphoma and resolved hepatitis B. J Clin Oncol 2013;31:2765–2772.
17 Mozessohn L, et al: Hepatitis B reactivation in HBsAg-negative/HBcAb-positive patients receiving rituximab for lymphoma: a meta-analysis. J Viral Hepat 2015;22:842–849.
18 Weinbaum CM, et al: Recommendations for identification and public health management of persons with chronic hepatitis B virus infection. MMWR Recomm Rep 2008;57:1–20.
19 Artz AS, et al: American Society of Clinical Oncology provisional clinical opinion: chronic hepatitis B virus infection screening in patients receiving cytotoxic chemotherapy for treatment of malignant diseases. J Clin Oncol 2010;28:3199–3202.
20 European Association for the Study of the Liver: EASL clinical practice guidelines: management of chronic hepatitis B virus infection. J Hepatol 2012;57:167–185.
21 Lok AS, McMahon BJ: Chronic hepatitis B: update 2009. Hepatology 2009;50:661–662.
22 Zurawska U, et al: Hepatitis B virus screening before chemotherapy for lymphoma: a cost-effectiveness analysis. J Clin Oncol 2012;30: 3167–3173.
23 Day FL, Karnon J, Rischin D: Cost-effectiveness of universal hepatitis B virus screening in patients beginning chemotherapy for solid tumors. J Clin Oncol 2011;29:3270–3277.
24 Hwang JP, et al: Hepatitis B virus screening for patients with cancer before therapy: American Society of Clinical Oncology Provisional Clinical Opinion Update. J Clin Oncol 2015;33:2212–2220.
25 Visram A, et al: Poor recognition of risk factors for hepatitis B by physicians prescribing immunosuppressive therapy: a call for universal rather than risk-based screening. PLoS One 2015;10:e0120749.
26 Gonzalez SA, Perrillo RP: Hepatitis B virus reactivation in the setting of cancer chemotherapy and other immunosuppressive drug therapy. Clin Infect Dis 2016;62(suppl 4):S306–S313.
27 Perrillo RP: Tumor necrosis factor inhibitor therapy for hepatitis B virus-infected individuals: how loud is the alarm bell? Hepatology 2015;62:16–18.
28 Collins JM, et al: Hepatitis B virus reactivation during successful treatment of hepatitis C virus with sofosbuvir and simeprevir. Clin Infect Dis 2015;61:1304–1306.
29 Wang C, et al: Hepatitis due to reactivation of hepatitis B virus in endemic areas among patients with hepatitis C treated with direct-acting antiviral agents. Clin Gastroenterol Hepatol 2017;15:132–136.
30 Gane EJ, et al: Ledipasvir and sofosbuvir for HCV infection in patients coinfected with HBV. Antivir Ther 2016;21:605–609.
31 Sulkowski MS, et al: No evidence of reactivation of hepatitis B virus among patients treated with ledipasvir-sofosbuvir for hepatitis C virus infection. Clin Infect Dis 2016;63:1202–1204.

Autoimmune Liver Disease

Digestive Diseases

Dig Dis 2017;35:359–366
DOI: 10.1159/000467547

What Comes after Ursodeoxycholic Acid in Primary Biliary Cholangitis?

Lin Lee Wong Vinod S. Hegade David E.J. Jones

NIHR Biomedical Research Centre, Newcastle University, Newcastle upon Tyne, UK

Keywords

Non response · Obeticholic acid · Primary biliary cirrhosis/cholangitis · Symptom · Ursodeoxycholic acid

Abstract

Primary biliary cholangitis (PBC) is a rare autoimmune liver disease characterized by chronic cholestasis. Treatment with the accepted primary therapy ursodeoxycholic acid (UDCA) has been shown to be associated with delayed disease progression probably through reduced impact of cholestatic injury on the target biliary epithelial cells. Patients with inadequate response to UDCA (which can be identified through validated biochemical criteria) are at increased risk of disease progression, need for liver transplantation, and death. Obeticholic acid (OCA) is a farnesoid X receptor (FXR) agonist which has been evaluated as a second-line therapy in PBC and has been recently licensed by the Food and Drug Administration and European Medicines Agency for use in patients showing an inadequate response to UDCA or who are unable to tolerate it. Although evidence for biochemical improvement by OCA is compelling, there is, as yet, no evidence that OCA improves hard clinical outcomes or quality of life. In addition, OCA may not be suitable for PBC patients with pruritus as it can worsen the symptom. Other novel agents currently in clinical development may have better side-effect profile. Fibrates have the potential but currently lack high quality evidence to support their routine clinical use in PBC. Symptom management of PBC is challenging and ASBT inhibitors and rituximab are being evaluated for pruritus and fatigue, respectively.

Introduction

Primary biliary cholangitis (PBC), previously known as primary biliary cirrhosis, is a rare chronic autoimmune cholestatic liver disease which is characterized by lymphocytic cholangitis, gradual destruction of the small intrahepatic bile ducts, and progression to fibrosis, cirrhosis, and ultimately liver failure. It has a female preponderance with female to male ratio of 10:1 and usually presents in the fourth to sixth decade [1].

Patients with PBC can present with symptoms of fatigue or pruritus or, rarely, features of portal hypertension and/or advanced liver disease (ascites, hepatic encephalopathy, and esophageal variceal bleeding). A quarter of the patients are, however, asymptomatic at presentation and are identified through cholestatic liver function tests found on routine testing. PBC is currently diagnosed based on the fulfillment of 2 out of 3 criteria (elevated serum alkaline phosphatase [ALP], positive anti-mitochondrial antibody [AMA] or PBC-specific antinuclear antibody reactivity, and liver histology compatible with PBC) [2, 3]. As AMA is detected in 90–95% of patients with PBC and in less than 1% of normal controls liver histology is no longer a prerequisite for diagnosis of PBC [4]. Non-invasive methods such as transient elastography have mostly replaced liver biopsy for assessment of disease progression. Liver biopsy would be indicated in the absence of AMA and when considering other differential diagnosis [3, 5].

Ursodeoxycholic acid (UDCA) is the established first-line therapy and the current standard of care for

Prof. David E.J. Jones
Institute of Cellular Medicine, Faculty of Medical Sciences
4th Floor, William Leech Building
Newcastle University, Newcastle upon Tyne NE2 4HH (UK)
E-Mail David.Jones@newcastle.ac.uk

PBC. However, up to 40% of patients have incomplete biochemical response to UDCA and this has been shown to be associated with the risk of progression to end-stage liver disease and worse transplant-free survival rates than UDCA-responsive patients [3, 6–9]. Additional therapeutic options are therefore needed to improve clinical outcomes for this group of patients. To this end, a number of second-line agents are being evaluated, and among them, obeticholic acid (OCA), a farnesoid X receptor (FXR) agonist, has been licensed as a second-line therapy in PBC by the Food and Drug Administration (FDA) and European Medicines Agency (EMA).

This review will elaborate on the development of UDCA as standard accepted therapy, UDCA treatment response criteria and associated prognostic factors, the development of OCA as second-line therapy. It will also touch on the role of fibrates and several new agents evaluated for symptoms of pruritus and fatigue.

UDCA as Standard Accepted Therapy in the Treatment of PBC

UDCA is the current standard of care for patients with PBC at the recommended adult dose range of 13–15 mg per kg/day [2, 3]. The mechanism of action of UDCA in PBC is thought to be through diluting toxic bile acids (BAs), promoting their excretion, upregulating the biliary bicarbonate "umbrella" which protects the biliary tract, and exerting immune modulatory and anti-inflammatory effects [8, 10].

UDCA was studied in 5 randomized, placebo-controlled trials in PBC patients (stages I–IV) with some positive or mixed findings. The first trial (n = 180 patients, Mayo Clinic) found that UDCA use was associated with delayed progression of the disease but there was a limited effect on symptoms, histology, and need for liver transplantation or survival [11]. A second multicenter trial (n = 222 patients, Canada) showed that UDCA significantly improved serum markers of cholestasis but had no effect on survival or need for liver transplantation [12]. A third trial in Europe (n = 145) found reduction in rates of disease progression, need for liver transplantation, and probability of death in the UDCA-treated group compared to placebo [13]. This was followed by a trial in the USA (n = 151) which found major improvements in liver biochemical parameters in patients with less severe PBC (bilirubin <2 mg/dL) as compared to patients with entry serum bilirubin more or equal to 2 mg/dL. Liver histology also improved in the former group but not in the latter group [14]. The Spanish trial (n = 192) found that UDCA improved liver histology, prevented histological stage progression but had no effect on survival or liver transplantation. The study concluded UDCA may be useful for preventing the progression of PBC [15].

However, the above studies did not show any survival benefit by UDCA treatment. Moreover, 2 meta-analyses of 11 and 16 randomized controlled trials (RCTs), respectively, did not show a positive effect on survival. This may be due to the inclusion of trials of short duration (3 months to 2 years) as well as studies using UDCA doses which are currently known to be ineffective [16, 17]. Further reports with long-term follow-up have, however, shown the beneficial effect of UDCA on long-term survival in patients with PBC on standard doses (13–15 mg/kg/day). The transplant-free survival for patients (with early-stage PBC) treated with UDCA were equivalent to an age- and gender-matched healthy control population [18–20]. Taken together, evidence suggests that UDCA improves biochemical markers of cholestasis, slows down the progression of PBC, and delays liver transplantation and death with improved survival [2, 3].

Non-Response to UDCA Increases Risk of PBC Disease Progression

UDCA is an effective treatment and UDCA treatment response has been shown to be strongly predictive of long-term outcome in PBC [21]. However, up to 40% of patients with PBC fail to respond adequately to UDCA and do not improve their liver biochemistry [6, 7, 9]. These patients with incomplete biochemical response to UDCA are referred to as "UDCA non-responders" and in comparison to UDCA responders, have poorer prognosis due to greater risk of disease progression, higher mortality risk, and likelihood to require liver transplantation [1]. Over the years, several treatment response criteria that have been developed based on various biochemical endpoints used in the clinical trials and are used as prognostic models (Table 1) [6, 22–24]. The Barcelona criteria for instance were developed following post-hoc analysis of the Spanish trial, evaluating patients based on their biochemical response to UDCA. This included total bilirubin, ALP, albumin, and prothrombin time. This analysis showed that in patients whose serum ALP reduced by 40% from baseline or normalized had similar survival to a standardized population. Patients who had incomplete

Table 1. Treatment response criteria

Criteria	Definition
Barcelona	Decrease in alkaline phosphatase level >40% of baseline level or a normal level
Paris I (all criteria met)	Alkaline phosphatase level ≤3 × ULN Aspartate aminotransferase level ≤2 × ULN Normal bilirubin level
Paris II (all criteria met)	Alkaline phosphatase level ≤1.5 × ULN Aspartate aminotransferase level ≤1.5 × ULN Normal bilirubin level
Toronto	Alkaline phosphatase level ≤1.67 × ULN

biochemical response had slightly better survival rates than predicted but worse than a comparable population group [23].

More recently, the United Kingdom PBC (UK-PBC) group studied a cohort of 2,353 patients and used all 4 treatment–response biochemical criteria (Barcelona, Paris I, Paris II, Toronto) to categorize patients as responders or non-responders to UDCA. Irrespective of the criteria used, there was a clear distinction in survival outcomes between responders and non-responders. Other predictive factors for nonresponse to UDCA include women diagnosed before age 50 years and men irrespective of age [7].

The same group compared 380 post-transplant patients and 2,300 non-transplant patients with PBC and found that more than 50% of patients presenting below the age of 50 had failed primary therapy (UDCA non-response) or already been transplanted at the time of the study. This further emphasized that PBC carries greater risk in younger patients and improved treatment options are urgently needed in this targeted group [25].

The Global PBC Study group, an international and multicenter collaboration between 15 liver centers in 8 North American and European countries performed a meta-analysis, combining individual patient data from major long-term follow-up cohorts. This showed the utility of serum levels of ALP and bilirubin as surrogate end points of outcomes in PBC. An elevated ALP greater than 1.67 × upper limit of normal (ULN) was independently associated with a 2–2.5 increase risk of transplantation or death compared to the risk associated with normal levels. A raised bilirubin above the ULN had a 5.1–10.7 times risk of liver transplantation or death compared to the risk associated with normal levels [26]. These 2 criteria (ALP >1.67 × ULN and bilirubin >ULN) have since been validated by the group and has become the de facto standard entry criteria for current trials of new treatments in PBC, notably the landmark POISE trial [27].

Obeticholic Acid

OCA (INT-747) is a semi-synthetic analog of the primary BA chenodeoxycholic acid that interferes with BA homeostasis through selective activation of the nuclear hormone receptor FXR [8, 28]. FXR activation reduces de novo synthesis of BAs in hepatocytes and increases transport of BAs out of hepatocytes leading to reduced exposure of the hepatocytes to BA. OCA has also been shown to have FXR-activation mediated anti-cholestatic, anti-inflammatory, and anti-fibrotic effects in pre-clinical and clinical studies [8, 28]. Due to these beneficial properties, it was postulated that OCA might exert a positive effect in patients with PBC.

OCA has been evaluated in both phase 2 and 3 trials. The first 12-week phase 2 trial (double-blind placebo-controlled parallel group dose–response study) randomized 59 patients with PBC (not on UDCA for 6 months with persistently raised ALP 1.5–10 × ULN) to placebo, OCA 10 mg, or 50 mg per day for 12 weeks. At the end of the study, the 10 mg group showed an ALP decrease from 3.9 × ULN pre-treatment to 1.9 × ULN. Pruritus was the most common adverse effect (AE; placebo – 30%, 10 mg – 70%, 50 mg – 94%) with severity and discontinuation rate increasing with dose [29]. The next key phase 2 trial (3-month duration with a 1-year open-label extension) randomized 165 patients with PBC who were on optimal UDCA dosage for 6 months and had an inadequate response to UDCA (persistently raised ALP 1.5–10 × ULN) to a range of OCA doses (10, 25, and 50 mg) or placebo. All OCA groups met the primary end point (relative percentage change in ALP values from baseline [day 0] to the end of the study [day 85] compared to placebo) with statistical significant reduction ($p < 0.0001$) of mean ALP values from baseline at the end of the study. The study concluded that daily OCA (10–50 mg) reduced ALP significantly compared with placebo in patients with PBC who had inadequate response to UDCA. Pruritus was again noted to be the main AE with incidence of 47% (no statistical significant difference), 87% ($p < 0.0003$), and 80% ($p < 0.006$) in the OCA 10, 25, and 50 mg group, respectively, compared to 50% in the placebo group [8].

More recently, a phase 3 randomized, double-blind, placebo-controlled trial (POISE trial) has been reported [27]. Patients were treated with OCA for over 12 months with open-label extension data of a further 1 year. This landmark study recruited 216 patients who had inadequate response to at least 1 year of UDCA monotherapy (at optimal dosage) or were intolerant to UDCA. The biochemical entry criteria were ALP level more than 1.67 × ULN or abnormal total bilirubin level not more than 2 × ULN. The patients were randomly assigned to 10 mg OCA, 5 mg OCA with adjustment to 10 mg if applicable (5–10 mg group), or placebo. The primary end point was an ALP level <1.67 × ULN with a reduction of at least 15% from baseline and a normal total bilirubin level, an end point validated in both the UK-PBC and Global PBC patient cohorts. Out of the 216 patients, 93% were on UDCA therapy. The primary end point was met in 47% of the OCA 10 mg group and 46% of the titration group (5–10 mg) compared to 10% in the placebo with UDCA group ($p < 0.0001$). Secondary end points included reduction in ALP level which was greater in the OCA groups compared to placebo, with significant reduction from baseline at 1 year (least squares mean ± SE reduction, –113 ± 14 U/L in the titration group, and –130 ± 15 U/L in the 10 mg group compared to –14 ± 15 U/L in the placebo group; $p < 0.001$ for both comparisons). With regards to symptom control, there was no improvement in the PBC-40 questionnaire scores with patients in the 10 mg group scoring significantly worse itch-domain scores than those in the placebo group (during the first 3 months of the study). Of those who continued into the open-label extension of the study after completing the 12-month double-blind phase (i.e., 193 of 198), a sustained decrease in ALP and total bilirubin levels was seen in the OCA group. Those in the placebo group who received OCA in the open-label extension also had similar efficacy as those in the OCA group. Non-invasive parameters for liver fibrosis (transient elastography/Fibroscan, hyaluronic acid, and TIMP-1) did not change significantly between baseline to 12 months for both treatment group and placebo group.

Pruritus was the main AE occurring more in the OCA group (56% in the titration group and 68% in the 10 mg group) compared to placebo (38%). Treatment discontinuation occurred in 10% of the OCA 10 mg group (n = 7) and 1% (n = 1) of the 5–10 mg group. The study concluded that OCA in combination with UDCA or as single therapy for 12 months in patients with PBC resulted in reduction in ALP and total bilirubin levels that were significantly different from the chances observed with placebo [27].

A further double-blind randomized controlled phase 3b trial (COBALT study, NCT02308111) is currently in recruitment to study the clinical outcomes of patients with PBC, comparing patients randomized to taking OCA vs. placebo (standard of care). The primary end point events include death, liver transplant, MELD score ≥15, uncontrolled ascites, hepatocellular carcinoma, and hospitalization for new onset or recurrence of either variceal bleed or encephalopathy or spontaneous bacterial peritonitis.

In the meantime, the FDA has approved OCA as a second-line therapy for adult patients with PBC who have inadequate response to UDCA, used in combination with UDCA or as monotherapy in patients intolerant to UDCA.

Other Agents

In addition to OCA, a number of other novel drugs are emerging as potential second-line agents to treat PBC patients with UDCA non-response. Some of these are already in phase 2 clinical development. For instance, LJN452 (Novartis pharmaceuticals), a non-BA FXR agonist is currently being investigated in a multicenter double-blind study to assess the safety and efficacy in PBC patients with UDCA non-response (NCT02516605). Similarly, a phase 2 placebo-controlled RCT of NGM-282 (NGM Biopharmaceuticals, Inc.), a FGF-19 analog administered in combination with UDCA for 28 days (NCT02026401), and a further phase 2b study to evaluate 3 different doses of NGM-282 administered for 24 weeks (NCT02135536) have been completed and results are pending.

In a recent phase 2 double-blind placebo-controlled study (NCT02609048), MBX-8025 (CymaBay Therapeutics, Inc.), an orally administered, potent, and selective peroxisome proliferator-activated receptor (PPAR) delta agonist has been shown to markedly improve biochemical markers of cholestasis in patients with PBC. The unblinded data from 26 patients completing at least 2 weeks of treatment with MBX-8025 (or placebo) showed mean decreases of 57 and 62% from baseline in ALP for the 50 and 200 mg dose groups, respectively (vs. 0.37% for placebo; $p < 0.0001$ for both). Also, the responder rates for the placebo, 50 and 200 mg groups were 10, 67, and 100%, respectively. These early results are encouraging and suggest that MBX-8025 produces a rapid and potent anti-cholestatic effect in patients with PBC. However, this study was terminated early as 3 cases of asymptomatic increases in transaminases were observed (2 in the 200 mg MBX-8025 and 1 in the 50 mg MBX-8025 cohorts).

Fibrates (fenofibrate and bezafibrate) have long been proposed as adjunctive treatment for UDCA non-response in PBC. The anti-cholestatic effect of fibrates is primarily due to the PPAR-mediated inhibition of hepatic BA synthesis. In addition, fibrates facilitate elimination of toxic BA, increase biliary phospholipid output, and exert immune modulator function via inhibition of NFκB [30]. A substantial body of circumstantial evidence (case series and small and/or short-term uncontrolled studies) have supported safety and efficacy of using fenofibrate and bezafibrate as adjunctive therapy to UDCA for up to a year in patients with PBC with incomplete response to UDCA [31, 32]. However, to date, there are no prospective RCTs of fibrates in PBC with hard end points and limited data exist on their use beyond 12 months [33]. Moreover, the effect of fibrates on disease progression is unclear. In a recent study, fenofibrate therapy was associated with significant improvements in decompensation-free and transplant-free survival in PBC patients with incomplete UDCA response but cirrhotic patients treated with fenofibrate had significantly higher elevation in serum bilirubin compared to the controls [34]. Therefore fenofibrate, should be used cautiously in PBC patients with cirrhosis with close monitoring for clinical/biochemical decompensation [34, 35]. Overall, there remains a considerable gap in our knowledge on fibrates in PBC and high quality RCTs are needed to address the effect of fibrates not only on biochemical markers, but also on histology, quality of life, need for transplantation, and survival [36]. Recently, bezafibrate has been subjected to a large multicenter, prospective, double-blind, placebo-controlled phase III study in combination with UDCA in PBC (BEZURSO study; NCT01654731) and results are pending.

New Treatments for PBC-Associated Symptoms

Pruritus and fatigue are the 2 most common symptoms of PBC, and their association with PBC is independent of biochemical severity or stage of the disease and seemingly unresponsive to both UDCA and OCA, the licensed therapies. Pruritus and fatigue are associated with significant impairment in the quality of life of PBC patients and they are often life altering when severe. The mechanisms driving these symptoms are complex and the treatment is challenging with few effective therapies available. UDCA, the primary therapy of PBC, has never been shown to reduce the severity of pruritus or fatigue. However, a cross-sectional study of 2,353 PBC patients showed that pruritus (but not fatigue) severity was significantly higher in patients who were unresponsive to UDCA therapy [37]. The same study also observed more severe pruritus and fatigue in patients presenting at an age younger than age 30 years.

Current pruritus treatment in PBC largely depends on the step-wise use of guideline recommended agents that include cholestyramine, rifampicin, naltrexone, and sertraline [3]. The potential newer agents for treating pruritus in PBC are ileal BA transporter (IBAT or ASBT) inhibitors and fibrates. The IBAT plays a key role in the enterohepatic circulation of BAs which are implicated in cholestatic pruritus [38]. Two RCTs of IBAT inhibitor drugs investigating their safety and efficacy in PBC patients with pruritus have been completed. The results of the CLARITY study ($n = 61$) where patients were randomized to daily oral lopixibat (LUM001) 10 mg, 20 mg, or placebo showed significant decrease in itch score from baseline in the within group comparison (26% lopixibat, $p < 0.0001$ and 23% placebo, $p < 0.0001$) but no significant difference between group comparison (lopixibat vs. placebo, $p = 0.47$) [39]. Another IBAT inhibitor drug GSK2330672 (GSK672) has been investigated in 21 PBC patients with pruritus. This was a phase 2 double-blind, randomized placebo-controlled crossover trial conducted over 14 days. No serious AEs were reported. GSK672 reduced itch intensity significantly more than placebo as measured by numeric rating scale (–23% [–1 to –45%]), PBC-40 itch domain (–14% [–1 to –26%]), and 5-D itch (–20% (–7 to –34%]). The study concluded that oral GSK672 was well tolerated and reduced itch intensity in PBC patients with pruritus. These results support further investigation of GSK672 as a potential treatment for cholestatic pruritus [38].

Although uncontrolled studies have suggested that fenofibrate and bezafibrate improve pruritus in PBC patients [40–42], there have been no prospective RCTs of fibrates with pruritus as the primary outcome. The BEZURSO study (NCT01654731) will hopefully shed more light on the effect of fibrates on pruritus associated with PBC.

OCA, although licensed for treating UDCA non-response PBC patients, is unfortunately not associated with significant abatement of symptoms as measured by the PBC-40 questionnaire. On the contrary, OCA therapy has been shown to be associated with dose-dependent increased frequency and severity of pruritus, as found in the phase 2 and 3 trials. Although the exact mechanism of pruritus related to OCA is unclear, TGR5 activation-induced pruritus (OCA is a weak TGR5 agonist) or activation of the autotaxin pathway have been proposed [8, 27].

Fatigue management in PBC is more challenging, and despite its high prevalence among PBC patients at present, there are no licensed treatments. Previous studies on oral supplementation with antioxidants (including coen-

Dig Dis 2017;35:359–366
DOI: 10.1159/000467547

zyme Q10) have shown mixed results at reducing fatigue levels [43, 44]. A strong association has been shown between abnormalities in sleep regulation, particularly excessive daytime somnolence and fatigue severity in PBC. Therefore, modafinil, a CNS-acting drug used in the treatment of excessive daytime somnolence in non-liver patients, has been investigated in PBC. An open-label study of 21 PBC patients treated with modafinil had shown objective, short-term benefit in daytime somnolence and fatigue [45] and a follow-up study of this cohort at 14 months showed sustained and statistically significant benefit in daytime somnolence but the fatigue scores were not significantly better than the baseline [46]. More recently, in a double-blind placebo-controlled study, PBC patients were randomized to receive modafinil (n = 20) or placebo (n = 20) for 12 weeks and fatigue was quantified by the Fisk Fatigue Impact Scale (FFIS). Although the treatment was found to be safe and well tolerated, modafinil did not significantly benefit fatigue as only 3 patients (17.6%) in the modafinil arm and 2 (12.5%) in the placebo arm (p = 1.00) met the primary end point of ≥50% reduction in FFIS score [47].

In the quest for effective treatment for fatigue, recent focus has been on rituximab, an anti-CD20 monoclonal antibody that selectively depletes B cell. Previously, 2 pilot studies that investigated rituximab (1,000 mg infusion) in UDCA non-responsive PBC showed it was safe and well tolerated in PBC and improved liver biochemistry [48, 49]. However, fatigue was not the primary outcome in these studies. A double-blind placebo-controlled study of rituximab (RIT-PBC study) aiming to investigate rituximab (given as two 1,000 mg intravenous infusion at 12 weeks apart) as a treatment for fatigue in PBC has been recently completed and a large number of PBC patients have been recruited in a single large UK center [50]. The first RCT of a treatment for fatigue in patients with PBC was likely to provide important data on the efficacy, safety, and tolerability of rituximab in PBC patients with significant fatigue.

Conclusion

The landscape of PBC therapy is changing rapidly with a recent surge in clinical trials of novel agents to treat UDCA non-response status and symptoms. OCA marks an important milestone in PBC and the data from phase 2 to 3 clinical trials on biochemical improvements are compelling, leading to its FDA approval for use in UDCA unresponsive patients. However, there is no evidence that OCA improves hard clinical outcomes or overall quality of life. In addition, OCA may not be suitable for PBC patients with pruritus as it may worsen the symptom. Other novel agents currently in clinical development may have better side effect profile. Fibrates have the potential but currently lack strong evidence to support their routine clinical use in PBC. Symptom management of PBC is challenging, and ASBT inhibitors and rituximab are being evaluated for pruritus and fatigue, respectively.

Disclosure Statement

L.L.W. declares no competing interests or financial disclosures.
V.S.H. reports personal fees and non-financial support from GSK. D.E.J.J. is an investigator on the UK-PBC consortium who has received research funding from GSK, Intercept, Pfizer. He has provided consultancy advice to Novartis, GSK and Intercept and has given sponsored lectures for Falk.

References

1 Selmi C, Bowlus CL, Gershwin ME, Coppel RL: Primary biliary cirrhosis. Lancet 2011; 377:1600–1609.
2 Lindor KD, Gershwin ME, Poupon R, Kaplan M, Bergasa NV, Heathcote EJ; American Association for Study of Liver Diseases: Primary biliary cirrhosis. Hepatology 2009;50:291–308.
3 European Association for the Study of the Liver: EASL clinical practice guidelines: management of cholestatic liver diseases. J Hepatol 2009;51:237–267.
4 Bowlus CL, Gershwin ME: The diagnosis of primary biliary cirrhosis. Autoimmun Rev 2014;13:441–444.
5 Corpechot C, Carrat F, Poujol-Robert A, Gaouar F, Wendum D, Chazouilleres O, Poupon R: Noninvasive elastography-based assessment of liver fibrosis progression and prognosis in primary biliary cirrhosis. Hepatology 2012;56: 198–208.
6 Corpechot C, Chazouilleres O, Poupon R: Early primary biliary cirrhosis: biochemical response to treatment and prediction of long-term outcome. J Hepatol 2011;55: 1361–1367.
7 Carbone M, Mells GF, Pells G, Dawwas MF, Newton JL, Heneghan MA, Neuberger JM, et al: Sex and age are determinants of the clinical phenotype of primary biliary cirrhosis and response to ursodeoxycholic acid. Gastroenterology 2013;144:560–569.e7; quiz e13–e14.
8 Hirschfield GM, Mason A, Luketic V, Lindor K, Gordon SC, Mayo M, Kowdley KV, et al: Efficacy of obeticholic acid in patients with primary biliary cirrhosis and inadequate response to ursodeoxycholic acid. Gastroenterology 2015;148:751–761. e758.
9 Kuiper EM, Hansen BE, de Vries RA, den Ouden-Muller JW, van Ditzhuijsen TJ, Haagsma EB, Houben MH, Witteman BJ, van Erpecum KJ, van Buuren HR; Dutch PBC Study Group: Improved prognosis of patients with primary biliary cirrhosis that have a biochemical response to ursodeoxycholic acid. Gastroenterology 2009;136: 1281–1287.

10 Hohenester S, Wenniger LM, Paulusma CC, van Vliet SJ, Jefferson DM, Elferink RP, Beuers U: A biliary HCO3- umbrella constitutes a protective mechanism against bile acid-induced injury in human cholangiocytes. Hepatology 2012;55:173–183.
11 Lindor KD, Dickson ER, Baldus WP, Jorgensen RA, Ludwig J, Murtaugh PA, Harrison JM, et al: Ursodeoxycholic acid in the treatment of primary biliary cirrhosis. Gastroenterology 1994;106:1284–1290.
12 Heathcote EJ, Cauch-Dudek K, Walker V, Bailey RJ, Blendis LM, Ghent CN, Michieletti P, et al: The Canadian multicenter double-blind randomized controlled trial of ursodeoxycholic acid in primary biliary cirrhosis. Hepatology 1994;19:1149–1156.
13 Poupon RE, Poupon R, Balkau B: Ursodiol for the long-term treatment of primary biliary cirrhosis. The UDCA-PBC Study Group. N Engl J Med 1994;330:1342–1347.
14 Combes B, Carithers RL Jr, Maddrey WC, Lin D, McDonald MF, Wheeler DE, Eigenbrodt EH, et al: A randomized, double-blind, placebo-controlled trial of ursodeoxycholic acid in primary biliary cirrhosis. Hepatology 1995; 22:759–766.
15 Pares A, Caballeria L, Rodes J, Bruguera M, Rodrigo L, Garcia-Plaza A, Berenguer J, et al: Long-term effects of ursodeoxycholic acid in primary biliary cirrhosis: results of a double-blind controlled multicentric trial. UDCA-cooperative group from the Spanish association for the study of the liver. J Hepatol 2000; 32:561–566.
16 Goulis J, Leandro G, Burroughs AK: Randomised controlled trials of ursodeoxycholic-acid therapy for primary biliary cirrhosis: a meta-analysis. Lancet 1999;354:1053–1060.
17 Gong Y, Huang ZB, Christensen E, Gluud C: Ursodeoxycholic acid for patients with primary biliary cirrhosis: an updated systematic review and meta-analysis of randomized clinical trials using Bayesian approach as sensitivity analyses. Am J Gastroenterol 2007;102: 1799–1807.
18 Corpechot C, Carrat F, Bahr A, Chrétien Y, Poupon RE, Poupon R: The effect of ursodeoxycholic acid therapy on the natural course of primary biliary cirrhosis. Gastroenterology 2005;128:297–303.
19 ter Borg PC, Schalm SW, Hansen BE, van Buuren HR: Prognosis of ursodeoxycholic acid-treated patients with primary biliary cirrhosis. Results of a 10-Yr cohort study involving 297 patients. Am J Gastroenterol 2006; 101:2044–2050.
20 Angulo P, Dickson ER, Therneau TM, Jorgensen RA, Smith C, DeSotel CK, Lange SM, et al: Comparison of three doses of ursodeoxycholic acid in the treatment of primary biliary cirrhosis: a randomized trial. J Hepatol 1999;30:830–835.
21 Carbone M, Sharp SJ, Flack S, Paximadas D, Spiess K, Adgey C, Griffiths L, et al: The UK-PBC risk scores: derivation and validation of a scoring system for long-term prediction of end-stage liver disease in primary biliary cholangitis. Hepatology 2016;63:930–950.
22 Corpechot C, Abenavoli L, Rabahi N, Chrétien Y, Andréani T, Johanet C, Chazouillères O, Poupon R: Biochemical response to ursodeoxycholic acid and long-term prognosis in primary biliary cirrhosis. Hepatology 2008; 48:871–877.
23 Pares A, Caballeria L, Rodes J: Excellent long-term survival in patients with primary biliary cirrhosis and biochemical response to ursodeoxycholic acid. Gastroenterology 2006;130: 715–720.
24 Kumagi T, Guindi M, Fischer SE, Arenovich T, Abdalian R, Coltescu C, Heathcote EJ, et al: Baseline ductopenia and treatment response predict long-term histological progression in primary biliary cirrhosis. Am J Gastroenterol 2010;105:2186–2194.
25 Pells G, Mells GF, Carbone M, Newton JL, Bathgate AJ, Burroughs AK, Heneghan MA, et al: The impact of liver transplantation on the phenotype of primary biliary cirrhosis patients in the UK-PBC cohort. J Hepatol 2013; 59:67–73.
26 Lammers WJ, van Buuren HR, Hirschfield GM, Janssen HL, Invernizzi P, Mason AL, Ponsioen CY, et al: Levels of alkaline phosphatase and bilirubin are surrogate end points of outcomes of patients with primary biliary cirrhosis: an international follow-up study. Gastroenterology 2014;147:1338–1349.e5; quiz e15.
27 Nevens F, Andreone P, Mazzella G, Strasser SI, Bowlus C, Invernizzi P, Drenth JP, et al: A placebo-controlled trial of obeticholic acid in primary biliary cholangitis. N Engl J Med 2016;375:631–643.
28 Mudaliar S, Henry RR, Sanyal AJ, Morrow L, Marschall HU, Kipnes M, Adorini L, et al: Efficacy and safety of the farnesoid X receptor agonist obeticholic acid in patients with type 2 diabetes and nonalcoholic fatty liver disease. Gastroenterology 2013;145:574–582.e1.
29 Jones D, Kowdley K, Chapman R, Burroughs A, Hirschfield G, Schramm C, Poupon R, et al: OP02 the first new monotherapy therapeutic PBC study in a decade? An international study evaluating the farnesoid X receptor agonist obeticholic acid in PBC. Gut 2011;60: A50–A50.
30 Ghonem NS, Assis DN, Boyer JL: On fibrates and cholestasis: a review. Hepatology 2015; 62:635–643.
31 Zhang Y, Li S, He L, Wang F, Chen K, Li J, Liu T, et al: Combination therapy of fenofibrate and ursodeoxycholic acid in patients with primary biliary cirrhosis who respond incompletely to UDCA monotherapy: a meta-analysis. Drug Des Devel Ther 2015;9:2757–2766.
32 Grigorian AY, Mardini HE, Corpechot C, Poupon R, Levy C: Fenofibrate is effective adjunctive therapy in the treatment of primary biliary cirrhosis: a meta-analysis. Clin Res Hepatol Gastroenterol 2015;39:296–306.
33 Hegade VS, Khanna A, Walker LJ, Wong LL, Dyson JK, Jones DE: Long-term fenofibrate treatment in primary biliary cholangitis improves biochemistry but not the UK-PBC risk score. Dig Dis Sci 2016;61:3037–3044.
34 Cheung AC, Lapointe-Shaw L, Kowgier M, Meza-Cardona J, Hirschfield GM, Janssen HL, Feld JJ: Combined ursodeoxycholic acid (UDCA) and fenofibrate in primary biliary cholangitis patients with incomplete UDCA response may improve outcomes. Aliment Pharmacol Ther 2016;43:283–293.
35 Jones DE, Hansen BE: Editorial: fenofibrate as second-line therapy in high risk PBC – more answers or more questions? Aliment Pharmacol Ther 2016;43:648–649.
36 Invernizzi P, Gershwin ME: New therapeutics in primary biliary cirrhosis: will there ever be light? Liver Int 2014;34:167–170.
37 Carbone M MG, Pells G, et al: Sex and age are determinants of the clinical phenotype of primary biliary cirrhosis and response to ursodeoxycholic acid. Gastroenterology 2013;144: 560–569.e7; quiz e13–e14.
38 Hegade VS, Kendrick S, Dobbins R, Miller S, Richards D, Dukes G, Hirschfield G, et al: A phase 2 randomised crossover trial of ileal bile acid transporter inhibitor GSK2330672 in patients with primary biliary cholangitis and symptoms of pruritus. Hepatology 2016;64: 108A.
39 Mayo MJ, Pockros P, Jones D, Bowlus C, Levy C, Patanwala I, Bacon B, Luketic V, Vuppalanchi R, Medendorp S, Dorenbaum A, Kennedy C, Novak P, Raychaudhuri A, Goyal S, Abi-Saab W, Hirschfield GM: CLARITY: A Phase 2, Randomized, Double-Blind, Placebo-Controlled Study of Lopixibat Chloride (Formerly LUM001), a Novel Apical Sodium-Dependent Bile Acid Transporter Inhibitor, in the Treatment of Primary Biliary Cirrhosis Associated with Itching. Journal of Hepatology, 2016 pp S183–S212.
40 Lens S, Leoz M, Nazal L, Bruguera M, Pares A: Bezafibrate normalizes alkaline phosphatase in primary biliary cirrhosis patients with incomplete response to ursodeoxycholic acid. Liver Int 2014;34:197–203.
41 Ohmoto K, Yoshioka N, Yamamoto S: Long-term effect of bezafibrate on parameters of hepatic fibrosis in primary biliary cirrhosis. J Gastroenterol 2006;41:502–503.
42 Han XF, Wang QX, Liu Y, You ZR, Bian ZL, Qiu DK, Ma X: Efficacy of fenofibrate in Chinese patients with primary biliary cirrhosis partially responding to ursodeoxycholic acid therapy. J Dig Dis 2012;13:219–224.
43 Prince MI, Mitchison HC, Ashley D, Burke DA, Edwards N, Bramble MG, James OF, et al: Oral antioxidant supplementation for fatigue associated with primary biliary cirrhosis: results of a multicentre, randomized, placebo-controlled, cross-over trial. Aliment Pharmacol Ther 2003;17:137–143.

44 Watson JP, Jones DE, James OF, Cann PA, Bramble MG: Case report: oral antioxidant therapy for the treatment of primary biliary cirrhosis: a pilot study. J Gastroenterol Hepatol 1999;14:1034–1040.
45 Jones DE, Newton JL: An open study of modafinil for the treatment of daytime somnolence and fatigue in primary biliary cirrhosis. Aliment Pharmacol Ther 2007;25:471–476.
46 Hardy T, MacDonald C, Jones DE, Newton JL: A follow-up study of modafinil for the treatment of daytime somnolence and fatigue in primary biliary cirrhosis. Liver Int 2010;30: 1551–1552.
47 Silveira MG, Gossard AA, Stahler AC, Jorgensen RA, Petz JL, Ali AH, Lindor KD: A randomized, placebo-controlled clinical trial of efficacy and safety: modafinil in the treatment of fatigue in patients with primary biliary cirrhosis. Am J Ther 2016, Epub ahead of print.
48 Myers RP, Swain MG, Lee SS, Shaheen AA, Burak KW: B-cell depletion with rituximab in patients with primary biliary cirrhosis refractory to ursodeoxycholic acid. Am J Gastroenterol 2013;108:933–941.
49 Tsuda M, Moritoki Y, Lian ZX, Zhang W, Yoshida K, Wakabayashi K, Yang GX, et al: Biochemical and immunologic effects of rituximab in patients with primary biliary cirrhosis and an incomplete response to ursodeoxycholic acid. Hepatology 2012;55: 512–521.
50 Jopson L, Newton JL, Palmer J, Floudas A, Isaacs J, Qian J, Wilkinson J, et al: RITPBC: B-cell depleting therapy (rituximab) as a treatment for fatigue in primary biliary cirrhosis: study protocol for a randomised controlled trial. BMJ Open 2015;5:e007985.

Autoimmune Liver Disease

Digestive Diseases

Dig Dis 2017;35:367–370
DOI: 10.1159/000456588

Can Understanding the Pathogenesis of Autoimmune Hepatitis Lead to Rational Therapy?

Ansgar W. Lohse Johannes Herkel Christina Weiler-Normann

I. Department of Medicine, University Medical Center Hamburg-Eppendorf, Hamburg, Germany

Keywords
Autoimmune hepatitis · Pathogenesis · Treatment

Abstract
The pathogenesis of autoimmune hepatitis is still poorly understood and therefore, the therapy administered to treat this condition is broadly targeted immunosuppression. However, the aim of therapy in the future should be more specific; it should be a therapy that interrupts the pathogenetic cascade at defined checkpoints. Even though these checkpoints are not yet defined, possible targets of immunotherapy are emerging. These are specifically enhancing the regulatory T-cell activity, anti-cytokine interventions, in particular targeting the tumor necrosis factor, and hopefully in the foreseeable future, defining the key T-cell receptors used and developing new therapies directed against these.

Autoimmune hepatitis (AIH) was the first liver disease to be shown to be amenable to effective therapy. Following a number of individual observations, several clinical trials showed very convincingly that treatment with corticosteroids leads not only to a usually rapid response but is actually life-saving [1]. While 5-year mortality of untreated icteric AIH was recorded to be around 75% in these trials, patients receiving prednisone or prednisolone therapy showed a survival of around 80% [2]. Prednisone or prednisolone have since been the mainstay of therapy in inducing remission in AIH, but side effects and need for long-term therapy have made additional immunosuppressive treatment necessary. Azathioprine was shown to be an excellent steroid-sparing drug in the management of AIH, and it was soon shown that while steroids are the drug of choice for remission induction, azathioprine is the drug of choice for maintenance of remission [3]. Subsequent debate concentrated on the most appropriate drug dosage and the relative role of each of these 2 drugs: some centres treat AIH with a high initial dose of prednisolone starting at 1 mg/kg body weight and tapering in weekly intervals, while others give only half or even less of this dosage. The relative advantages and disadvantages of these 2 approaches are obvious: higher initial doses induce faster remission but cause more (short-term) side effects. Similarly, while for many patients 1 mg/kg azathioprine is sufficient to achieve stable remission and lead to the withdrawal of steroids, in other patients, either low-dose steroids need to be added or azathioprine doses need to be increased to around 2 mg/kg body weight, similarly to how those with inflammatory bowel disease are treated. Individual centre and

KARGER

E-Mail karger@karger.com
www.karger.com/ddi

Prof. Dr. Ansgar W. Lohse
I. Department of Medicine
University Medical Center Hamburg-Eppendorf
Martinistrasse 52, DE–20246 Hamburg (Germany)
E-Mail alohse@uke.de

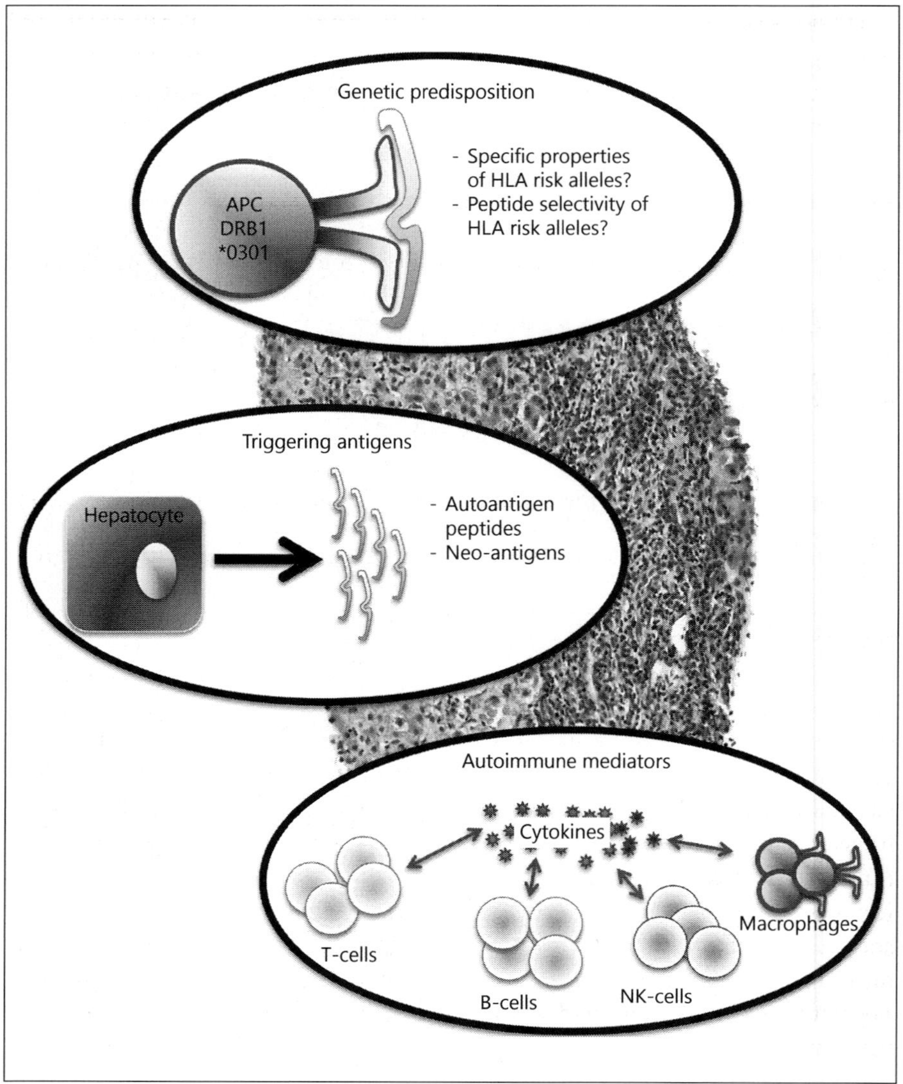

Color version available online

Fig. 1. Contributors to pathogenesis in autoimmune hepatitis.

patient preferences may decide upon individual management of the patient. Response to treatment and doses needed for maintaining remission may differ considerably between patients as may the individual side effects [4].

Some patients are intolerant to azathioprine, and some patients may fail to achieve sufficient remission despite optimum therapy. Even though these problematic cases constitute probably less than 10% of the whole AIH patient population, it is particularly these patients who require a more specific and more effective therapy [5]. Furthermore, long-term immunosuppression with non-specific agents such as steroids and azathioprine carries long-term risks that are only poorly defined as of now. Finally, long-term treatment, as presently required for a vast majority of AIH patients [6], is not very popular with patients, and non-adherence is a major problem in the long-term management of this patient population [7]. In particular, in adolescence, adherence to recommended drug therapy is often rather poor [8], leading to considerable morbidity and even mortality. So far, second-line drugs such as cyclosporine [9], tacrolimus [10] or even cyclophosphamide [11] have primarily been more potent immunosuppressive agents. Thus, we possess an armamentarium of potent immunosuppressive drugs, but these are non-specific and are associated with a number of side effects. Moreover, these drugs suppress AIH effectively, but they only very rarely cure the disease, thus necessitating life-long therapy for a majority of patients [12].

Options of More Specific Immune Interventions

Various options for more specific immune interventions spring to mind considering the possible pathogenesis of the disease. The key for effective immunotherapy is a better understanding of the exact pathogenesis, both the initiating and the perpetuating factors of the disease process. These fall into the following categories (Fig. 1):

- Genetic predisposition,
- Triggering antigen(s),
- Autoimmune mediators (cells, cytokines, etc.).

Genetic Predisposition

Like in other autoimmune diseases, there is a strong genetic risk association, and this is primarily linked to defined HLA-alleles [13]. The DR0301 allele is the most common risk factor in Caucasian populations, and is associated with more severe AIH; it occurs more likely in younger patients. The second strongly associated allele, DR0401, is more associated with disease in older patients and is more often a milder disease form. It is also commonly found in Asian patients [14]. The very strong association with these 2 HLA-DR alleles makes it very likely that HLA-DR-restricted CD4+ cells are key mediators of the disease. Conceivably, there are 2 reasons for this HLA-association: these HLA-alleles are also associated with a number of other autoimmune diseases, and it must therefore be assumed that thymic selection, negative or positive, linked to these alleles leads to an immune phenotype more likely to allow aberrant autoimmune reactions [15]. Understanding these immunoregulatory phenomena might be an approach not specific for AIH, but an approach specific for autoimmunity in general, and thus of high clinical relevance. Investigations into the role of regulatory T-cells have so far yielded contradictory results [16, 17], and there clearly is not a simple phenotype associated with these HLA-alleles. Nonetheless, this avenue of research appears promising.

The second pathogenetic factor that might be closely related to these HLA risk alleles is related to the function of HLA molecules: these molecules bind the peptide antigens that antigen-presenting cells present to CD4+ cells. It is very likely that the key autoantigenic peptide(s) underlying the autoimmune reaction in AIH is bound by these risk-associated DR-molecules. In the search for the possible causative antigen, looking for these HLA-restrictions might be very helpful. In turn, specific immune intervention at the interface DR3 – T-cell receptor interaction might allow specific immunotherapy even without the identification of the causative antigenic peptide.

Triggering Antigens

As outlined, the triggering antigen or antigens are very likely to include antigenic peptides presented by the risk HLA-DR molecules. What kind of antigens could this be? The high degree of specificity of AIH for hepatocytes, and the few and rare extra-hepatic aspects of the disease, make it very likely that we are dealing with a hepatocyte-specific antigen. It should therefore be a molecule only present in hepatocytes. It could either be one of the many metabolic molecules such as enzymes of hepatocytes not present in other cells in the body, or it could indeed be a neo-autoantigen, that is, an external factor that is metabolized in the liver to an antigen metabolite and thus functioning as a hapten. In other words, it could well be that AIH, just as celiac disease, is not purely autoimmune, but the immune reaction is directed against an antigen that only becomes antigenic by metabolism or synthesis in the liver. The analogy to drug-induced immunoallergic hepatitis is obvious [18]. If indeed this is the case, the triggering factor, again like in celiac disease, could be removed and the disease cured. Thus far, careful history taking and association studies have failed to suggest such external triggering antigens, but it is conceivable that these are components of everyday food, or of intestinal microbes, and thus very difficult to identify. A search for such triggers would be a highly valuable initiative.

Autoimmune Mediators

Whatever triggers the disease, the actual disease process is mediated by a number of players that can be seen on liver biopsy in the injured tissue [19]: lymphocytes of both T- and B-cell lineage, NK-cells, macrophages, and so on. All of these are orchestrated and they themselves orchestrate a complex inflammatory response by secreting cytokines, chemokines and other factors. The complexity of such an inflammatory response makes it extremely difficult to identify key players. It is very likely that a better understanding of the inflammatory mediators in AIH is the easiest way to make immunotherapy more specific and more effective. For example, unpublished data suggest that, among the various cytokines expressed in patients with active AIH, tumor necrosis factor (TNF) alpha is particularly prominent. This seems to apply to the analysis of both peripheral as well as intrahepatic immune cells. Most intriguingly, autoantigen-specific CD4 cells isolated from liver biopsies of patients seem to overexpress TNF most prominently. In view of clinical data showing the effectiveness of anti-TNF therapy in difficult-to-treat AIH [20], these findings could provide a pathophysiological explanation for the therapeutic potential of anti-TNF and warrant further confirmation. Disappointingly, many centres report frustrating results with anti-B-cell therapy with rituximab – one might have thought that in view of the marked hypergammaglobulinaemia in AIH, and the presence of plasma cells in the inflammatory infiltrate, anti-B-cell therapy might be effective and specific. However, rituximab is not an anti-plasma cell antibody and the mediators leading to increased IgG-secretion are likely to arise from T cells or other immune cells rather than B cells. So here again, a better understanding of the underlying pathophysiology of AIH might lead to more specific therapy or perhaps also simply to the elimination of ineffective treatment trials.

Disclosure Statement

The authors have nothing to disclose.

References

1 Cook GC, Mulligan R, Sherlock S: Controlled prospective trial of corticosteroid therapy in active chronic hepatitis. Q J Med 1971;40: 159–185.

2 Kirk AP, Jain S, Pocock S, Thomas HC, Sherlock S: Late results of the royal free hospital prospective controlled trial of prednisolone therapy in hepatitis B surface antigen negative chronic active hepatitis. Gut 1980;21:78–83.

3 Mackay IR: Chronic hepatitis: effect of prolonged suppressive treatment and comparison of azathioprine with prednisolone. Q J Med 1968;37:379–392.

4 European Association for the Study of the Liver: EASL clinical practice guidelines: autoimmune hepatitis. J Hepatol 2015;63:971–1004.

5 Czaja AJ: Difficult treatment decisions in autoimmune hepatitis. World J Gastroenterol 2010;16:934–947.

6 van Gerven NM, Verwer BJ, Witte BI, et al: Relapse is almost universal after withdrawal of immunosuppressive medication in patients with autoimmune hepatitis in remission. J Hepatol 2013;58:141–147.

7 Sockalingam S, Blank D, Abdelhamid N, Abbey SE, Hirschfield GM: Identifying opportunities to improve management of autoimmune hepatitis: evaluation of drug adherence and psychosocial Factors. J Hepatol 2012;57: 1299–1304.

8 Osterberg L, Blaschke T: Adherence to medication. N Engl J Med 2005;353:487–497.

9 Alvarez F, Ciocca M, Canero-Velasco C, et al: Short-term cyclosporine induces a remission of autoimmune hepatitis in children. J Hepatol 1999;30:222–227.

10 Larsen FS, Vainer B, Eefsen M, Bjerring PN, Adel Hansen B: Low-dose tacrolimus ameliorates liver inflammation and fibrosis in steroid refractory autoimmune hepatitis. World J Gastroenterol 2007;13:3232–3236.

11 Kanzler S, Gerken G, Dienes HP, Meyer zum Buschenfelde KH, Lohse AW: Cyclophosphamide as alternative immunosuppressive therapy for autoimmune hepatitis – report of three cases. Z Gastroenterol 1997;35:571–578.

12 Weiler-Normann C, Lohse AW: Autoimmune hepatitis: a life-long disease. J Hepatol 2013;58:5–7.

13 van Gerven NM, de Boer YS, Zwiers A, et al: HLA-DRB1*03:01 and HLA-DRB1*04:01 modify the presentation and outcome in autoimmune hepatitis type-1. Genes Immun 2015;16:247–252.

14 Yoshizawa K, Ota M, Katsuyama Y, et al: Genetic analysis of the HLA region of Japanese patients with type 1 autoimmune hepatitis. J Hepatol 2005;42:578–584.

15 Ridgway WM, Fasso M, Fathman CG: A new look at MHC and autoimmune disease. Science 1999;284:749, 751.

16 Peiseler M, Sebode M, Franke B, et al: FOXP3+ regulatory T cells in autoimmune hepatitis are fully functional and not reduced in frequency. J Hepatol 2012;57:125–132.

17 Longhi MS, Ma Y, Bogdanos DP, Cheeseman P, Mieli-Vergani G, Vergani D: Impairment of CD4(+)CD25(+) regulatory T-cells in autoimmune liver disease. J Hepatol 2004;41:31–37.

18 Weiler-Normann C, Schramm C: Drug induced liver injury and its relationship to autoimmune hepatitis. J Hepatol 2011;55:747–749.

19 Lohr HF, Schlaak JF, Gerken G, Fleischer B, Dienes HP, Meyer zum Buschenfelde KH: Phenotypical analysis and cytokine release of liver-infiltrating and peripheral blood T lymphocytes from patients with chronic hepatitis of different etiology. Liver 1994;14:161–166.

20 Weiler-Normann C, Schramm C, Quaas A, et al: Infliximab as a rescue treatment in difficult-to-treat autoimmune hepatitis. J Hepatol 2013;58:529–534.

Metabolic Liver Disease

Digestive Diseases

Dig Dis 2017;35:371–376
DOI: 10.1159/000456589

The Role of a Dedicated Non-Alcoholic Fatty Liver Disease Clinic in 2016

Sarah A. Townsend[a, b] Philip N. Newsome[a, b]

[a]National Institute for Health Research (NIHR) Birmingham Liver Biomedical Research Unit and Centre for Liver Research, University of Birmingham, and [b]Liver Unit, University Hospital Birmingham NHS Foundation Trust, Birmingham, UK

Keywords
Non-alcoholic fatty liver disease · Service provision · Management · Clinic

Abstract
Background: Non-alcoholic fatty liver disease (NAFLD) is the commonest cause of liver disease in the United Kingdom, and is predicted to become the leading indication for liver transplantation (LT) within the next 10 years. ***Key Messages:*** With rising demands on liver services, identifying those at risk of developing significant liver disease is important, so that risk factors for disease progression can be addressed. Emerging diagnostic techniques make it possible to diagnose significant fibrosis without the need for liver biopsy, and while there are currently no approved therapies for NAFLD, a specialist clinic can also provide access to clinical trials. For patients who develop cirrhosis, the presence of multiple comorbidities necessitates expertise in the selection and management of individuals requiring LT. ***Conclusions:*** A dedicated multidisciplinary NAFLD clinic facilitates rationalisation of services, improves patient outcomes, and provides access to emerging diagnostics and therapies.

Introduction

Non-alcoholic fatty liver disease (NAFLD) has become the commonest cause of liver disease in Western countries, affecting 25% of the UK population [1], and up to 90% of obese individuals with diabetes and other features of the metabolic syndrome [2]. Moreover, its prevalence is expected to continue to rise in parallel with the obesity epidemic [3]; in the United States, NAFLD is expected to become the leading pointer to liver transplantation (LT) within the next 10 years [4]. Ensuing demands on liver services will continue to increase for those with chronic liver disease [5], as will the discrepancy between the number of liver organs available and those on the waiting list awaiting transplantation.

There are no approved pharmacological interventions for NAFLD, and current management strategies aim to identify and treat features of the metabolic syndrome, in order to reduce long-term cardiovascular and liver-related morbidity and mortality [6]. Indeed, it has long been established that cardiovascular disease is the commonest cause of death in NAFLD [7]. Patients may be seen across a range of medical and hepatology clinics, where expertise is lacking. Treatment decisions may be made on the basis

KARGER

E-Mail karger@karger.com
www.karger.com/ddi

Dr. Sarah Townsend and Professor Philip Newsome
NIHR Birmingham Liver Biomedical Research Unit and Centre for Liver Research
5th Floor Institute of Biomedical Research
University of Birmingham, Birmingham B15 2TT (UK)
E-Mail s.a.townsend@bham.ac.uk and P.N.Newsome@bham.ac.uk

of liver function tests, which fail to capture disease severity in NAFLD [8]. A dedicated NAFLD clinic can provide expert management targeted towards those at highest risk of progressive liver disease, as well as access to emerging diagnostics and clinical trials.

The Challenge

The assessment and management of NAFLD patients can be challenging; patients tend to be older than for other types of liver disease [9, 10] and often have multiple comorbidities such as obstructive sleep apnoea, cardiovascular disease or features of the metabolic syndrome (obesity, hypertension, hyperlipidaemia and diabetes). With increasing patient numbers and burgeoning demands on liver services, it is increasingly important to identify and streamline those patients who are at greater risk of liver or cardiovascular mortality, and require more aggressive intervention and follow-up. Liver fibrosis is believed to be the most important factor for progression to cirrhosis [11], but as yet there is no ideal tool for assessing its presence. Liver biopsy remains the gold standard for both diagnosis and staging of disease, but is not without risk. Non-invasive alternatives are not without their flaws; the NAFLD fibrosis score is easily accessible but often indeterminate, transient elastography using the FibroScan® machine is less widely available and not always reliable in obese patients [12], and the more sensitive enhanced liver fibrosis (ELF) test [13], which combines 3 candidate serum biomarkers for fibrosis, is not yet available outside secondary or even tertiary care.

Once those patients with fibrosis have been identified, the emphasis is on halting progression to cirrhosis and reducing long-term cardiovascular mortality. Features of the metabolic syndrome should be aggressively managed, with a focus on weight loss. This in itself is notoriously difficult to achieve in this population; even in highly supervised randomised clinical trials (RCTs), less than 50% participants have been shown to achieve the ideal 7% total body weight reduction [14].

The final challenge in NAFLD is the management of those who become cirrhotic. While weight loss will have been desirable for a majority of patients during disease progression, the onset of sarcopenia and protein malnutrition, particularly in the presence of obesity, can be problematic. LT may be indicated for those patients with end-stage liver disease, and aforementioned comorbidities such as cardiovascular disease, obesity and diabetes, which are far less commonly seen in those transplanted for other indications, bring an additional complexity both peri-operatively and post procedure [15–17].

Key Components of an NAFLD Clinic

Reflecting the needs of patients with NAFLD, a dedicated clinic should incorporate input from hepatologists, diabetologists/weight loss physicians, diabetes specialist nurses (DSN), dieticians and practitioners proficient in non-invasive modalities such as FibroScan® use. Figure 1 outlines a suggested pathway for patients referred to NAFLD clinic.

What a Dedicated NAFLD Clinic Allows You to Do

Provides Holistic Care Reducing Need for Attendance at Multiple Clinics

Nearly one third of patients with NAFLD have diabetes; hypertension and hyperlipidaemia are seen in approximately 40 and 70% of patients respectively [18]. The prevalence of all features of the metabolic syndrome, including obesity, is yet higher in subjects who demonstrate non-alcoholic steatohepatitis (NASH) at liver biopsy [18]. Each of these features are addressed in clinics and reinforced in primary care. Blood pressure, weight, and body mass index are measured at each visit, and serum lipid profile assessed annually. Lifestyle advice and/or treatments are recommended for those with hypertension or hyperlipidaemia, and a close relationship is maintained with our specialists in metabolic disorders who provide advice to those with refractory hyperlipidaemia.

Diabetic patients are reviewed by the DSN who will often arrange regular follow-up through telephone consultation and later in Diabetic clinics where necessary. Complex diabetic patients or patients who are likely to benefit from intensive weight loss management can be discussed with the Diabetic consultant who also runs a separate weight management clinic. This is turn facilitates access to expert dietetic advice, medications such as orlistat, which promote weight loss and, where appropriate, referral for bariatric surgery.

The dietician shows a specialist interest towards liver disease and also works in parallel with the clinic to provide dietetic advice and support for improved diabetic control, weight loss regimens, and patients with end-stage liver disease. Approximately two-thirds of appointments are pre-booked and the remaining time slots are retained as a "walk-in" service for patients to be referred and seen on the same day.

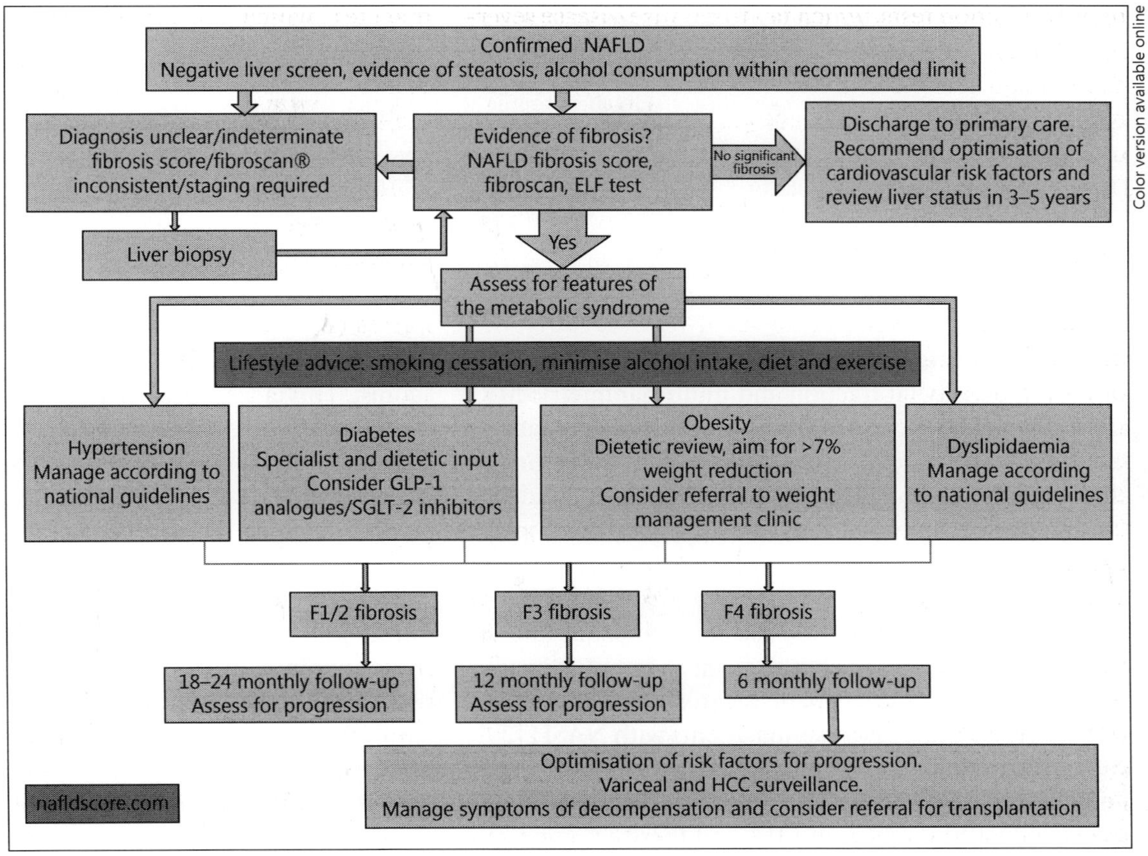

Fig. 1. Algorithm for the suggested management of non-alcoholic fatty liver disease. ELF, enhanced liver fibrosis; HCC, hepatocellular carcinoma.

Ensures Management of Co-Morbidities Is Undertaken with Consideration of Possible Effect on NAFLD

Weight loss is currently the most effective treatment for NAFLD, and a loss of >7% total body weight is associated with a reduction in NASH, with a possible reduction in fibrosis in those who achieve >10% reduction [14, 19]. Patients are therefore given a goal of achieving a 5–10% weight reduction.

In diabetic patients, there is emphasis on avoiding drugs that cause weight gain, such as thiazolidinediones and insulin secretagogues. Metformin is used in keeping with national guidelines [20]; thereafter, the use of glucagon-like peptide-1 (GLP-1) inhibitors or sodium-glucose cotransporter 2 inhibitors, which can promote weight loss and improve insulin sensitivity [21–23], is encouraged. Furthermore, one study has demonstrated that the GLP-1 inhibitor liraglutide has additional benefits in improving NASH in both diabetic and non-diabetic patients [24].

Hypertension and dyslipidaemia are managed according to national guidelines, with a preference for pravastatin in those undergoing LT due to interaction with calcineurin inhibitors [24].

Early Adoption of New Diagnostics and Treatments

Transient elastography, or the Fibroscan® is available in many secondary care centres for the assessment of liver fibrosis, and studies have shown a sensitivity of 91% and a specificity of 75% in for the detection of significant fibrosis using a cut off of >7.9 kPa [25] and a sensitivity and specificity of 90% in those with a BMI ≥30 using a cut off of 7.2 kPa [26]. There remains a proportion of patients in whom the presence of fibrosis is unclear.

The ELF test combines 3 candidate serum biomarkers for fibrosis; hyaluronic acid, procollagen III amino terminal peptide, and tissue inhibitor of metalloproteinase 1. A cut-off of 10.51 has been demonstrated to have a sensitivity of 100% and a specificity of 98% for detecting advanced fibrosis, and can be used in patients in whom transient elec-

Table 1. Potential treatment options for NAFLD. Glucagon-like peptide (GLP-1) inhibitors, sodium-glucose co-transporter-2 (SGLT-2) inhibitors, dipeptidyl peptidase-4 (DDP4) inhibitor

Ineffective treatment	Uncertain efficacy/side-effect profile	Efficacy seen in phase 2 trials	Phase 2 trials incomplete
Metformin	Vitamin E	Obeticholic acid	CCR2/CCR5 antagonist
DDPIV inhibition	Pioglitazone	GFT505/elafibrinor	Anti-VAP-1 therapy
	Omega 3 fatty acids	GLP-1 analogues	

trography is unsuccessful or unreliable [13]. MRI-estimated proton density fat fraction and multi-parametric MRI are also being developed for the evaluation of liver fat and fibrosis but are currently only available with the setting of clinical trials. It is hoped that both the Fibroscan® and ELF testing may become available within primary care in the United Kingdom over the next 5 years, so that the presence of fibrosis can be assessed by general practitioners [28].

Some specialists favour the use of pioglitazone and vitamin E. Pioglitazone has been shown to improve insulin sensitivity and reduce hepatic steatosis, inflammation, and to a lesser degree fibrosis in patients with NASH [29], and reduce cardiovascular morbidity and mortality in patients with type 2 diabetes [30]. However, its use has been associated with weight gain [31], and there are concerns regarding increased risk of heart failure [32], bladder cancer [33], and osteoporosis [34]. Similarly vitamin E, a widely investigated antioxidant, has been shown to improve steatosis and inflammation in several RCTs in both diabetic and non-diabetic children and adults [35], but one study suggested an increased risk of prostate cancer [36], and another an increased risk of haemorrhagic stroke [37]. Risks and benefits of using such agents must therefore be carefully considered and discussed with each patient in detail before they can be recommended.

Table 1 illustrates potential treatment options for NAFLD. Some treatments have been demonstrated ineffective while others have poor side effect profiles and unclear efficacy. New treatment methods may emerge from phase 2 trials.

Access to Clinical Trials

While there is currently a dearth of treatment for NAFLD-related fibrosis, several phase 3 trials are underway and currently recruiting patients [38]. The team of hepatology consultants and trainees are all investigators or those involved in recruiting to clinical trials and are supported by a research nurse who attends clinic. The centre has previously undertaken a phase 2 for liraglutide and we are currently recruiting for imaging studies and phase 3 trials of obeticholic acid and GFT505, a dual PPARα and δ receptors agonist. This facilitates early access to potentially beneficial therapies for some patients, with the objective that effective therapies will become available to all over the next few years.

Well-Defined Pathway from Primary to Secondary Care and Pathway in Clinic

Newly referred patients have usually had an ultrasound scan and non-invasive liver screen prior to their clinic appointment as part of the referral pathway. On arrival to clinic, a FibroScan® is carried out prior to consultation with the hepatologist. The results of this scan, in addition to a calculated NAFLD fibrosis score, allow the presence of fibrosis to be assessed. A liver biopsy may be requested for those in whom there is diagnostic uncertainty or when the presence of fibrosis is unclear. ELF testing can be performed where a biopsy is contraindicated or declined by the patient.

In this manner, those patients with significant fibrosis can be directed towards appropriate services at an early stage, and features contributing to their disease are recognised and treated. Those patients who have no evidence of liver fibrosis and few risk factors for disease progression can be discharged back to primary care for modification of cardiovascular risk factors and advice that the patients' liver status should be reviewed in 5 years' time.

Patients who are found to have fibrosis or who are at high risk of progression are followed up on a 6 monthly, one or 2 yearly basis according to individual needs. Patients with early-stage fibrosis and well-controlled diabetes, hypertension or hyperlipidaemia may be seen annually or even biennially, given the slowly progressive nature of NAFLD. Those with cirrhosis, or advanced fibrosis and poorly controlled metabolic risk factors are seen on a 6-monthly basis.

This results in a cost-efficient service and high quality of care, and is supported by a recent study demonstrating improved cardiovascular risk factors and sustained weight loss in a cohort of patients attending a multidisciplinary NAFLD clinic [39].

NAFLD and End-Stage Liver Disease

Cirrhosis is estimated to occur in 5% of patients with NAFLD and 11% of those with NASH [10, 37, 40]. Patients who develop cirrhosis and end-stage liver disease are managed in the same manner as for other causes of liver disease, and require regular screening for varices and hepatocellular carcinoma. Some patients may meet liver transplant criteria, and selection of patients suitable for liver transplant assessment can require considerable expertise in the context of significant comorbidities such as cardiovascular disease, obstructive sleep apnoea and diabetes. For patients on the transplant waiting list, specialised dietetic input is crucial at this stage in order to maintain adequate nutritional fitness for surgery, which is particularly challenging where there is sarcopenic obesity and/or coexistent diabetes.

In the post-transplant follow-up years, expertise in NAFLD is helpful; rates of renal impairment can be higher in this cohort and immunosuppression should be carefully supervised with early referral to renal services and use of alternative agents where necessary [17]. Diabetic control often deteriorates in the setting of steroid therapy used in the initial 3 months following transplantation and patients often require considerable augmentation of their anti-diabetic medication and close supervision by the diabetic team. Patients often return to the NAFLD clinic earlier than usual (3 months) post-operatively to facilitate this and earlier tapering of steroids where possible. Disease recurrence in the graft is not uncommon [41] and should be recognised early by ultrasound surveillance and confirmed with a liver biopsy [15]. However, clinicians must be aware that coexistent graft issues such as rejection, biliary complications and vascular disorders, can mimic some of the histological features of NASH [42, 43], and therefore exercise caution when attributing graft dysfunction solely to disease recurrence, particularly if there is clinical doubt.

Finally, cardiovascular mortality is known to be elevated in transplant recipients, compounding the risk for those with NAFLD. Patients who have features of the metabolic syndrome post-transplantation have significantly more cardiovascular events than those without (30 vs. 8%) [44, 45]; thus, patients must be screened regularly for hypertension, hyperlipidaemia and glucose intolerance and treated appropriately according to UK guidelines [28].

Conclusion

A dedicated multidisciplinary NAFLD clinic facilitates rationalisation of services, improves patient outcomes, and provides access to emerging diagnostics and therapies.

Disclosure Statement

Sarah A. Townsend has no disclosures. Philip N. Newsome is a consultancy on behalf of the University of Birmingham for: Boehringer Ingelheim, Shire, Novo Nordisk, Pfizer.

Grant Support

P.N.N. and S.A.T. are supported by the NIHR Birmingham Liver Biomedical Research Unit based at University Hospitals Birmingham and the University of Birmingham. The views expressed are those of the author(s) and not necessarily those of the NHS, the NIHR or the Department of Health.

References

1 Armstrong MJ, Houlihan DD, Bentham L, et al: Presence and severity of non-alcoholic fatty liver disease in a large prospective primary care cohort. J Hepatol 2012;56:234–240.

2 Smits MM, Ioannou GN, Boyko EJ, et al: Nonalcoholic fatty liver disease as an independent manifestation of the metabolic syndrome: results of a US national survey in three ethnic groups. J Gastroenterol Hepatol 2013;28:664–670.

3 Visscher TL, Heitmann BL, Rissanen A, et al: A break in the obesity epidemic? Explained by biases or misinterpretation of the data? Int J Obes (Lond) 2015;39:189–198.

4 Wong RJ, Aguilar M, Cheung R, et al: Nonalcoholic steatohepatitis is the second leading etiology of liver disease among adults awaiting liver transplantation in the United States. Gastroenterology 2015;148:547–555.

5 Annual Report of the Chief Medical Officer (CMO), Volume 1, 2011.

6 Than NN, Newsome PN: Non-alcoholic fatty liver disease: when to intervene and with what. Clin Med (Lond) 2015;15:186–90.

7 Musso G, Gambino R, Cassader M, Pagano G: Prognosis and non-invasive methods to assess liver disease severity in non-alcoholic fatty liver disease (NAFLD): systematic review and meta-analysis. Ann Med 2011;43:617–649.

8 Mofrad P, Contos MJ, Haque M, Sargeant C, Fisher RA, Luketic VA, et al: Clinical and histologic spectrum of nonalcoholic fatty liver disease associated with normal ALT values. Hepatology 2003;37:1286–1292.

9 Adams LA, Lymp JF, St Sauver J, et al: The natural history of nonalcoholic fatty liver disease: a population-based cohort study. Gastroenterology 2005;129:113–121.

10 Bhala N, Angulo P, van der Poorten D, et al: The natural history of nonalcoholic fatty liver disease with advanced fibrosis or cirrhosis: an international collaborative study. Hepatology 2011;54:1208–1216.

11 Angulo P, Kleiner DE, Dam-Larsen S, et al: Liver fibrosis, but no other histologic features, is associated with long-term outcomes of patients with nonalcoholic fatty liver disease. Gastroenterology 2015;149:389–397.e10.

12 Brener S: Transient elastography for assessment of liver fibrosis and steatosis: an evidence-based analysis. Ont Health Technol Assess Ser 2015;15:1–45.
13 Nobili V, Parkes J, Bottazzo G, et al: Performance of ELF serum markers in predicting fibrosis stage in pediatric non-alcoholic fatty liver disease. Gastroenterology 2009;136:160–167.
14 Musso G, Cassader M, Rosina F, et al: Impact of current treatments on liver disease, glucose metabolism and cardiovascular risk in non-alcoholic fatty liver disease (NAFLD): a systematic review and meta-analysis of randomised trials. Diabetologia 2012;55:885–904.
15 Newsome PN, Allison ME, Andrews PA: Guidelines for liver transplantation for patients with non-alcoholic steatohepatitis. Gut 2012;61:484–500.
16 Wang X, Li J, Riaz DR, Shi G, Liu C, Dai Y: Outcomes of liver transplantation for nonalcoholic steatohepatitis: a systematic review and meta-analysis. Clin Gastroenterol Hepatol 2014;12:394–402.e1.
17 Houlihan DD, Armstrong MJ, Davidov Y, et al: Renal function in patients undergoing transplantation for nonalcoholic steatohepatitis cirrhosis: time to reconsider immunosuppression regimens? Liver Transpl 2011;17:1292–1298.
18 Younossi ZM, Koenig AB, Abdelatif D, Fazel Y, Henry L, Wymer M: Global epidemiology of nonalcoholic fatty liver disease-meta-analytic assessment of prevalence, incidence and outcomes. Hepatology 2016;64:73–84.
19 Vilar-Gomez E, Martinez-Perez Y, Calzadilla-Bertot L, et al: Weight loss through lifestyle modification significantly reduces features of nonalcoholic steatohepatitis. Gastroenterology 2015;149:367–378.e5; quiz e14–e15.
20 National Institute for Clinical Excellence (NICE): Type 2 Diabetes in Adults: Management, 2015.
21 Astrup A, Carraro R, Finer N: Safety, tolerability and sustained weight loss over 2 years with the once-daily human GLP-1 analog, liraglutide. Int J Obes (Lond). 2012;36:843–854.
22 Vasilakou D, Karagiannis T, Athanasiadou E, Mainou M, Liakos A, Bekiari E, Sarigianni M, et al: Sodium-glucose cotransporter 2 inhibitors for type 2 diabetes: a systematic review and meta-analysis. Ann Intern Med 2013;159:262–274.
23 Armstrong MJ, Hull D, Guo K, et al: Glucagon-like peptide 1 decreases lipotoxicity in non-alcoholic steatohepatitis. J Hepatol 2016;64:399–408.
24 Armstrong MJ, Gaunt P, Aithal GP, et al: Liraglutide safety and efficacy in patients with non-alcoholic steatohepatitis (LEAN): a multicentre, double-blind, randomised, placebo-controlled phase 2 study. Lancet 2016;387:679–690.
25 Mells G, Neuberger J: Long-term care of the liver allograft recipient. Semin Liver Dis 2009;29:102–120.
26 Wong VW, Vergniol J, Wong GL, et al: Diagnosis of fibrosis and cirrhosis using liver stiffness measurement in nonalcoholic fatty liver disease. Hepatology 2010;51:454–462.
27 Wong VW, Vergniol J, Wong GL, et al: Liver stiffness measurement using XL probe in patients with nonalcoholic fatty liver disease. Am J Gastroenterol 2012;107:1862–1871.
28 National Institute for Clinical Excellence (NICE): Non-Alcoholic Fatty Liver Disease. Assessment and Management of Non-Alcoholic Fatty Liver Disease (NAFLD) in Children, Adults and Young People, 2016.
29 Boettcher E, Csako G, Pucino F, Wesley R, Loomba R: Meta-analysis: pioglitazone improves liver histology and fibrosis in patients with non-alcoholic steatohepatitis. Aliment Pharmacol Ther 2012;35:66–75.
30 Lincoff AM, Wolski K, Nicholls SJ, Nissen SE: Pioglitazone and risk of cardiovascular events in patients with type 2 diabetes mellitus: a meta-analysis of randomized trials. JAMA 2007;298:1180–1188.
31 Sanyal AJ, Chalasani N, Kowdley KV, et al: Pioglitazone, vitamin E, or placebo for nonalcoholic steatohepatitis. N Engl J Med 2010;362:1675–1685.
32 Lago RM, Singh PP, Nesto RW: Congestive heart failure and cardiovascular death in patients with prediabetes and type 2 diabetes given thiazolidinediones: a meta-analysis of randomised clinical trials. Lancet 2007;370:1129–1136.
33 Piccinni C, Motola D, Marchesini G, Poluzzi E: Assessing the association of pioglitazone use and bladder cancer through drug adverse event reporting. Diabetes Care 2011;34:1369–1371.
34 Lecka-Czernik B: Bone loss in diabetes: use of antidiabetic thiazolidinediones and secondary osteoporosis. Curr Osteoporos Rep 2010;8:178–184.
35 Lavine JE, Schwimmer JB, Van Natta ML, et al: Effect of vitamin E or metformin for treatment of nonalcoholic fatty liver disease in children and adolescents: the TONIC randomized controlled trial. JAMA 2011;305:1659–1668.
36 Chan JM, Darke AK, Penney KL, et al: Selenium- or vitamin E-related gene variants, interaction with supplementation, and risk of high-grade prostate cancer in SELECT. Cancer Epidemiol Biomarkers Prev 2016;25:1050–1058.
37 Schürks M, Glynn RJ, Rist PM, Tzourio C, Kurth T: Effects of vitamin E on stroke subtypes: meta-analysis of randomised controlled trials. BMJ 2010;341:c5702.
38 Townsend SA, Newsome PN: Non-alcoholic fatty liver disease in 2016. Br Med Bull 2016;119:143–156.
39 Cobbold JF, Raveendran S, Peake CM, et al: Piloting a multidisciplinary clinic for the management of non-alcoholic fatty liver disease: initial 5-year experience. Piloting a multidisciplinary clinic for the management of non-alcoholic fatty liver disease. Frontline Gastroenterol 2013;0:1–7.
40 Ekstedt M, Franzén LE, Mathiesen UL, Thorelius L, Holmqvist M, Bodemar G, et al: Long-term follow-up of patients with NAFLD and elevated liver enzymes. Hepatology 2006;44:865–873.
41 Yalamanchili K, Saadeh S, Klintmalm GB, et al: Nonalcoholic fatty liver disease after liver transplantation for cryptogenic cirrhosis or nonalcoholic fatty liver disease. Liver Transpl 2010;16:431–439.
42 Demetris AJ, Adeyi O, Bellamy CO, et al: Liver biopsy interpretation for causes of late liver allograft dysfunction. Hepatology 2006;44:489–501.
43 Hübscher SG: Transplantation pathology. Semin Liver Dis 2009;29:74–90.
44 Johnston SD, Morris JK, Cramb R, et al: Cardiovascular morbidity and mortality after orthotopic liver transplantation. Transplantation 2002;73:901–906.
45 Laryea M, Watt KD, Molinari M, et al: Metabolic syndrome in liver transplant recipients: prevalence and association with major vascular events. Liver Transpl 2007;13:1109–1114.

Metabolic Liver Disease

Digestive Diseases

Dig Dis 2017;35:377–383
DOI: 10.1159/000456590

The Gut Microbiota and the Hepatologist: Will Our Bugs Prove to be the Missing Link?

Mark J. Pallen[b] Mohammed N. Quraishi[a]

[a]University Hospital Birmingham NHS Foundation Trust, University of Birmingham, Birmingham, and
[b]University of Warwick, Coventry, UK

Keywords
Gut microbiota · Chronic liver disease

Abstract
The advent of next-generation sequencing has enabled in-depth analysis to study the composition and function of the gut microbiota in a culture-independent manner. Consequently, this has led to rapid interest in understanding the pathogenesis and progression of chronic liver disease in relation to perturbations of the gut microbiota. Animal models and human studies have demonstrated its crucial role in contributing to disease mechanisms in alcoholic and non-alcoholic liver disease and more recently in primary sclerosing cholangitis. There is increasing evidence to suggest that the gut microbiota and its components influence the development and modulation of chronic liver damage through direct communication via the portal system, metabolite production, alterations in gut barrier integrity, liver/gut immune axis and bile acid metabolism. The impact of microbiota-directed therapies for liver disease is still in its infancy. Better understanding of its role in disease mechanisms will lead to a more targeted approach in modulation of gut microbiota to influence both progression and complications of liver disease. This review discusses the current evidence for the gut microbiota-liver axis and its role in the development, progression and treatment of liver disease.

Introduction

The human gastrointestinal tract harbours a complex microbial community, encompassing over a 1,000 bacterial species and at least a 100-times more genes than are found in the human genome. This community of microorganisms (the gut microbiota) – with which its genes and genomes make up the gut microbiome – plays a central role in health and disease, regulating many aspects of host physiology, metabolism and immunology [1]. The gut microbiome and its human host evolve together from birth. Its core composition generally remains stable throughout adulthood, although some components respond to changes in environment and nutrition. Disruption of the gut microbiota, often referred to as dysbiosis, can disturb the balance between health and disease.

The influence of the gut microbiota is not constrained to the gastrointestinal tract. The gut and liver are intimately connected, with constant communication through the portal vein and biliary system. As a result, the liver encounters gut-derived translocated bacteria and their pathogen-associated molecular patterns (PAMPs). The liver and the gut microbiota are linked in both directions: (i) by the effects of gut microbes and their products on the liver and (ii) by the effects of the liver and biliary system on the gut microbiota.

Gram-negative bacteria from the gut release lipopolysaccharide (LPS), which, when bound to LPS-binding

KARGER

E-Mail karger@karger.com
www.karger.com/ddi

Mark J. Pallen
University of Warwick
Coventry CV4 7AL (UK)
E-Mail m.pallen@warwick.ac.uk

protein (LBP), causes Kupffer cells (specialised macrophages found in the liver) to activate inflammatory pathways in the liver involving mitogen-activated protein kinase and the NF-κB [2]. In addition, gut barrier integrity is compromised in liver disease, both through direct effects of the underlying pathology (e.g., alcohol-induced damage) and through the secretion of inflammatory mediators by an activated mucosal immune system [3]. In cirrhosis, the enhanced translocation of gut microbiota and PAMPs impacts on an already compromised hepatic immune system.

Liver disease can also directly influence the composition of gut microbiota. Bile acids have been shown to have a direct impact on the gut microbiota: observations from murine models and human subjects show that obstruction of biliary outflow results in dysbiosis and a compromised gut barrier [4]. These effects can be reversed by the administration of bile acids. In addition, the bile acid pool can be modified by intestinal microbiota. Microbial conversion of primary to secondary bile acids can exacerbate liver diseases through the farnesoid X receptor (FXR), a nuclear receptor for bile acids [5]. This receptor has been shown to induce enteroprotection genes and inhibit bacterial overgrowth and translocation; as a result, therapeutic modulation of FXR is under evaluation in liver disease.

Understanding the links between gut dysbiosis, integrity of the gut barrier and the hepatic immune response to gut-derived factors is crucial to the development of new therapies to treat chronic liver diseases. Below, we provide an overview of the laboratory techniques to study the gut microbiota and review microbiota-associated pathogenic mechanisms and microbiota-targeted therapies in common liver diseases.

Techniques for Studying the Gut Microbiota

Although it is often said that most gut microbes cannot be cultured in the laboratory, this assumption has recently been challenged by some recent heroic efforts [6]. However, it remains clear that culture-independent, sequence-based methods are much more tractable and scalable when applied to the identification and quantitation of microbes in large numbers of samples. Broadly, 2 approaches have been used [7]. The first is based on amplification and high-throughput sequencing of a molecular barcode common to all cellular life forms, the gene sequences encoding the small-subunit ribosomal RNA (represented by the 16S ribosomal RNA in bacteria). This approach allows a rapid census of bacterial taxa within a sample but lacks the resolution needed to identify and characterise bacterial species and strains. A second less established but more powerful approach is shotgun metagenomics, that is, the sequencing en masse of all DNA molecules within a sample, without target-specific culture, capture or amplification. This approach can be used diagnostically and allows detailed reconstruction of the virulence, metabolic and resistance phenotypes associated with strains in the microbiota [8]. In both approaches, an important goal is not just to work out the strains that are already present but how it varies from one sample to another, using tools and concepts drawn from microbial ecology [9].

Although sequenced-based approaches to the characterisation of microbial communities have become much easier and cost effective in recent years, this results in problems. A potential concern is the growth of a wild frontier of microbiome analyses performed by non-experts, hand-cranking data through pipelines that they do not fully understand and then naively interpreting results without engaging the healthy scepticism of the seasoned expert. This problem particularly applies to contamination from sequencing reagents but also to mistaking correlation for causation [10, 11].

The Gut Microbiota in Alcoholic Liver Disease

The gut microbiota plays a crucial role in the pathogenesis of alcoholic liver disease (ALD). Alcohol consumption itself has shown to cause dysbiosis and small intestinal bacterial overgrowth, as well as increasing gut permeability and translocation of microbial products. In a mouse model, intragastric infusion of alcohol led to increased abundance of 2 bacterial phyla, the *Bacteroidetes* and *Verrucomicrobia* and a reduced abundance of the phylum *Firmicutes*, particularly the genus *Lactobacillus*, compared to control mice [12]. The mice fed alcohol showed downregulation of bactericidal c-type lectins Reg3g in the small intestine; interestingly, treatment with prebiotics partially restored Reg3g expression, decreased bacterial overgrowth and led to a reduction in alcoholic steatohepatitis [13]. Another study elegantly demonstrated that the probiotic *Lactobacillus rhamnosus* GG prevented alcohol-induced pathogenic changes in the microbiome and the liver [14].

Studies characterizing gut microbiota in patients with ALD have demonstrated a decreased abundance of the phylum *Bacteroidetes* and a relative increase in the phylum *Proteobacteria* compared to healthy subjects; importantly, these alterations correlate with serum endotoxinaemia [15]. In one study, patients with alcoholic hepatitis showed an increased abundance of *Streptococci*, *Bifidobacteria* and *Enterobacteria*, but a decrease in anti-inflammatory species such as *Clostridium leptum* or *Faecalibacterium prausnitzii* [16]. A postmortem study of cirrhotic alcoholics showed a 27-fold increase in the abundance of the *Enterobacteriaceae* in stools, compared to healthy controls, with significant translocation into the cirrhotic liver and ascites, confirming a role of bacterial translocation in the pathogenesis of ALD [17].

Disruption of the gut microbiota by alcohol should not be dismissed as an inconsequential epiphenomenon: instead, there is evidence that it actually drives the progression of ALD. For example, Llopis et al. [16] showed that when an intestinal microbiota from a patient with severe alcoholic hepatitis was administered to mice, they developed severe liver inflammation and necrosis, greater intestinal permeability and higher bacterial translocation. Some components of the microbiota probably protect against ALD, as evidenced by the observation that germ-free mice show more severe liver injury, steatosis and inflammation after oral gavage with alcohol, than do conventional C57Bl/6 mice [18].

Wang et al. [13] showed that the administration of alcohol to mice caused intestinal deficiency in Reg3 lectins, which led to an increase in mucosa-associated bacteria, enhanced translocation of gut bacteria to the liver and mesenteric lymph nodes and promoted progression from fatty liver disease to steatohepatitis.

Bacterial endotoxin, also known as LPS, plays an integral role in ALD. Patients with ALD and mice models of the disease show higher serum levels of LPS [19]. LPS binds to toll-like receptor 4 (TLR4), activating Kupffer cells. The consequent upregulation of pro-inflammatory cytokines contributes to liver injury and modulation of hepatocyte function. Further support for the hypothesis that gut-derived endotoxin plays a role in ethanol-induced liver disease comes from studies on mice deficient in TLR4 or its co-receptor CD14, where these mice are protected from alcoholic liver damage [20].

Diet also plays a major role in modulating gut bacteria and potentially influences alcoholic liver disease. In a mouse model of ALD, saturated and unsaturated dietary fats differentially modulated ethanol-Induced changes, so that mice fed with an unsaturated fat diet experienced a reduction in abundance of the *Bacteroidetes* and an increase in the *Proteobacteria* and *Actinobacteria* and experienced more severe alcohol-induced endotoxaemia, liver steatosis and injury [21].

Accumulating evidence that the gut microbiota influences the course of alcoholic liver disease has led to interest in developing novel therapies targeting the microbial ecology of the gut, including consideration of probiotics, manipulation of the diet and even faecal microbiota transplants as promising strategies for altering the course and severity of ALD and alcoholic hepatitis.

Non-Alcoholic Fatty Liver Disease

Non-alcoholic fatty liver disease (NAFLD) has a very strong association with diabetes and obesity and presents as a spectrum that ranges from hepatic steatosis alone to non-alcoholic steatohepatitis (NASH). Alteration of the gut microbiota plays a crucial role in the initiation and progression of NAFLD. Sequence-based surveys of the faecal microbiota in NALFD patients have revealed an overrepresentation of selected taxa within the phylum *Firmicutes*, including *Lachnospiraceae*, *Lactobacillus*, *Dorea*, *Robinsoniella* and *Roseburia* and a reduced abundance of *Oscillibacter ruminantium* [22].

In one survey, obese children with NAFLD had a greater abundance of *Gammaproteobacteria* and *Prevotella* in the stool microbiome and significantly higher levels of ethanol in the stool metabolome compared to lean healthy children [23]. In another survey, the phylum *Proteobacteria*, and in particular, the taxa *Enterobacteriaceae* and *Escherichia* were increased in abundance in the gut microbiota of children with NASH compared to obese individuals, while obese and NASH children showed greater abundance of *Bacteroidetes*, predominantly *Prevotella*, compared to lean children [24].

Research on mouse models and humans has provided evidence of a causal role for gut dysbiosis in the pathogenesis of obesity and NAFLD. An elegant study by Turnbaugh et al. [25] demonstrated that germ-free lean mice gavaged with microbiota from an obese-mouse developed increased body fat and weight compared to mice supplied with lean-mouse microbiota. Similarly, when the microbiota from a mouse that had developed hyperglycemia and a pro-inflammatory response on a high-fat diet was transferred into germ-free mice, this led to hepatic macrovesicular steatosis and increased expression of genes involved in lipogenesis in the new host, together with overrepresentation of *Barnesiella intestinihominis* and *Lachnospiraceae* [26].

Small intestinal bacterial overgrowth is more common in patients with obesity and has been shown to be associated with severe hepatic steatosis. In a study of patients fed a choline-depleted diet, a higher baseline abundance of *Gammaproteobacteria* was correlated with a lower risk of developing fatty liver, whereas a higher baseline abundance of *Erysipelotrichia* was linked to a higher risk of fatty liver [27].

The inflammation seen in NASH is the result of several factors including endogenous production of alcohol, serum endotoxaemia and release of pro-inflammatory mediators, with the gut microbiota contributing to each of these processes. NASH patients exhibit significantly elevated blood ethanol levels due to production of alcohol by bacteria such as *Escherichia* [24].

As highlighted in the earlier section, alcohol-induced dysbiosis has been shown to increase hepatocyte triglyceride accumulation, generate reactive oxygen species and bring about gut barrier integrity. In patients with NALFD and in murine models of NASH, there is increased intestinal permeability and alteration of tight junction proteins [28]. This promotes LPS translocation, liver injury and inflammation. Patients on the NAFLD/NASH spectrum have significantly higher LPS levels and this correlates with higher tumour necrosis factor (TNF)-alpha gene expression in hepatocytes [29]. Obese mice given the probiotic VSL#3 or anti-TNF antibodies had significantly improved liver histology and biochemistry, as well as reduced hepatic fat content [30]. This information supports the hypothesis that the gut microbiota and its products contribute to the pathogenesis of NAFLD.

One way in which microorganisms can promote an inflammatory response is through the induction of a protein complex termed the inflammasome. Defective inflammasome function in mouse models has been shown to result in dysbiosis and contribute to NAFLD development and progression to NASH [31]. Furthermore, cohousing these mice with wild-type mice results in worsening of hepatic steatosis.

Although evidence for a contribution of the gut microbiota to development of NAFLD is growing, the next stage is more ambitious mechanistic studies that will prove crucial in the design of microbiota therapies targeted against NAFLD and NASH, which are likely to impact more generally on the management of obesity and diabetes.

Autoimmune Liver Disease

The 3 main categories of autoimmune liver disease are primary sclerosing cholangitis (PSC), autoimmune hepatitis (AIH) and primary biliary cirrhosis (PBC). Although these diseases are well-defined entities and contribute to 5% of all chronic liver diseases, the aetiology and environmental triggers for these conditions remain obscure. With the advent of high-throughput sequencing, novel associations between the gut microbiota and known mechanisms of disease pathogenesis are being identified, implicating aberrant lymphocyte trafficking, bile acid signalling and molecular mimicry.

Primary Sclerosing Cholangitis

PSC is closely associated with inflammatory bowel disease (IBD), which in turn is closely linked to the gut microbiota, raising the suspicion that gut microbiota might also play a role in the pathogenesis of PSC. In support of this supposition, several recent studies have shown that patients with PSC and PSC-IBD have a distinct gut microbiota compared to IBD patients and healthy controls. Sabino et al. [32] demonstrated that the faecal microbiota in patients with PSC is characterized by decreased microbial diversity, together with an increased abundance of *Enterococcus*, *Fusobacterium* and *Lactobacillus*.

Similar dysbiosis was present in patients with both PSC and PSC-IBD and was distinct from IBD and independent of treatment with ursodeoxycholic acid. An increased abundance of *Enterococcus* was associated with increased levels of serum alkaline phosphatase. Similar findings were reported by Kummen et al. [33], who found that the abundance of the genus *Veillonella* was markedly increased in PSC compared to healthy controls and patients with ulcerative colitis. In our own study, we found a distinctive population of mucosa-adherent bacteria in patients with PSC-IBD, showing significant increases in *Escherichia*, *Lachnospiraceae* and *Megasphera* along with a reduced abundance of *Prevotella* and *Roseburia* and a near-absence of *Bacteroides* [34]. Yet another study observed a significant increase in *Barnesiellaceae* and shifts in the abundance of *Clostridiales* and *Bacteroidales* in intestinal mucosal biopsies from patients with PSC [35].

There is clearly a need to take these findings beyond just associations, so that we can link up dysbiosis causally to known mechanisms of disease. Genetic association studies in PSC have identified genetic risk variants in FUT-2 gene, which is implicated in the handling of translocated gut bacteria and antigens associated with PSC and IBD [36]. Murine models have shown that compromised mucosal integrity in an inflamed gut results in biliary disease and impaired epithelial barrier function is associated with biliary infection [37]. Interestingly, in a germ-free murine model of PSC (multidrug-resistance-2 knockout mice), secondary bile acids were absent and the mice showed biochemical and histological features of PSC [38].

The genus *Veillonella* shows an increased abundance in patients with PSC. This bacterium contains genes for copper amine oxidase proteins, which may influence the expression of vascular adhesion protein-1, an adhesion molecule implicated in aberrant trafficking of gut-homing lymphocytes to the liver in patients with PSC [39]. In addition, bacteria that produce biogenic amines or possess amine oxidase activity show an increased abundance in PSC patients and may contribute, via their metabolites, to pathogenesis of disease [40]. Oral vancomycin significantly improves liver biochemistry in patients with PSC, presumably by modulating the gut microbiota [41].

Large-scale prospective studies are now needed for us to understand the contribution of the gut microbiota to pathophysiology of PSC-IBD, linking functional and metabolic properties of microorganisms to disease pathways to develop novel microbiota-targeted treatment strategies.

PBC and AIH

There have been few studies investigating the role of gut microbiota in patients with PBC or AIH. However, it is believed that the autoimmunity is probably triggered by environmental factors through molecular mimicry. Nearly 95% of patients with PBC produce antimitochondrial antibodies and these antibodies show cross reactivity to PDC-E2 and bacterial proteins of *E. coli*, *Lactobacillus delbrueckii*, and *Novosphingobium aromaticivorans* [42]. There are also changes in the microbiota in these patients. For example, gram-positive cocci were found more frequently in bile samples from patients with PBC than in samples from patients without primary hepatobiliary disease [43].

A study on 24 patients with AIH showed a decrease in the abundance of *Bifidobacterium* and *Lactobacillus* in patients compared to controls [44]. These patients also had a significant reduction of tight junction protein expression in duodenal mucosa, along with elevated serum LPS levels.

Microbiota-Targeted Therapies

Hepatologists have been targeting the microbiota for some time now, using lactulose as a prebiotic, as well as antibiotics such as rifaximin and ciprofloxacin, to influence the abundance of the urease-producing bacteria linked to hepatic encephalopathy. Several studies have examined the potential for targeted modulation of the gut microbiota using probiotics in patients with complications of cirrhosis. In a study that randomized patients with minimal hepatic encephalopathy (MHE) to receive a symbiotic (probiotic and fermentable fibre) or placebo, half the patients in the test group showed a significant reversal of MHE and improvement in the Child-Turcotte-Pugh class [45]. A significant reduction in blood ammonia levels and endotoxaemia was directly correlated with an increase in the faecal abundance of the non-urease-producing taxon, *Lactobacillus*.

Another randomised controlled trial demonstrated a significant reduction in fasting ammonia serum levels and improvement in psychometric and neurophysiological scores in patients with MHE, following treatment with *Bifidobacterium longum* and *fructo-oligosaccharide* [46]. Similar findings were demonstrated with probiotic yogurt supplementation in cirrhotics.

A meta-analysis has shown that probiotics given in NAFLD produce significant reductions in abnormal liver biochemistry, lower serum levels of cholesterol and TNF-α and improve insulin resistance [47]. An important mechanistic study showed that the administration of probiotic mixture VSL#3 resulted in significant reductions of the hepatic venous pressure gradient, cardiac index and heart rate, with increases in systemic vascular resistance, mean arterial pressure and serum sodium [48]. These changes were, however, unrelated to the detection of serum bacterial DNA or to the levels of LBP.

There has not yet been any randomised controlled trial evaluating the efficacy of faecal microbiota transplantation (FMT) to treat liver disease, although numerous animal studies and clinical reports have suggested a role [26]. For example, when the intestinal microbiota from lean donors was infused into male recipients with metabolic syndrome, the recipients showed a significant increase in peripheral, but not hepatic, insulin sensitivity and this was associated with an increase in butyrate-producing intestinal microbiota [49]. A case report published in 2015 on a patient with alcohol and hepatitis C induced cirrhosis showed a significant subjective and objective improvement in hepatic encephalopathy following 4 infusions of FMT [50]. However, this beneficial effect did not persist after FMT was discontinued.

Registered trials are ongoing to assess the efficacy of FMT in treating patients with NAFLD, PSC and recurrent hepatic encephalopathy. Although FMT is unlikely to become a main therapeutic option in patients with liver disease, these studies will help identify disease mechanisms and facilitate modulation of disease processes with specific candidate bacteria.

Conclusion

As research on the gut microbiota progresses at an extraordinary pace, we are documenting the pathways linking the gut microbiota and liver disease. It is clear that there are distinctive gut microbiotas in various liver diseases. However, the challenge now is to move from observations and correlations to a detailed understanding of mechanisms to pave the way for targeted microbiota-based therapies to prevent and ameliorate liver disease. We just need to find those missing links!

Disclosure Statement

The authors have nothing to disclose.

References

1 Marchesi JR, et al: The gut microbiota and host health: a new clinical frontier. Gut 2016; 65:330–339.
2 Wu D, Cederbaum A: Cytochrome P4502E1 sensitizes to tumor necrosis factor alpha-induced liver injury through activation of mitogen-activated protein kinases in mice. Hepatology 2008;47:1005–1017.
3 Wang L, et al: Methods to determine intestinal permeability and bacterial translocation during liver disease. J Immunol Methods 2015;421:44–53.
4 White JS, Hoper M, Parks RW, Clements WD, Diamond T: Patterns of bacterial translocation in experimental biliary obstruction. J Surg Res 2006;132:80–84.
5 Sayin SI, et al: Gut microbiota regulates bile acid metabolism by reducing the levels of tauro-beta-muricholic acid, a naturally occurring FXR antagonist. Cell Metab 2013;17:225–235.
6 Browne HP, et al: Culturing of 'unculturable' human microbiota reveals novel taxa and extensive sporulation. Nature 2016;533:543–546.
7 Walker AW: Studying the human microbiota. Adv Exp Med Biol 2016;902:5–32.
8 Pallen MJ: Diagnostic metagenomics: potential applications to bacterial, viral and parasitic infections. Parasitology 2014;141:1856–1862.
9 Seksik P, Landman C: Understanding microbiome data: a primer for clinicians. Dig Dis 2015;33(suppl 1):11–16.
10 Hanage WP: Microbiology: microbiome science needs a healthy dose of scepticism. Nature 2014;512:247–248.
11 Salter SJ, et al: Reagent and laboratory contamination can critically impact sequence-based microbiome analyses. BMC Biol 2014;12:87.
12 Yan AW, et al: Enteric dysbiosis associated with a mouse model of alcoholic liver disease. Hepatology 2011;53:96–105.
13 Wang L, et al: Intestinal REG3 lectins protect against alcoholic steatohepatitis by reducing mucosa-associated microbiota and preventing bacterial translocation. Cell Host Microbe 2016;19:227–239.
14 Bull-Otterson L, et al: Metagenomic analyses of alcohol induced pathogenic alterations in the intestinal microbiome and the effect of Lactobacillus rhamnosus GG treatment. PLoS One 2013;8:e53028.
15 Mutlu EA, et al: Colonic microbiome is altered in alcoholism. Am J Physiol Gastrointest Liver Physiol 2012;302:G966–G978.
16 Llopis M, et al: Intestinal microbiota contributes to individual susceptibility to alcoholic liver disease. Gut 2016;65:830–839.
17 Tuomisto S, et al: Changes in gut bacterial populations and their translocation into liver and ascites in alcoholic liver cirrhotics. BMC Gastroenterol 2014;14:40.
18 Chen P, et al: Microbiota protects mice against acute alcohol-induced liver injury. Alcohol Clin Exp Res 2015;39:2313–2323.
19 Fukui H, Brauner B, Bode JC, Bode C: Plasma endotoxin concentrations in patients with alcoholic and non-alcoholic liver disease: reevaluation with an improved chromogenic assay. J Hepatol 1991;12:162–169.
20 Hritz I, et al: The critical role of toll-like receptor (TLR) 4 in alcoholic liver disease is independent of the common TLR adapter MyD88. Hepatology 2008;48:1224–1231.
21 Kirpich IA, et al: Saturated and unsaturated dietary fats differentially modulate ethanol-induced changes in gut microbiome and metabolome in a mouse model of alcoholic liver disease. Am J Pathol 2016;186:765–776.
22 Raman M, et al: Fecal microbiome and volatile organic compound metabolome in obese humans with nonalcoholic fatty liver disease. Clin Gastroenterol Hepatol 2013;11:868–875. e1–e3.
23 Michail S, et al: Altered gut microbial energy and metabolism in children with non-alcoholic fatty liver disease. FEMS Microbiol Ecol 2015;91:1–9.
24 Zhu L, et al: Characterization of gut microbiomes in nonalcoholic steatohepatitis (NASH) patients: a connection between endogenous alcohol and NASH. Hepatology 2013;57:601–609.
25 Turnbaugh PJ, et al: An obesity-associated gut microbiome with increased capacity for energy harvest. Nature 2006;444:1027–1031.
26 Le Roy T, et al: Intestinal microbiota determines development of non-alcoholic fatty liver disease in mice. Gut 2013;62:1787–1794.
27 Spencer MD, et al: Association between composition of the human gastrointestinal microbiome and development of fatty liver with choline deficiency. Gastroenterology 2011; 140:976–986.
28 Luther J, et al: Hepatic injury in nonalcoholic steatohepatitis contributes to altered intestinal permeability. Cell Mol Gastroenterol Hepatol 2015;1:222–232.
29 Harte AL, et al: Elevated endotoxin levels in non-alcoholic fatty liver disease. J Inflamm (Load) 2010;7:15.
30 Li Z, et al: Probiotics and antibodies to TNF inhibit inflammatory activity and improve nonalcoholic fatty liver disease. Hepatology 2003;37:343–350.
31 Henao-Mejia J, et al: Inflammasome-mediated dysbiosis regulates progression of NAFLD and obesity. Nature 2012;482:179–185.
32 Sabino J, et al: Primary sclerosing cholangitis is characterised by intestinal dysbiosis independent from IBD. Gut 2016;65:1681–1689.
33 Kummen M, et al: The gut microbial profile in patients with primary sclerosing cholangitis is distinct from patients with ulcerative colitis without biliary disease and healthy controls. Gut 2016 pii:gutjnl-2015-310500.
34 Quraishi MN, et al: The gut-adherent microbiota of PSC-IBD is distinct to that of IBD. Gut 2017;66:386–388.
35 Torres J, et al: The features of mucosa-associated microbiota in primary sclerosing cholangitis. Aliment Pharmacol Ther 2016;43:790–801.
36 Goto Y, et al: Innate lymphoid cells regulate intestinal epithelial cell glycosylation. Science 2014;345:1254009.
37 Kawaguchi T, et al: Cholestasis with altered structure and function of hepatocyte tight junction and decreased expression of canalicular multispecific organic anion transporter in a rat model of colitis. Hepatology 2000;31: 1285–1295.

38 Tabibian JH: Absence of the intestinal microbiota exacerbates hepatobiliary disease in a murine model of primary sclerosing cholangitis. Hepatology 2016;63:185–196.

39 Trivedi PJ, Adams DH: Gut-liver immunity. J Hepatol 2016;64:1187–1189.

40 Pessione E, et al: A proteomic approach to studying biogenic amine producing lactic acid bacteria. Proteomics 2005;5:687–698.

41 Tabibian JH, Talwalkar JA, Lindor KD: Role of the microbiota and antibiotics in primary sclerosing cholangitis. Biomed Res Int 2013; 2013:389537.

42 Bogdanos DP, et al: Primary biliary cirrhosis is characterized by IgG3 antibodies cross-reactive with the major mitochondrial autoepitope and its Lactobacillus mimic. Hepatology 2005;42:458–465.

43 Hiramatsu K, et al: Amplification and sequence analysis of partial bacterial 16S ribosomal RNA gene in gallbladder bile from patients with primary biliary cirrhosis. J Hepatol 2000;33:9–18.

44 Lin R, Zhou L, Zhang J, Wang B: Abnormal intestinal permeability and microbiota in patients with autoimmune hepatitis. Int J Clin Exp Pathol 2015;8:5153–5160.

45 Liu Q, et al: Synbiotic modulation of gut flora: effect on minimal hepatic encephalopathy in patients with cirrhosis. Hepatology 2004;39: 1441–1449.

46 Malaguarnera M, et al: Bifidobacterium longum with fructo-oligosaccharide (FOS) treatment in minimal hepatic encephalopathy: a randomized, double-blind, placebo-controlled study. Dig Dis Sci 2007;52:3259–3265.

47 Ma YY, et al: Effects of probiotics on nonalcoholic fatty liver disease: a meta-analysis. World J Gastroenterol 2013;19:6911–6918.

48 Rincón D, et al: Oral probiotic vsl#3 attenuates the circulatory disturbances of patients with cirrhosis and ascites. Liver Int 2014;34: 1504–1512.

49 Vrieze A, et al: Transfer of intestinal microbiota from lean donors increases insulin sensitivity in individuals with metabolic syndrome. Gastroenterology 2012;143:913–916.e7.

50 Kao D, et al: Fecal microbiota transplantation in the management of hepatic encephalopathy. Hepatology 2016;63:339–340.

Liver and Bile Duct Cancer

Digestive Diseases

Dig Dis 2017;35:384–386
DOI: 10.1159/000456591

Treating Hepatobiliary Cancers: The Oncology Way

Peter Robert Galle

I. Medical Department, University Medical Center Mainz, Mainz, Germany

Keywords
Hepatobiliary cancer · Intrahepatic cholangiocarcinoma

Abstract
Hepatocellular carcinoma (HCC) is the third most common cause of cancer-related deaths worldwide. HCC represents more than 90% of primary liver cancers. There is growing incidence of HCC worldwide. In the western world, HCC arises in a cirrhotic background in up to 90% of cases, and cirrhosis itself is a progressive disease that affects patient survival. Thus, outcome in patients with HCC and the chances for anti-tumor treatment and it is results are dependent not only on tumor-associated factors but also on the liver function. Cholangio carcinoma is the second most common primary liver tumor with an estimated incidence of 1:100,000. Cholangiocarcinoma can be sub-classified as intrahepatic (iCCA), perihilar or distal where iCCA arises within the liver parenchyma. Overall, the incidence of iCCA seems to be increasing globally. This may be attributed to a global increase of risk factors shared between HCC and iCCA, such as viral hepatitis, liver cirrhosis, diabetes mellitus, obesity, NASH, and others.

Recommendations regarding screening, diagnosis and treatment of hepatocellular carcinoma (HCC) in western countries have been summarized in international guidelines, such as those endorsed by the American Association for the Study of Liver Diseases (AASLD) and the European Association of the Study of the Liver (EASL)/European Organization for Research and Treatment of Cancer (EORTC) [1, 2].

Guidelines for the diagnosis and management of intrahepatic cholangiocarcinoma (CCA) have been developed as a result of a preconference workshop of the International Liver Cancer Association [3].

This short review gives an overview of the current recommendations.

Hepatocellular Carcinoma

Screening

Guidelines of the American, European and German Liver/Gastroenterology associations (i.e., AASLD, EASL) universally recommend screening in all patients with liver cirrhosis, regardless of the etiology [1, 2]. In addition, EASL guidelines recommend HBV patients with chronic

KARGER

E-Mail karger@karger.com
www.karger.com/ddi

Peter Robert Galle
I. Medical Department
University Medical Center Mainz
Langenbeckstrasse 1, DE–55131 Mainz (Germany)
E-Mail galle@uni-mainz.de

active HBV or a family history of HCC as candidates for screening. Screening for HCC is cost effective when using abdominal ultrasound. The optimal screening interval seems to be 6 months.

Diagnosis

Diagnosis in most patients can be achieved by non-invasive measures. The finding of wash-in in the arterial phase and wash-out in the portal-venous or delayed phase of a dynamic contrast-enhanced imaging technique (CT, MRI, or US) in nodules larger than 1–2 cm is considered diagnostic.

Pathologic diagnosis is required only for suspicious lesions with inconclusive findings on imaging. However, in recent discussions, this non-invasive approach has been challenged: it clearly results in lack of biopsies in a majority of patients, which may result in a certain level of false positive patients (data from transplanted patients), in a lack of clinically relevant data (grading etc.) and is preventive with respect to the development of new diagnostic and predictive biomarkers.

Treatment

Assessment of tumor extension is critical for defining staging and treatment strategy and needs to be complemented by an assessment of liver function. The current EASL-EORTC clinical practice guidelines endorse the Barcelona-Clínic Liver Cancer (BCLC) classification. It includes prognostic variables related to tumor status, liver function and health performance status along with treatment-dependent variables.

Early HCC (BCLC stage A) is defined in patients presenting single tumors >2 cm or 3 nodules <3 cm of diameter, ECOG-0 and Child–Pugh class A or B. Median survival of patients with early HCC reaches 50–70% at 5 years after resection, liver transplantation or local ablation in selected candidates.

Intermediate HCC (BCLC stage B): untreated patients at an intermediate stage – BCLC B class (multinodular asymptomatic tumors without a vascular invasive pattern) present a median survival of 16 months or 49% at 2 years. Chemoembolization extends the survival of these patients to a median of up to 19–20 months.

Advanced HCC (BCLC stage C): patients with cancer-related symptoms (symptomatic tumors, ECOG 1–2), macro-vascular invasion (either segmental or portal invasion) or extra-hepatic spread (lymph node involvement or metastases) bear a dismal prognosis, with expected median survival times of 6 months, or 25% at 1 year. This outcome varies according to the liver functional status and other variables. The only available systemic treatment option to date is the TK inhibitor Sorafenib, which improves overall survival in the western population by about 3 months.

Recently, results of a phase III trial in second line (RESORCE) have been presented, demonstrating an improved overall survival for regorafenib-treated HCC patients with documented radiological progression during sorafenib treatment. Approval of regorafenib in HCC is expected by late 2017.

Future Perspective

After a series of phase III trial failures, future trials will have to pay more attention to drug toxicity and – most importantly – on patient selection. The former "all-comer-approach" resulting in a molecularly heterogeneous group of patients needs to be replaced by biomarker-driven trial design, linking targeted therapy to appropriate patient subgroups. Promising trials are on the way. In addition, novel immunotherapeutic approaches in early phase trials have yielded first positive results and are further elaborated in several phase II and III trials with the perspective to change the field in systemic therapy. The positive RESORCE trial will broaden our systemic armamentarium.

Intrahepatic Cholangiocarcinoma

Diagnosis

The clinical presentation of intrahepatic cholangiocarcinoma (iCCA) is non-specific and insufficient to establish a diagnosis. Most patients are asymptomatic. In patients with PSC or hepatolithiasis, any degradation in the performance status should be taken as a possible indication of CCA.

Radiographic imaging is non-specific. Pathological diagnosis is recommended for all patients who are considered for therapeutic intervention.

Treatment

Surgical resection is the treatment of choice for CCA. Patients demonstrating intrahepatic metastases, vascular invasion or obvious lymph node metastases should not undergo resection. There is no established adjuvant therapy after resection.

TACE and TARE have shown anti-tumor effects with acceptable toxicities in patients with iCCA but require further examination in appropriately designed clinical trials and therefore cannot be recommended as standard therapy.

Cisplatin and Gemcitabine constitute a systemic therapy practice standard for CCA in patients with ECOG performance status 0 or 1.

Disclosure Statement

The author received lecture fees and honoraria for advisory boards from Bayer, BMS, MSD, Lilly, AstraZeneca, Sillajen, Sirtex.

References

1 European Association for the Study of the Liver; European Organisation for Research and Treatment of Cancer: EASL-EORTC clinical practice guidelines: management of hepatocellular carcinoma. J Hepatol 2012;56:908–943.

2 Bruix J, Sherman M; American Association for the Study of Liver Diseases: Management of hepatocellular carcinoma: an update. Hepatology 2011;53:1020–1022.

3 Bridgewater J, Galle PR, Khan SA, Llovet JM, Park JW, Patel T, Pawlik TM, Gores GJ: Guidelines for the diagnosis and management of intrahepatic cholangiocarcinoma. J Hepatol 2014;60:1268–1289.

Liver and Bile Duct Cancer

Digestive Diseases

Dig Dis 2017;35:387–389
DOI: 10.1159/000456592

Stemness in Liver Cancer

Snorri S. Thorgeirsson

Laboratory of Human Carcinogenesis, Center for Cancer Research, National Cancer Institute, NIH, Bethesda, MD, USA

Keywords
Liver · Cancer · Stemness · Cancer stem cells

Abstract
Cancer cells possessing "stemness," or stem-cell properties, are referred to as cancer stem cells (CSC) or cancer-initiating cells. The concept that these cells rest at the apex of the cancer hierarchy is an evolving theme in cancer research. These cells are by definition primarily responsible for the initiation and propagation of tumors as well as relapse after therapy, and they are therefore of major scientific interest. Several studies indicate that hepatocellular carcinomas that harbor phenotypic features of stem cells and progenitor cells constitute a subclass of therapeutically challenging cancers that are associated with a particularly poor prognosis. We recently demonstrated that any cell type in the mouse hepatic lineage can undergo oncogenic reprogramming into a CSC by activating different cell type–specific pathways [1]. Identification of common and cell of origin-specific phenotypic and genetic changes could provide new therapeutic targets for liver cancer.

Introduction

The biological similarity that exists between cancer and stem cells has long been recognized, and consequently, the concept of cancer as a disease of abnormal stem cells is not new [2]. Furthermore, the extensive confirmation of the cancer stem cell (CSC) concept in multiple tumor types has decisively established the importance of the CSC paradigm in both experimental and human neoplasia [3]. In this context, it is worth emphasizing the importance of the discovery of Takahashi and Yamanaka demonstrating that introduction and expression of only four genes (e.g., Oct-3/4, Sox2, c-Myc, and KLF4) into adult mouse fibroblasts, and later other cell types such as hepatocytes, could reprogram these cells into functional embryonic stem cells entitled induced pluripotent stem cells (iPSCs) for the cancer field [4]. It is noteworthy that most of the effective reprogramming factors have an established role in oncogenesis (e.g., c-Myc, Oct-4, Sox-2, Nanog, Lin28, and p53). These discoveries strongly indicate that differentiated cells (e.g., hepatocytes) could be the source of CSC and are capable of supporting both inter- and intratumoral phenotypic and genetic heterogeneity seen in most human cancers [5].

KARGER

E-Mail karger@karger.com
www.karger.com/ddi

Snorri S. Thorgeirsson, MD, PhD
Laboratory of Human Carcinogenesis, Center for Cancer Research
National Cancer Institute, NIH, 37 Convent Drive MSC 4262
Building 37, Room 4128B, Bethesda, MD 20892-4262 (USA)
E-Mail snorri_thorgeirsson@nih.gov

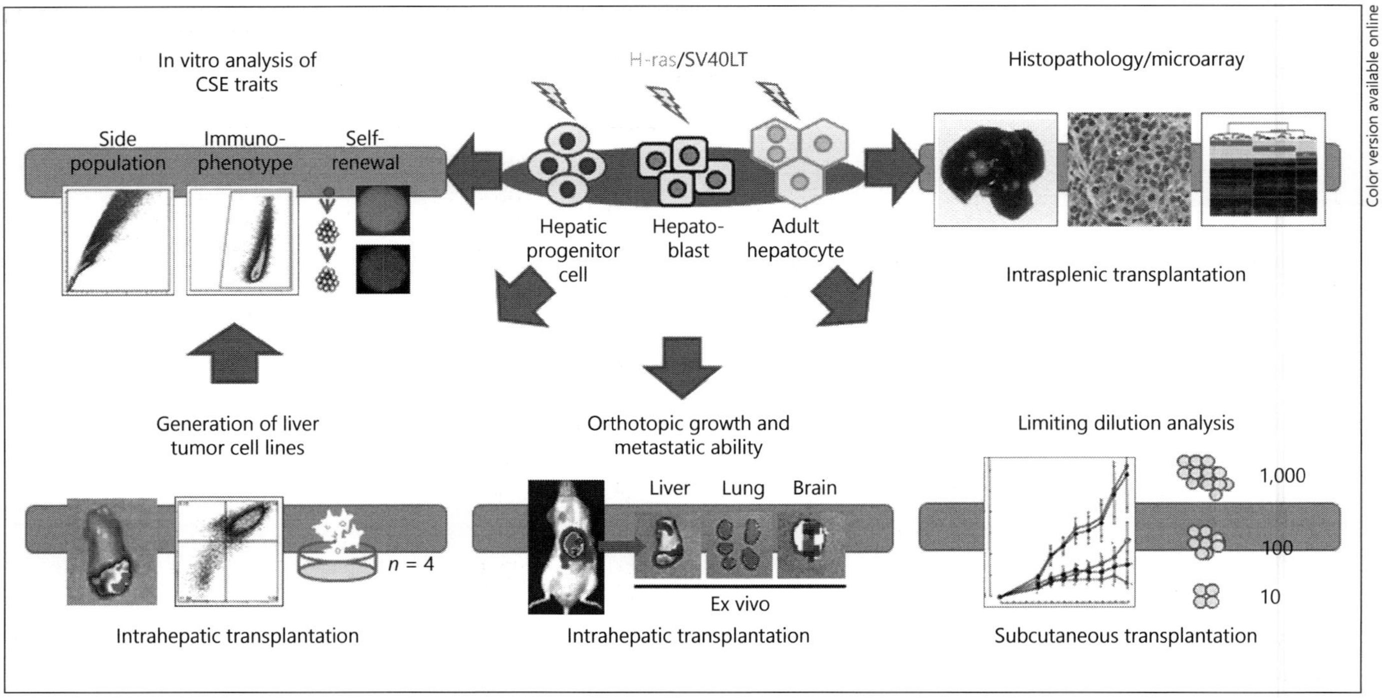

Fig. 1. Schematic representation of the experimental designs.

The evolution of CSCs from cells at different stages of differentiation may contribute, at least in part, to the phenotypic and genetic heterogeneity seen in liver cancer. However, whether a lineage stage may be a factor in acquisition of stemness properties at the cellular and molecular levels is not yet understood. We have recently addressed whether the differentiation stage of distinct hepatic lineage cells (a) dictates the acquisition of CSC properties and (b) contributes to the phenotypic and genetic heterogeneity of liver cancer [1]. These data will be summarized and discussed here.

Results and Discussion

Three cell types from mouse liver were used (i.e., adult hepatocytes (AH) hepatoblasts (HB) and hepatic progenitor cells (HPCs)) to perform a systematic side-by-side comparison of tumorigenesis after oncogeneic transformation. The cell types were isolated at high purity and subjected to lentiviral transduction with vectors encoding oncogenic H-ras and SV40LT (experimental procedures summarized in Figure 1). All three lineages gave rise to tumors with varying hepatocellular carcinomas (HCCs) and cholangiocarcinoma (CCA) content, that is, AH- tumors showed mostly HCC, HB-tumors mostly CCA, and HPC-tumors mostly anaplastic histopathology, indicating an epithelial-to-mesenchymal transition. Since HCCs, CCAs, and anaplastic tumors were generated in the model and produced by the same initial oncogenetic drivers, multiple side-by-side comparisons were possible, independent of confounding factors caused by different oncogenic drivers. The key observations included (1) a 590-gene signature with significant common dysregulation in all 3 tumor types; (2) hierarchical clustering of common genes separated the tumors in accordance with the originally transformed cell type; (3) the identified gene signature was able to separate human HCCs from CCAs and combined hepatocellular CCAs; (4) AH-derived iPSC gene signature was enriched in AH-derived but not in HB- and HPC-derived tumors; and (5) c-myc was strongly induced only in AH-derived tumors, and RNA-mediated knockdown re-affirmed the central role of c-myc in reprogramming and oncogenic transformation of AH [6].

In conclusion, this study provides the first comprehensive and systematic comparison of hepatocarcinogenesis initiated by controlled oncogenic transformation of cells at specific stages of hepatic lineage. Differentiated hepatocytes, HB, and adult HPCs were isolated at high purity and efficiently transduced with the same combination of H-ras and SV40LT oncogenes. This permitted

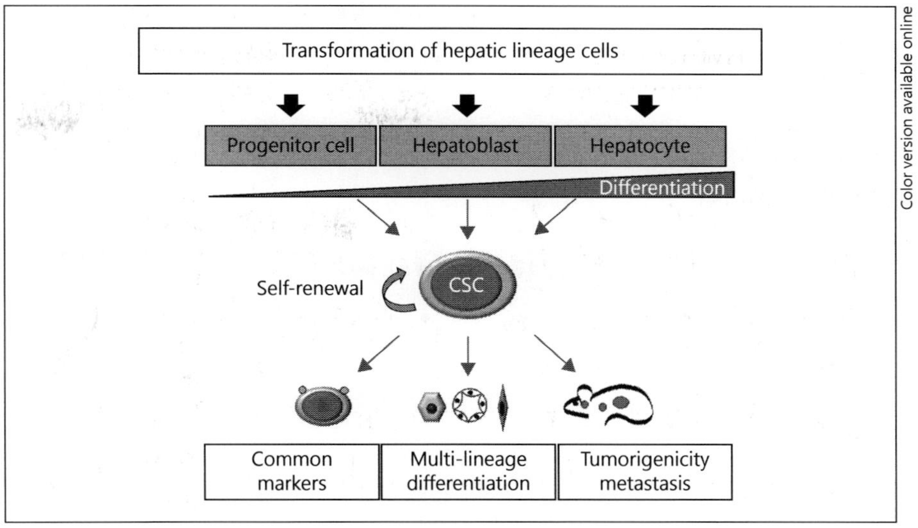

Fig. 2. Schematic illustration of the transformation of hepatic lineage cells.

a unique and direct side-by-side comparison of cellular and molecular characteristics of transformed cells both in vitro and in vivo. The study formally showed that any hepatic lineage cell can be reprogrammed into CSC by activating diverse cell type–specific pathways (Fig. 2). It also described common and cell of origin–specific phenotypic and genetic changes that correctly identified the murine tumors according to their cellular origin, providing an important means to phenotypically classify morphologically diverse human primary hepatocellular cancers. Accordingly, identification of cells that are both susceptible to oncogenic transformation and relevant to molecular pathways is essential for a deeper understanding of the origin of liver cancer and development of more effective therapeutic strategies.

Disclosure Statement

Nothing to declare.

References

1 Holczbauer A, Factor VM, Andersen JB, Marquardt JU, Kleiner DE, Raggi C, Kitade M, Seo D, Akita H, Durkin ME, Thorgeirsson SS: Modeling pathogenesis of primary liver cancer in lineage-specific mouse cell types. Gastroenterology 2013;145:221–231.

2 Sell S: Stem cell origin of cancer and differentiation therapy. Crit Rev Oncol Hematol 2004;51:1–28.

3 Plaks V, Kong N, Werb Z: The cancer stem cell niche: how essential is the niche in regulating stemness of tumor cells? Cell Stem Cell 2015;16:225–238.

4 Campos-Sanchez E, Cobaleda C: Tumoral reprogramming: plasticity takes a walk on the wild site. Biochim Biophys Acta 2015;1849:436–447.

5 Marquardt JU, Andersen JB, Thorgeirsson SS: Functional and genetic deconstruction of the cellular origin in liver cancer. Nat Rev Cancer 2015;15:653–667.

6 Kaposi-Novak P, et al: Central role of c-Myc during malignant conversion in human hepatocarcinogenesis. Cancer Res 2009;69:2775–2782.

Liver and Bile Duct Cancer

Digestive Diseases

Dig Dis 2017;35:390–396
DOI: 10.1159/000456593

Treating Hepatobiliary Cancer: The Immunologic Approach

A.G. Duffy T.F. Greten

Gastrointestinal Malignancies Section, Thoracic-GI Oncology Branch, Center for Cancer Research, National Cancer Institute, National Institutes of Health, Bethesda, MD, USA

Keywords
Immune · Inflammation · Immune-evasion · Hepatobiliary · Cholangiocarcinoma

Abstract
Hepatobiliary cancer comprises a heterogeneous group of malignancies in which the standard treatments for advanced disease are minimally effective and evolve slowly over time. Like the majority of gastrointestinal cancers, with some notable exceptions, the impact of immune-based approaches is yet to be experienced. Notwithstanding this, the etiological background of hepatobiliary cancer – overlapping in almost every known causative or associated factor with inflammation – provides a strong clue that these approaches may have an impact on this group of diseases. This review seeks to put the management of hepatobiliary cancers in the context of its inflammation-based etiology, with the aim of pointing to the therapeutic opportunities in immune-based approaches currently entering the clinic or those that are about to do so.

Introduction

The term hepatobiliary cancer refers to primary malignancies, which develop in the liver, either hepatocellular carcinoma (HCC), or the intra- and extra-hepatic biliary ductal system giving rise to biliary tract carcinomas (BTC). Hepatobiliary cancers have in common trends in global prevalence where striking peaks in incidence in certain regional hotspots contrast with relative rarity in western countries. For example, gallbladder cancer is a leading cause of cancer mortality in Chile but has an incidence of approximately in 5,000 people in the United States [1]. The practical consequence of this is that standard of care evolves slowly with a general paucity of randomized studies. For advanced metastatic disease, the modest standard of care comprises either sorafenib (for HCC) or gemcitabine-based chemotherapy (for BTC), based on the so-called SHARP and ABC-02 trials respectively [2, 3]. Beyond that there is no outright standard second-line option and clearly there is an unmet need here to improve the treatment options at every stage for patients with this group of malignancies.

Austin G. Duffy
Gastrointestinal Malignancies Section, Thoracic-GI Oncology Branch,
Center for Cancer Research, National Cancer Institute, National Institutes
of Health, 9000 Rockville Pike, 10/12N224, Bethesda, MD 20892 (USA)
E-Mail duffya@mail.nih.gov

The past number of years have seen much progress for immune-based approaches in solid tumor malignancies, with FDA approvals for various strategies, including dendritic cell vaccination as well as so-called immune checkpoint inhibition [4–6]. The next frontier is for these treatments to prove themselves in diseases that have thus far proved refractory. So far, with notable exceptions, this has included cancers of the gastrointestinal tract, including hepatobiliary cancers as a group. One of the first studies evaluating PD1/programmed death ligand (PD-L1)-directed therapy was disappointing from a GI cancer viewpoint [7]. Similarly negative results for GI cancers were seen in other studies of checkpoint inhibition when used as a single modality [8–10].

Inflammation and Predisposition to Hepatobiliary Cancer

The causative link between inflammation and cancer development stretches back to the 19th-century observations of Rudolph Virchow. Chronic inflammation can greatly facilitate cancer development through a number of means, culminating in an immunosuppressed microenvironment containing dysfunctional "exhausted" T cells, high expression of inhibitory receptors (e.g., CTLA4) and cytokine milieu weighted towards suppression versus activation [11, 12]. This broad and sometimes paradoxical relationship between cancer and inflammation is particularly relevant in hepatobiliary cancers, a group of malignancies whose predominantly associated predisposing conditions have chronic inflammation as their common underlying pathological denominator (Fig. 1). The dominant known risk factor for HCC is cirrhosis induced by long-standing inflammation from a variety of causes – viral hepatitis, environmental factors such as alcohol, metabolic syndromes and, more appreciably, non-alcoholic steatohepatitis. Similarly, for biliary tract cancers gallbladder carcinoma – the most common subtype of BTC in the United States – cholelithiasis-induced chronic inflammation, whereas – worldwide – infestation of the biliary ducts by parasites or persistent hepatolithiasis are important predisposing factors for intrahepatic cholangiocarcinoma (ICC) [13]. In the United States and Europe, primary biliary cirrhosis and sclerosing cholangitis are all established risk factors for BTC, as are causes of intrahepatic inflammation, for example, obesity [14]. Recent studies have linked liver disease associated with the same increasing incidence of chronic hepatitis C virus infection, which explains much of the increase in HCC rates with ICC [15].

Immunogenicity of Hepatobiliary Cancer

The acknowledgement of an immune role in the etiology of hepatobiliary cancer is important because it raises the possibility of an immune-based remedy where the predisposition and pathogenesis can be manipulated for therapeutic gains. The success of immune checkpoint inhibition is dependent upon the presence of an existing endogenous anti-tumor immune response. Spontaneous immune responses including T-cell responses [16] as well as humoral responses to different tumor-associated antigens [17] have been described in HCC. A number of studies have described that tumor infiltrating CD4+ regulatory T-cells correlate with poor outcome in patients who undergo surgical resection [18, 19]. Likewise, spontaneous immune responses also occur in BTC. This was illustrated in a dramatic manner by Tran and colleagues who performed whole-exomic-sequencing on the resected tumor of a patient with metastatic chemo-refractory cholangiocarcinoma [20]. By generating tandem minigene constructs of each of the somatic tumor mutations and co-culturing with expanded populations of isolated tumor infiltrating lymphocytes (TIL), they identified a reactive population of CD4+ cells, an enriched population of which the investigators were able to adoptively transfer to produce tumor regression. It has been postulated that the degree to which these anti-tumor responses exist is related to the mutagenic burden of the tumor. Hepatobiliary cancers in general are not highly mutated. In HCC, the median number of mutations is 39 [21]. The number is similarly low in BTC. Whole-exome sequencing of 239 cases of BTC revealed median numbers of mutations across the ICC, extrahepatic cholangiocarcinoma and gallbladder cancer subtypes of 39, 35, and 64 [22]. This relatively average degree of mutagenicity in the setting of spontaneous anti-tumor immunity challenges somewhat the direct relationship between mutagenicity and immunogenicity, which is clearly relevant but not absolute. Indeed, Tran and colleagues have recently suggested that this relationship is more nuanced, with the finding of immunoreactive TIL even in the setting of low mutational burden [23].

Perhaps the best indicator of an existing antitumor immunity is the presence of TIL. In HCC, the presence of TIL has been shown to be prognostic [24, 25]. In BTC, the prevalence and prognostic relevance of TIL have also been documented. Sabbatino et al. [26] evaluated lymphocyte infiltration in 27 cases of ICC. All tumors had TIL, and this correlated with HLA expression. Nakakubo et al. [27] investigated the significance of TIL pres-

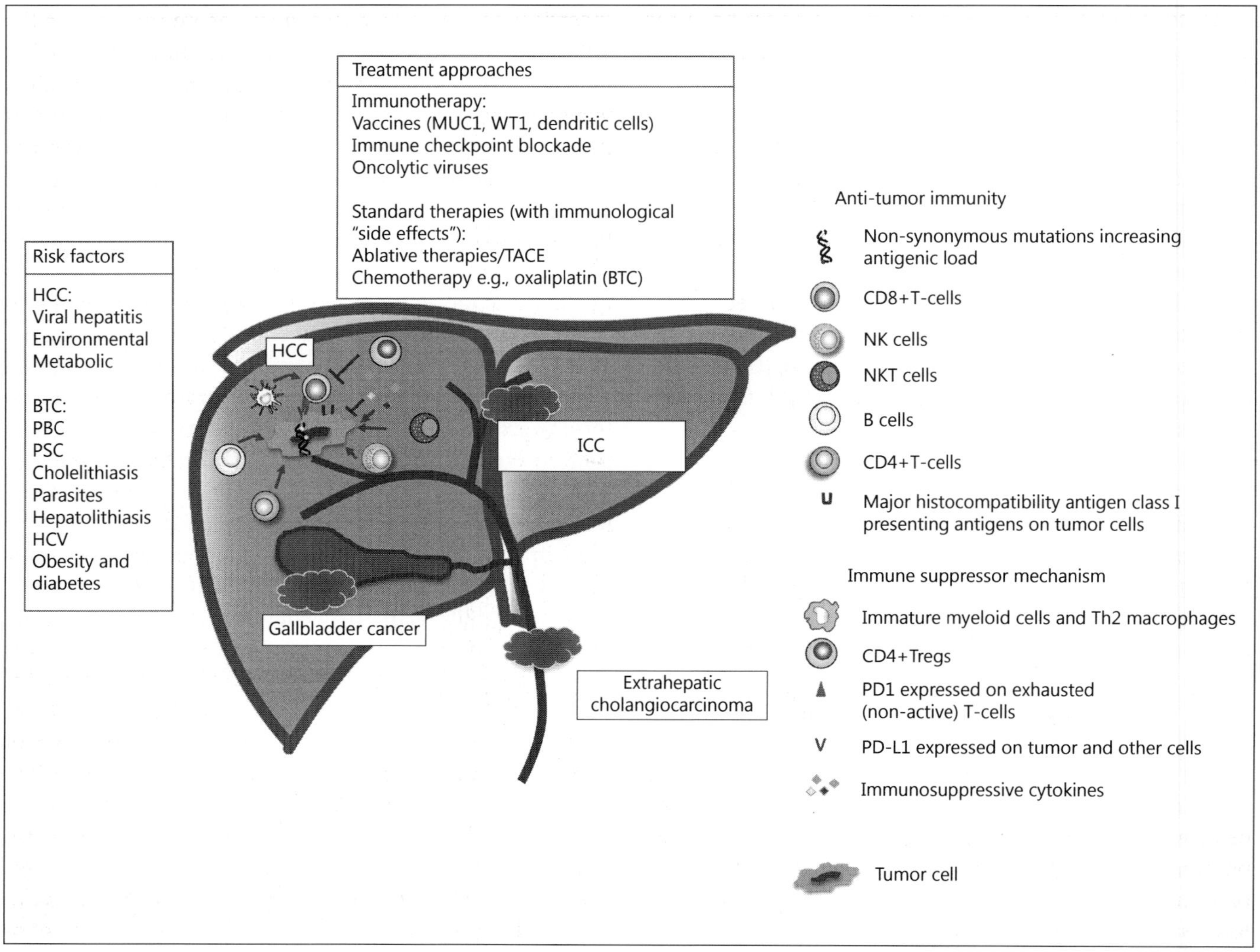

Fig. 1. Immunological events described in hepatobiliary cancer: risk factors, immune-based approaches, immune-activating and immunosuppressive events.

ence in 110 resected gallbladder specimens and found that both CD4+ and CD8+ T cell infiltration correlated with decreasing tumour invasion and survival. Goeppert et al. [28] evaluated immune cell infiltration in 375 cases of BTC following resection. Approximately half the number of patients had some degree of TIL and this was also found to correlate with survival. Interestingly, patients who had higher total regulatory T lymphocyte counts had a better survival outcome. The prognostic value of Tregs in other GI tumor types has been varying in terms of whether it was a favorable or adverse factor [29].

Another method of immune evasion by tumors is achieved by changes in the expression downregulation of MHC I [30–32]. HCCs express low levels of MHC class I molecules in addition to costimulatory molecules [33]. Similarly, in BTC, Goeppert et al. [34] analysed the impact of MHC expression on survival in a large series of patients ($n = 334$) as well as the relationship of this to TIL. MHC I expression was assessed semi-quantitatively and divided into 2 groups of high and low expression. There was a trend for higher MHC I expression in lower disease stages and an association between MHC I expression and the number of TIL. Interestingly, the investigators found that associations differed based on the BTC subtype, with the prognostic significance of MHC I expression, being by trend stronger in extrahepatic disease compared with intrahepatic disease, suggesting that mechanisms of immune escape may vary with anatomical subtype.

In addition to evasive mechanisms, tumors have the ability to suppress antitumor immunity in a variety of ways. Myeloid-derived suppressor cells, a heterogeneous cell population that suppress T-cell responses, have been shown to accumulate in the blood of patients with hepatobiliary malignancies [35, 36]. A separate mechanism results from the expression by tumors of PD-L1, which also inhibits T-cell reactivity. PD-L1 is heavily expressed in HCC and has been shown to be of prognostic significance [37, 38]. Similarly, in BTC, Ye et al. [39] evaluated the expression of PD-L1 and its ligand PD-1 in n = 31 surgically resected cases in addition to the corresponding cancer-adjacent tissues. Expression of PD-L1 was found to be upregulated in cholangiocarcinoma tissues compared with the cancer-adjacent tissues. Tumor-related PD-L1 expression was significantly correlated with both tumor differentiation and pTNM stage and was inversely correlated with CD8+ tumor-infiltrating lymphocytes. In the analysis by Sabbatino et al. [26] 8 of 27 ICC cases expressed PD-L1.

Translational Immune-Based Approaches in Hepatobiliary Cancers

Immunotherapy has been tested in hepatobiliary cancers for many years, particularly HCC. Most studies in the past have either used cytokine-based or antigen-based approaches [35]. While these studies have generally proven to be safe with induction – in peripheral blood or serum – of tumor-specific immune responses, a majority have failed to show that this translates into clinical efficacy. In more recent times, however, evidence of efficacy has been demonstrated in a number of immune modalities, mainly in HCC.

Hepatocellular Carcinoma

The use of immune-based approaches is especially attractive for HCC, given the invariable underlying existence of cirrhosis and related problems such as thrombocytopenia. The development of conventional cytotoxic regimens, particularly those requiring hepatic metabolism, is therefore an additional challenge in this cancer over others. The most promising immune-based approaches tested in HCC have been oncolytic viruses and immune checkpoint inhibitors. The use of oncolytic virus as a treatment strategy in HCC is a recent development. JX-594 is an oncolytic poxvirus modified by the insertion of β-galactosidase, a surrogate marker for the detection of viral gene expression and human GM-CSF to stimulate anti-tumor immune responses. The vaccinia virus replicates in cancer cells dependent on cellular thymidine kinase activity [40]. Intra-tumoral application of JX-594 was shown to be safe in a phase I study in HCC [41]. Results from a second study in 30 patients with advanced HCC were subsequently reported in which patients were randomized for treatment with low-dose (10^8 PFU) or high-dose (10^9 PFU) JX-594 administered by intra-tumoral injection [42]. Objective responses rates were 15% in both groups and an intrahepatic disease control of 50% was achieved. It should be noted that disease control rates were equivalent in injected and distant untreated tumors suggesting the presence of a systemic immune response. There was a clear dose relationship with regard to overall survival (6.7 months in the low and 14.1 months in the high dose). Immune-monitoring studies demonstrated that at least 11 of 16 patients developed HCC-specific antibody responses as determined by the analysis of complement-dependent cytotoxicity of patients' serum against HCC cell lines. Cellular immune responses were studied by ELISpot analysis against β-gal and they demonstrated the induction of β-gal specific T cells, which were found in one patient 18 months after treatment.

The other strategy that has shown promise in HCC recently is immune checkpoint inhibition. Tremelimumab – a fully human monoclonal antibody that binds to CTLA-4 expressed on the surface of activated T lymphocytes and results in inhibition of B7-CTLA-4-mediated downregulation of T-cell activation – was initially tested in a pilot clinical trial in 20 patients with advanced HCC and HCV infection [43]. Tremelimumab, at a dose of 15 mg/kg every 90 days i.v., was tolerated well and showed evidence of activity. Three out of 17 evaluable patients developed confirmed partial responses and 10 patients had stable disease as the best response to treatment. HCV-specific T-cell responses were studies conducted in these patients as a surrogate marker for the anti-CTLA4-induced immune responses. Recently, preliminary results for a representative agent of the other most prominent class of immune checkpoint inhibitors currently in clinic, PD1 blockade, were presented [44]. In this study, n = 47 patients with preserved liver function but advanced HCC were treated with nivolumab, with impressive, preliminary evidence of activity. Out of 39 evaluable patients, there were 2 complete responses and 7 partial responses.

One of the unique features of HCC is the reliance upon interventional radiologic procedures in everyday

Dig Dis 2017;35:390–396
DOI: 10.1159/000456593

patient management, either for the purposes of curative intent (heat-based or cryo-ablation) or disease control (TACE). Systemic therapy plays a comparatively modest role. Following ablation, tumor antigens from necrotic tumor are taken up by antigen-presenting cells (mainly DCs), resulting in activating tumor-specific immune responses [45, 46]. Ablated tumor tissue has been shown to promote DC maturation [47, 48]. A tumor-specific immune response may prevent recurrent disease in addition to treating distant metastases. Several preclinical and clinical studies have documented an increase in peripheral immunity following ablation [47, 49–52]. We are currently conducting a study evaluating subtotal RFA in combination with anti-CTLA4 therapy (NCT01853618) in patients with HCC and BTC. Provisionally, this approach is feasible and safe, with some early evidence of efficacy, which needs to be confirmed with more number of patients and more mature follow-up [53].

Biliary Tract Carcinomas

In terms of published clinical data for immune approaches in BTC, the experience is dominated by peptide vaccines. These small studies have been well tolerated without showing a strong signal of efficacy [54, 55]. For example, Aruga et al. [56] conducted a small phase I clinical trial evaluating multiple-peptide vaccination for patients with advanced BTC. Peptide-specific T-cell immune responses and disease stability were observed in some patients. Dendritic cell–based vaccines have also been evaluated, most commonly in combination with standard modalities, which complicates assessment of efficacy [57, 58]. The experience with checkpoint inhibitors is very preliminary. Documented response to anti-CTLA-4 therapy has been observed, manifesting as a delayed response after initial disease progression [59]. The early data for anti-PD1 inhibition has been recently presented, showing encouraging evidence of efficacy, and which seems consistent with use of this agent in other solid tumor studies [60].

One of the advantages of immune-based approaches is the potential role of their combination with standard therapies – cytotoxic agents, radiation or interventional radiologic procedures [61]. Certain chemotherapeutics can activate rather than suppress the immune system and a robust immune response is a necessary component determining tumor response [62]. Gemcitabine is a nucleoside analogue that is part of the standard treatment, and probably the most common chemotherapeutic agent used in BTC [3, 63]. The immune effects of gemcitabine have been studied perhaps more than for any other drug used in GI cancer. Its effects on the immune system are diverse [61]. With regard to BTC, Koido et al. [65] demonstrated that in ICC cells isolated from a patient with malignant ascites, immunogenic modulation of the cells could be induced by gemcitabine with the upregulation of MHC class I and II, calreticulin – a modulator or immunogenic cell death – MUC1 and WT1 mRNA [64]. Interestingly, the authors found that gemcitabine also induced the upregulation of immunosuppressive PD-L1, suggesting a potential rationale for combination therapy.

Conclusions

The advantages of immune-based treatments are clear, such that the initial results of the checkpoint inhibitors in particular have captured the imaginations of physicians and the general public alike. While the benefit seen thus far is real, hepatobiliary malignancies have not been among the banner group of malignancies to have so far shown dramatic and durable evidence of efficacy. This is beginning to change with the presentation of what so far is a relatively small volume of clinical experience, albeit encouraging. The close etiological relationship between hepatobiliary cancer and inflammation speaks to an important role for the immune system in these diseases, as do the data discussed showing by almost any measure – TIL, MHC downregulation, PD-L1 expression – evidence of a reactive surveillance, which can be potentially manipulated by the new drugs and technologies that are making their way in the clinic.

Disclosure Statement

The authors report no financial conflicts of interest to declare.

Financial Support

This research was supported by the Intramural Research Program of the NIH, National Cancer Institute, Center for Cancer Research. The content of this publication does not necessarily reflect the views or policies of the Department of Health and Human Services, nor does mention of trade names, commercial products, or organizations imply endorsement by the US Government.

References

1 Nogueira L, Foerster C, Groopman J, et al: Association of aflatoxin with gallbladder cancer in Chile. JAMA 2015;313:2075–2077.
2 Llovet JM, Ricci S, Mazzaferro V, et al: Sorafenib in advanced hepatocellular carcinoma. N Engl J Med 2008;359:378–390.
3 Valle J, Wasan H, Palmer DH, et al: Cisplatin plus gemcitabine versus gemcitabine for biliary tract cancer. N Engl J Med 2010;362: 1273–1281.
4 Kantoff PW, Higano CS, Shore ND, et al: Sipuleucel-T immunotherapy for castration-resistant prostate cancer. N Engl J Med 2010; 363:411–422.
5 Hodi FS, O'Day SJ, McDermott DF, et al: Improved survival with ipilimumab in patients with metastatic melanoma. N Engl J Med 2010;363:711–223.
6 Robert C, Thomas L, Bondarenko I, et al: Ipilimumab plus dacarbazine for previously untreated metastatic melanoma. N Engl J Med 2011;364:2517–2526.
7 Brahmer JR, Tykodi SS, Chow LQ, et al: Safety and activity of anti-PD-L1 antibody in patients with advanced cancer. N Engl J Med 2012;366:2455–2465.
8 Topalian SL, Hodi FS, Brahmer JR, et al: Safety, activity, and immune correlates of anti-PD-1 antibody in cancer. N Engl J Med 2012; 366:2443–2454.
9 Chung KY, Gore I, Fong L, et al: Phase II study of the anti-cytotoxic T-lymphocyte-associated antigen 4 monoclonal antibody, tremelimumab, in patients with refractory metastatic colorectal cancer. J Clin Oncol 2010;28:3485–3490.
10 Royal RE, Levy C, Turner K, et al: Phase 2 trial of single agent Ipilimumab (anti-CTLA-4) for locally advanced or metastatic pancreatic adenocarcinoma. J Immunother 2010;33: 828–833.
11 Jiang Y, Li Y, Zhu B: T-cell exhaustion in the tumor microenvironment. Cell Death Dis 2015;6:e1792.
12 Trinchieri G: Cancer and inflammation: an old intuition with rapidly evolving new concepts. Annu Rev Immunol 2012;30:677–706.
13 Rizvi S, Gores GJ: Pathogenesis, diagnosis, and management of cholangiocarcinoma. Gastroenterology 2013;145:1215–1229.
14 Chang JS, Tsai CR, Chen LT: Medical risk factors associated with cholangiocarcinoma in Taiwan: a population-based case-control study. PLoS One 2013;8:e69981.
15 El-Serag HB, Engels EA, Landgren O, et al: Risk of hepatobiliary and pancreatic cancers after hepatitis C virus infection: a population-based study of U.S. veterans. Hepatology 2009;49:116–123.
16 Mizukoshi E, Nakamoto Y, Arai K, et al: Comparative analysis of various tumor-associated antigen-specific t-cell responses in patients with hepatocellular carcinoma. Hepatology 2011;53:1206–1216.
17 Korangy F, Ormandy LA, Bleck JS, et al: Spontaneous tumor-specific humoral and cellular immune responses to NY-ESO-1 in hepatocellular carcinoma. Clin Cancer Res 2004;10:4332–4341.
18 Fu J, Xu D, Liu Z, et al: Increased regulatory T cells correlate with CD8 T-cell impairment and poor survival in hepatocellular carcinoma patients. Gastroenterology 2007;132: 2328–2339.
19 Gao Q, Qiu SJ, Fan J, et al: Intratumoral balance of regulatory and cytotoxic T cells is associated with prognosis of hepatocellular carcinoma after resection. J Clin Oncol 2007;25: 2586–2593.
20 Tran E, Turcotte S, Gros A, et al: Cancer immunotherapy based on mutation-specific CD4+ T cells in a patient with epithelial cancer. Science 2014;344:641–645.
21 Vogelstein B, Papadopoulos N, Velculescu VE, Zhou S, Diaz LA Jr, Kinzler KW: Cancer genome landscapes. Science 2013;339:1546–1558.
22 Nakamura H, Arai Y, Totoki Y, et al: Genomic spectra of biliary tract cancer. Nat Genet 2015;47:1003–1010.
23 Tran E, Ahmadzadeh M, Lu YC, et al: Immunogenicity of somatic mutations in human gastrointestinal cancers. Science 2015;350: 1387–1390.
24 Garnelo M, Tan A, Her Z, et al: Interaction between tumour-infiltrating B cells and T cells controls the progression of hepatocellular carcinoma. Gut 2017;66:342–351.
25 Chew V, Tow C, Teo M, et al: Inflammatory tumour microenvironment is associated with superior survival in hepatocellular carcinoma patients. J Hepatol 2010;52:370–379.
26 Sabbatino F, Villani V, Yearley JH, et al: PD-L1 and HLA class I antigen expression and clinical course of the disease in intrahepatic cholangiocarcinoma. Clin Cancer Res 2016; 22:470–478.
27 Nakakubo Y, Miyamoto M, Cho Y, et al: Clinical significance of immune cell infiltration within gallbladder cancer. Br J Cancer 2003; 89:1736–1742.
28 Goeppert B, Frauenschuh L, Zucknick M, et al: Prognostic impact of tumour-infiltrating immune cells on biliary tract cancer. Br J Cancer 2013;109:2665–2674.
29 Zhuo C, Xu Y, Ying M, et al: FOXP3+ Tregs: heterogeneous phenotypes and conflicting impacts on survival outcomes in patients with colorectal cancer. Immunol Res 2015;61:338–347.
30 Campoli M, Ferrone S: HLA antigen changes in malignant cells: epigenetic mechanisms and biologic significance. Oncogene 2008;27: 5869–5885.
31 Campoli M, Ferrone S: Tumor escape mechanisms: potential role of soluble HLA antigens and NK cells activating ligands. Tissue Antigens 2008;72:321–334.
32 Ryschich E, Nötzel T, Hinz U, et al: Control of T-cell-mediated immune response by HLA class I in human pancreatic carcinoma. Clin Cancer Res 2005;11(2 pt 1):498–504.
33 Fujiwara K, Higashi T, Nouso K, et al: Decreased expression of B7 costimulatory molecules and major histocompatibility complex class-I in human hepatocellular carcinoma. J Gastroenterol Hepatol 2004;19: 1121–1127.
34 Goeppert B, Frauenschuh L, Zucknick M, et al: Major histocompatibility complex class I expression impacts on patient survival and type and density of immune cells in biliary tract cancer. Br J Cancer 2015;113:1343–1349.
35 Greten TF, Duffy AG, Korangy F: Hepatocellular carcinoma from an immunologic perspective. Clin Cancer Res 2013;19:6678–6685.
36 Xu XD, Hu J, Wang M, et al: Circulating myeloid-derived suppressor cells in patients with pancreatic cancer. Hepatobiliary Pancreat Dis Int 2016;15:99–105.
37 Gao Q, Wang XY, Qiu SJ, et al: Overexpression of PD-L1 significantly associates with tumor aggressiveness and postoperative recurrence in human hepatocellular carcinoma. Clin Cancer Res 2009;15:971–979.
38 Zeng Z, Shi F, Zhou L, et al: Upregulation of circulating PD-L1/PD-1 is associated with poor post-cryoablation prognosis in patients with HBV-related hepatocellular carcinoma. PLoS One 2011;6:e23621.
39 Ye Y, Zhou L, Xie X, Jiang G, Xie H, Zheng S: Interaction of B7-H1 on intrahepatic cholangiocarcinoma cells with PD-1 on tumor-infiltrating T cells as a mechanism of immune evasion. J Surg Oncol 2009;100:500–504.
40 Kirn DH, Thorne SH: Targeted and armed oncolytic poxviruses: a novel multi-mechanistic therapeutic class for cancer. Nat Rev Cancer 2009;9:64–71.
41 Park BH, Hwang T, Liu TC, et al: Use of a targeted oncolytic poxvirus, JX-594, in patients with refractory primary or metastatic liver cancer: a phase I trial. Lancet Oncol 2008;9: 533–542.
42 Heo J, Reid T, Ruo L, et al: Randomized dose-finding clinical trial of oncolytic immunotherapeutic vaccinia JX-594 in liver cancer. Nat Med 2013;19:329–336.
43 Sangro B, Gomez-Martin C, de la Mata M, et al: A clinical trial of CTLA-4 blockade with tremelimumab in patients with hepatocellular carcinoma and chronic hepatitis C. J Hepatol 2013;59:81–88.
44 El-Khoueiry AB, Melero I, Crocenzi TS, et al: Phase I/II safety and antitumor activity of nivolumab in patients with advanced hepatocellular carcinoma (HCC): CA209-040. J Clin Oncol 2015;33:LBA101.
45 Greten TF, Korangy F: Radiofrequency ablation for the treatment of HCC–maybe much more than simple tumor destruction? J Hepatol 2010;53:775–776.

46 den Brok MH, Sutmuller RP, Nierkens S, et al: Efficient loading of dendritic cells following cryo and radiofrequency ablation in combination with immune modulation induces anti-tumour immunity. Br J Cancer 2006;95: 896–905.
47 Zerbini A, Pilli M, Penna A, et al: Radiofrequency thermal ablation of hepatocellular carcinoma liver nodules can activate and enhance tumor-specific T-cell responses. Cancer Res 2006;66:1139–1146.
48 Zerbini A, Pilli M, Fagnoni F, et al: Increased immunostimulatory activity conferred to antigen-presenting cells by exposure to antigen extract from hepatocellular carcinoma after radiofrequency thermal ablation. J Immunother 2008;31:271–282.
49 Hansler J, Wissniowski TT, Schuppan D, et al: Activation and dramatically increased cytolytic activity of tumor specific T lymphocytes after radio-frequency ablation in patients with hepatocellular carcinoma and colorectal liver metastases. World J Gastroenterol 2006; 12:3716–3721.
50 Hiroishi K, Eguchi J, Baba T, et al: Strong CD8(+) T-cell responses against tumor-associated antigens prolong the recurrence-free interval after tumor treatment in patients with hepatocellular carcinoma. J Gastroenterol 2010;45:451–458.
51 Johnson EE, Yamane BH, Buhtoiarov IN, et al: Radiofrequency ablation combined with KS-IL2 immunocytokine (EMD 273066) results in an enhanced antitumor effect against murine colon adenocarcinoma. Clin Cancer Res 2009;15:4875–4884.
52 Nijkamp MW, Borren A, Govaert KM, et al: Radiofrequency ablation of colorectal liver metastases induces an inflammatory response in distant hepatic metastases but not in local accelerated outgrowth. J Surg Oncol 2010; 101:551–556.
53 Duffy AG, Makarova-Rusher OV, Kerkar SP, et al: A pilot study of tremelimumab – a monoclonal antibody against CTLA-4 – in combination with either trans catheter arterial chemoembolization (TACE) or radiofrequency ablation (RFA) in patients with hepatocellular carcinoma (HCC). J Clin Oncol 2015;33:4081.
54 Kaida M, Morita-Hoshi Y, Soeda A, et al: Phase 1 trial of Wilms tumor 1 (WT1) peptide vaccine and gemcitabine combination therapy in patients with advanced pancreatic or biliary tract cancer. J Immunother 2011;34:92–99.
55 Yamamoto K, Ueno T, Kawaoka T, et al: MUC1 peptide vaccination in patients with advanced pancreas or biliary tract cancer. Anticancer Res 2005;25:3575–3579.
56 Aruga A, Takeshita N, Kotera Y, et al: Phase I clinical trial of multiple-peptide vaccination for patients with advanced biliary tract cancer. J Transl Med 2014;12:61.
57 Kobayashi M, Sakabe T, Abe H, et al: Dendritic cell-based immunotherapy targeting synthesized peptides for advanced biliary tract cancer. J Gastrointest Surg 2013;17: 1609–1617.
58 Lepisto AJ, Moser AJ, Zeh H, et al: A phase I/II study of a MUC1 peptide pulsed autologous dendritic cell vaccine as adjuvant therapy in patients with resected pancreatic and biliary tumors. Cancer Ther 2008;6:955–964.
59 Shimomura A, Fujiwara Y, Kondo S, et al: Tremelimumab-associated tumor regression following after initial progression: two case reports. Immunotherapy 2016;8:9–15.
60 Bang YJ, Doi T, De Braud F, Piha-Paul S, Hollebecque A, Abdul Razak AR, Lin CC, Ott PA, He AR, Yuan SS, Koshiji M, Lam B, Aggarwal R: Safety and efficacy of pembrolizumab (MK-3475) in patients (pts) with advanced biliary tract cancer: Interim results of KEYNOTE-028. Eur J Cancer 2015;51(suppl 3):S112.
61 Duffy AG, Greten TF: Immunological off-target effects of standard treatments in gastrointestinal cancers. Ann Oncol 2014;25:24–32.
62 Liu WM, Fowler DW, Smith P, Dalgleish AG: Pre-treatment with chemotherapy can enhance the antigenicity and immunogenicity of tumours by promoting adaptive immune responses. Br J Cancer 2010;102:115–123.
63 Burris H, Storniolo AM: Assessing clinical benefit in the treatment of pancreas cancer: gemcitabine compared to 5-fluorouracil. Eur J Cancer 1997;33(suppl 1):S18–S22.
64 Koido S, Kan S, Yoshida K, et al: Immunogenic modulation of cholangiocarcinoma cells by chemoimmunotherapy. Anticancer Res 2014;34:6353–6361.

Complications of Liver Disease

Digestive Diseases

Dig Dis 2017;35:397–401
DOI: 10.1159/000456594

Novel Approaches to Reducing the Risk of Variceal Hemorrhage

Frederik Nevens

Department of Gastroenterology and Hepatology, University Hospitals KU Leuven, Leuven, Belgium

Keywords

Portal hypertension · Variceal bleeding · Elastography · FXR agonist · Non-selective beta blockers · Self-expanding stent

Abstract

Background: Complications of advanced liver disease occur at the moment of clinical significant portal hypertension. Nitric oxide (NO) dysfunction and fibrosis play an important role in the pathophysiology of PH, but other mechanisms are also involved. Non-selective beta blockers (NSBB) stay the cornerstone in the primary and secondary prevention of variceal bleeding, but their safety in advanced cirrhosis has been recently debated and new drugs are under investigation. Transjugular intrahepatic portosystemic shunt and balloon tamponade are the standard therapy in case of refractory variceal bleeding, but both interventions have drawbacks. ***Key Message:*** Transelastography under certain conditions and the presence of collateral circulation on imaging allow to rule-in CSPH, which makes patients open at risk for variceal hemorrhage. FXR agonists are intrahepatic NO donors; they reduce fibrosis and prevent bacterial translocation, which make them promising drugs for the treatment of PH. NSBB should be used with caution in patients with refractory ascites and certainly in those with hepatorenal syndrome. Preliminary clinical data suggest that simvastatin and enoxaparin improve the prognosis of patients with cirrhosis. Finally, covered esophageal metallic stents are safer and more effective than balloon tamponade in the case of refractory variceal bleeding. ***Conclusions:*** Liver stiffness measurements enable the selection of patients for endoscopic screening for esophageal varices. In the case of tense ascites, the dose of NSBB should be adapted to the hemodynamic condition of the patient. Self-expanding, covered esophageal metallic stents replace balloon tamponade in the treatment of massive variceal hemorrhage.

One of the most frequent complications of chronic advanced liver disease is portal hypertension (PH), since it is the main cause of death and it triggers liver transplantation. More than in the case of ascites and hepatic encephalopathy, variceal rupture and bleeding are directly linked to the level of portal pressure [1].

Diagnosis of Clinical Significant PH

Variceal bleeding occurs when the portal pressure gradient increases ≥10 mm Hg and this is called clinical significant PH (CSPH) [2]. However, a marked reduction of the risk of variceal bleeding can also be achieved with less marked reduction of the portal pressure gradient [3]. Hepatic venous pressure measurement is the gold-standard method to assess the presence of CSPH. It should be measured with the occlusion-balloon technique [4].

KARGER

E-Mail karger@karger.com
www.karger.com/ddi

Frederik Nevens, MD, PhD
Hepatology – Liver Transplantation
University Hospitals KU Leuven
Herestraat 49, BE–3000 Leuven (Belgium)
E-Mail frederik.nevens@uzleuven.be

In patients with virus-related compensated advanced chronic liver disease and in the absence of ALT flares, non-invasive methods are sufficient to rule-in CSPH, defining the group of patients at risk of having endoscopic signs of PH, such as gastroesophageal varices and congestive gastropathy. The last Baveno consensus meeting defined this non-invasive method as a liver stiffness by transelastography of ≥20–25 kPa (at least 2 measurements on different days in fasting conditions) in patients with viral-induced cirrhosis. Also, imaging showing collateral circulation is sufficient to rule-in CSPH in patients of all etiologies [5]. In these patients, endoscopy should be performed to rule out large varices and if this is the case, prophylaxis to prevent variceal hemorrhage has to be started (Table 1).

Table 1. Non-invasive methods to rule-in clinical significant portal hypertension [5]

In patients with viral induced cirrhosis:
Transelastography ≥20–25 kPa (≥2 measurements on different days in fasting conditions)
In patients with all etiologies:
Collateral circulation on imaging

Treatment of PH

Evolution of the Treatment Strategies

Whereas direct reduction of portal pressure by portosystemic shunts, initially surgical and later on by transjugular intrahepatic portosystemic shunt (TIPS), resulted in improved outcome of our patients with variceal bleeding [6], understanding of the pathophysiology of PH led to other successful treatment plans (Table 2). Demonstration that increased portal inflow was an important contributor to PH led to the use of non-selective beta blockers (NSBB) in chronic conditions and vasoconstrictors (terlipressin, somatostatin, and analogues) in acute conditions with a significant decrease in mortality [7, 8]. Further understanding that there was a partial reversible increased intrahepatic resistance in which nitric oxide (NO) dysfunction played a major role, resulted in the treatment of vasodilating nitrates in combination with NSBB [9, 10]. Fibrosis is one of the main reasons of the increased intrahepatic resistance. In this regard, reversal of fibrosis has been demonstrated after control or cure of the cause of the disease, leading to an improvement of the PH. Nevertheless, Hepatitis C patients with CSPH remain at risk for variceal bleeding, irrespective of the patient's response to antiviral therapy [11]. Finally, recent advances in the knowledge of the pathophysiology of PH have led to the discovery of intrahepatic vascular thrombosis and bacterial translocation as factors worsening PH [12]. In this regard, FXR agonists, which improve in rats PH, reduce fibrosis and prevent bacterial translocation, are promising drugs in the treatment of PH [13–16].

Old Strategies with New Insights

The NSBBs propranolol and nadolol have been used in the management of cirrhosis and PH for over 25 years. Carvedilol, an NSBB with weak anti-α adrenergic (vasodilator) activity has been shown to have a significant hemodynamic response rate in propranolol non-responders. In a lower dose as previously used (median 12.5 mg/day), it was better tolerated (no drop in mean arterial pressure and no fluid retention) [17, 18]. In contrast to propranolol/nadolol, carvedilol was effective in one study in preventing the progression of small to large varices [19]. However, the overall quality of evidence is still low to replace systematically carvedilol instead of propranonol/nadolol [20].

It has recently been suggested that patients with refractory ascites on NSBB have a higher mortality than those without [21–23]. Other retrospective studies and meta analyses could not confirm this [24–26], but it is nevertheless possible that in a subset of patients with refractory ascites in whom the cardiac response to hypotension may be inadequate, NSBB may lead to a disturbance in the circulatory status, and therefore the Baveno consensus meeting recommended that for the given time, NSBB should be used cautiously in case of a systolic blood pressure <90 mm Hg, serum sodium <130 mEq/L or acute kidney injury [5]. In this regard, a recent study demonstrated that there was no clinical or hemodynamic rebound after abrupt interruption of NSBB in patients with cirrhosis [27]. Finally, prophylactic NSBB treatment is not an aggravating factor for the short-term mortality in case of variceal bleeding [28].

New Drugs to Improve PH

Preclinical data suggested that simvastatin modifies hepatic vascular tone by acting on NO signaling and improves liver fibrogenesis. A clinical study could not confirm an additional beneficial effect on top of the standard therapy on the risk of rebleeding, but an improved survival was observed [29]. Probably, a reduction in the bleeding-related mortality due to a better microcircula-

Table 2. Treatment of portal hypertension

Mechanism	Treatment
Invasive reduction of portal pressure	TIPS
Reduction of increased portal inflow	Acute conditions: – Terlipressin, somatostatin and analogues Chronic conditions: – NSBB – Carvedilol
Reduction of intrahepatic resistance	Intrahepatic NO donors: – Nitrates in combination with NSBB – Simvastatin – FXR agonists? Prevention of intrahepatic vascular thrombosis: – Enoxaparin Antifibrotic: – Simvastatin – FXR agonists? Prevention of bacterial translocation: – FXR agonists?

tion and the attenuation of the liver inflammation in relation with the hemorrhage, resulted in a survival benefit.

With regard to the role of thrombosis on the development of PH, a recent clinical paper, which showed a potential beneficial effect of enoxaparin in subgroups of patients with cirrhosis, supports this concept [30]. In this regard, anticoagulation does not have an important impact on the outcome of an upper gastrointestinal bleeding in patients with cirrhosis [31].

Advances in the Treatment of Acute Esophageal Bleeding

TIPS became the standard therapy for variceal bleeding in case endoscopic and vasoactive therapy failed [6, 32]. Long-term improved patency with covered versus bare stents has been established [33]. This results in a lower risk of rebleeding and reduced costs [34]. In this regard, covered TIPS was superior to endoscopic variceal ligation + NSBB for reduction of variceal rebleeding but was still associated with higher rates of early hepatic encephalopathy [35, 36].

Finally, self-expanding, covered esophageal metallic stents achieve similar or greater hemostatic rates, can be left in place for much longer periods (up to 7 days), cause fewer severe complications and are safer than balloon tamponade [37].

Disclosure Statement

Frederik Nevens received a consultancy fee from Intercept Pharmaceuticals.

References

1 Nevens F, Bustami R, Scheys I, Lesaffre E, Fevery J: Variceal pressure is a factor predicting the risk of a first variceal bleeding: a prospective cohort study in cirrhotic patients. Hepatology 1998;27:15–19.

2 Groszmann RJ, Garcia-Tsao G, Bosch J, Grace ND, Burroughs AK, Planas R, Escorsell A, Garcia-Pagan JC, Patch D, Matloff DS, Gao H, Makuch R; Portal Hypertension Collaborative Group: Beta-blockers to prevent gastroesophageal varices in patients with cirrhosis. N Engl J Med 2005;353:2254–2261.

3 D'Amico G, Garcia-Pagan JC, Luca A, Bosch J: Hepatic vein pressure gradient reduction and prevention of variceal bleeding in cirrhosis: a systematic review. Gastroenterology 2006;131:1611–1624.

4 Maleux G, Willems E, Fieuws S, Heye S, Vaninbroukx J, Laleman W, Cassiman D, Verslype C, Nevens F: Prospective study comparing different indirect methods to measure portal pressure. J Vasc Interv Radiol 2011;22:1553–1558.

5 de Franchis R; Baveno VI Faculty: Expanding consensus in portal hypertension: report of the Baveno VI Consensus Workshop: stratifying risk and individualizing care for portal hypertension. J Hepatol 2015;63:743–752.

6 García-Pagán JC, Caca K, Bureau C, Laleman W, Appenrodt B, Luca A, Abraldes JG, Nevens F, Vinel JP, Mössner J, Bosch J; Early TIPS (Transjugular Intrahepatic Portosystemic Shunt) Cooperative Study Group: Early use of TIPS in patients with cirrhosis and variceal bleeding. N Engl J Med 2010;362:2370–2379.
7 Lebrec D, Nouel O, Corbic M, Benhamou JP: Propranolol – a medical treatment for portal hypertension? Lancet 1980;2:180–182.
8 Avgerinos A, Nevens F, Raptis S, Fevery J: Early administration of somatostatin and efficacy of sclerotherapy in acute oesophageal variceal bleeds: the European Acute Bleeding Oesophageal Variceal Episodes (ABOVE) randomised trial. Lancet 1997;350:1495–1499.
9 Van de Casteele M, Omasta A, Janssens S, Roskams T, Desmet V, Nevens F, Fevery J: In vivo gene transfer of endothelial nitric oxide synthase decreases portal pressure in anaesthetised carbon tetrachloride cirrhotic rats. Gut 2002;51:440–445.
10 Laleman W, Van Landeghem L, Van der Elst I, Zeegers M, Fevery J, Nevens F: Nitroflurbiprofen, a nitric oxide-releasing cyclooxygenase inhibitor, improves cirrhotic portal hypertension in rats. Gastroenterology. 2007; 132:709–719.
11 Lens S, Rincón D, García-Retortillo M, Albillos A, Calleja JL, Bañares R, Abraldes JG, Bosch J, Sanchez-Tapias JM, Forns X, García-Pagán JC: Association between severe portal hypertension and risk of liver decompensation in patients with hepatitis C, regardless of response to antiviral therapy. Clin Gastroenterol Hepatol 2015;13:1846–1853.
12 Wanless IR, Wong F, Blendis LM, Greig P, Heathcote EJ, Levy G: Hepatic and portal vein thrombosis in cirrhosis: possible role in development of parenchymal extinction and portal hypertension. Hepatology 1995;21:1238–1247.
13 Nevens F, Andreone P, Mazzella G, Strasser SI, Bowlus C, Invernizzi P, Drenth JP, Pockros PJ, Regula J, Beuers U, Trauner M, Jones DE, Floreani A, Hohenester S, Luketic V, Shiffman M, van Erpecum KJ, Vargas V, Vincent C, Hirschfield GM, Shah H, Hansen B, Lindor KD, Marschall HU, Kowdley KV, Hooshmand-Rad R, Marmon T, Sheeron S, Pencek R, MacConell L, Pruzanski M, Shapiro D; POISE Study Group: A placebo-controlled trial of obeticholic acid in primary biliary cholangitis. N Engl J Med 2016;375: 631–643.
14 Verbeke L, Farre R, Verbinnen B, Covens K, Vanuytsel T, Verhaegen J, Komuta M, Roskams T, Chatterjee S, Annaert P, Vander Elst I, Windmolders P, Trebicka J, Nevens F, Laleman W: The FXR agonist obeticholic acid prevents gut barrier dysfunction and bacterial translocation in cholestatic rats. Am J Pathol 2015;185:409–419.
15 Verbeke L, Farre R, Trebicka J, Komuta M, Roskams T, Klein S, Elst IV, Windmolders P, Vanuytsel T, Nevens F, Laleman W: Obeticholic acid, a farnesoid X receptor agonist, improves portal hypertension by two distinct pathways in cirrhotic rats. Hepatology 2014; 59:2286–2298.
16 Verbeke L, Mannaerts I, Schierwagen R, Govaere O, Klein S, Vander Elst I, Windmolders P, Farre R, Wenes M, Mazzone M, Nevens F, van Grunsven LA, Trebicka J, Laleman W: FXR agonist obeticholic acid reduces hepatic inflammation and fibrosis in a rat model of toxic cirrhosis. Sci Rep 2016;6:33453.
17 Reiberger T, Ulbrich G, Ferlitsch A, Payer BA, Schwabl P, Pinter M, Heinisch BB, Trauner M, Kramer L, Peck-Radosavljevic M; Vienna Hepatic Hemodynamic Lab: Carvedilol for primary prophylaxis of variceal bleeding in cirrhotic patients with haemodynamic nonresponse to propranolol. Gut 2013;62:1634–1641.
18 Sinagra E, Perricone G, D'Amico M, Tinè F, D'Amico G: Systematic review with meta-analysis: the haemodynamic effects of carvedilol compared with propranolol for portal hypertension in cirrhosis. Aliment Pharmacol Ther 2014;39:557–568.
19 Bhardwaj A, Kedarisetty CK, Vashishtha C, Bhadoria AS, Jindal A, Kumar G, Choudhary A, Shasthry SM, Maiwall R, Kumar M, Bhatia V, Sarin SK: Carvedilol delays the progression of small oesophageal varices in patients with cirrhosis: a randomised placebo-controlled trial. Gut 2016, Doi: 10.1136/gutjnl-2016-311735 [Epub ahead of print].
20 Li T, Ke W, Sun P, Chen X, Belgaumkar A, Huang Y, Xian W, Li J, Zheng Q: Carvedilol for portal hypertension in cirrhosis: systematic review with meta-analysis. BMJ Open 2016;6:e010902.
21 Sersté T, Melot C, Francoz C, Durand F, Rautou PE, Valla D, Moreau R, Lebrec D: Deleterious effects of beta-blockers on survival in patients with cirrhosis and refractory ascites. Hepatology 2010;52:1017–1022.
22 Sersté T, Francoz C, Durand F, Rautou PE, Melot C, Valla D, Moreau R, Lebrec D: Beta-blockers cause paracentesis-induced circulatory dysfunction in patients with cirrhosis and refractory ascites: a cross-over study. J Hepatol 2011;55:794–799.
23 Mandorfer M, Bota S, Schwabl P, Bucsics T, Pfisterer N, Kruzik M, Hagmann M, Blacky A, Ferlitsch A, Sieghart W, Trauner M, Peck-Radosavljevic M, Reiberger T: Nonselective β blockers increase risk for hepatorenal syndrome and death in patients with cirrhosis and spontaneous bacterial peritonitis. Gastroenterology 2014; 146: 1680–1690.
24 Leithead JA, Rajoriya N, Tehami N, Hodson J, Gunson BK, Tripathi D, Ferguson JW: Nonselective β-blockers are associated with improved survival in patients with ascites listed for liver transplantation. Gut 2015;64:1111–1119.
25 Bossen L, Krag A, Vilstrup H, Watson H, Jepsen P: Nonselective β-blockers do not affect mortality in cirrhosis patients with ascites: post hoc analysis of three randomized controlled trials with 1198 patients. Hepatology 2016;63:1968–1976.
26 Chirapongsathorn S, Valentin N, Alahdab F, Krittanawong C, Erwin PJ, Murad MH, Kamath PS: Nonselective β-blockers and survival in patients with cirrhosis and Ascites: a systematic review and meta-analysis. Clin Gastroenterol Hepatol 2016;14:1096–1104.
27 Payancé A, Bissonnette J, Roux O, Elkrief L, Gault N, Francoz C, Nekachtali O, Soubrane O, Lebrec D, Valla D, Durand F, Rautou PE: Lack of clinical or haemodynamic rebound after abrupt interruption of beta-blockers in patients with cirrhosis. Aliment Pharmacol Ther 2016;43:966–973.
28 de Souza AR, La Mura V, Berzigotti A, García-Pagán JC, Abraldes JG, Bosch J: Prognosis of acute variceal bleeding: is being on beta-blockers an aggravating factor? A short-term survival analysis. Hepatology 2015;62:1840–1846.
29 Abraldes JG, Villanueva C, Aracil C, Turnes J, Hernandez-Guerra M, Genesca J, Rodriguez M, Castellote J, García-Pagán JC, Torres F, Calleja JL, Albillos A, Bosch J; BLEPS Study Group: Addition of simvastatin to standard therapy for the prevention of variceal rebleeding does not reduce rebleeding but increases survival in patients with cirrhosis. Gastroenterology 2016;150:1160–1170.
30 Villa E, Cammà C, Marietta M, Luongo M, Critelli R, Colopi S, Tata C, Zecchini R, Gitto S, Petta S, Lei B, Bernabucci V, Vukotic R, De Maria N, Schepis F, Karampatou A, Caporali C, Simoni L, Del Buono M, Zambotto B, Turola E, Fornaciari G, Schianchi S, Ferrari A, Valla D: Enoxaparin prevents portal vein thrombosis and liver decompensation in patients with advanced cirrhosis. Gastroenterology 2012;143:1253–1260.
31 Cerini F, Gonzalez JM, Torres F, Puente Á, Casas M, Vinaixa C, Berenguer M, Ardevol A, Augustin S, Llop E, Senosiaín M, Villanueva C, de la Peña J, Bañares R, Genescá J, Sopeña J, Albillos A, Bosch J, Hernández-Gea V, Garcia-Pagán JC: Impact of anticoagulation on upper-gastrointestinal bleeding in cirrhosis. A retrospective multicenter study. Hepatology 2015;62:575–583.
32 Garcia-Pagán JC, Di Pascoli M, Caca K, Laleman W, Bureau C, Appenrodt B, Luca A, Zipprich A, Abraldes JG, Nevens F, Vinel JP, Sauerbruch T, Bosch J: Use of early-TIPS for high-risk variceal bleeding: results of a post-RCT surveillance study. J Hepatol 2013;58: 45–50.
33 Geeroms B, Laleman W, Laenen A, Heye S, Verslype C, van der Merwe S, Nevens F, Maleux G: Expanded polytetrafluoroethylene-covered stent-grafts for transjugular intrahepatic portosystemic shunts in cirrhotic patients: long-term patency and clinical outcome results. Eur Radiol 2016, September 15 [Epub ahead of print].

34 Perarnau JM, Le Gouge A, Nicolas C, d'Alteroche L, Borentain P, Saliba F, Minello A, Anty R, Chagneau-Derrode C, Bernard PH, Abergel A, Ollivier-Hourmand I, Gournay J, Ayoub J, Gaborit C, Rusch E, Giraudeau B; STIC-TIPS Group: Covered vs. uncovered stents for transjugular intrahepatic portosystemic shunt: a randomized controlled trial. J Hepatol 2014;60:962–968.
35 Sauerbruch T, Mengel M, Dollinger M, Zipprich A, Rössle M, Panther E, Wiest R, Caca K, Hoffmeister A, Lutz H, Schoo R, Lorenzen H, Trebicka J, Appenrodt B, Schepke M, Fimmers R; German Study Group for Prophylaxis of Variceal Rebleeding: Prevention of rebleeding from esophageal varices in patients with cirrhosis receiving small-diameter stents versus hemodynamically controlled medical therapy. Gastroenterology 2015;149:660–668.
36 Holster IL, Tjwa ET, Moelker A, Wils A, Hansen BE, Vermeijden JR, Scholten P, van Hoek B, Nicolai JJ, Kuipers EJ, Pattynama PM, van Buuren HR: Covered transjugular intrahepatic portosystemic shunt versus endoscopic therapy + β-blocker for prevention of variceal rebleeding. Hepatology 2016;63:581–589.
37 Escorsell À, Pavel O, Cárdenas A, Morillas R, Llop E, Villanueva C, Garcia-Pagán JC, Bosch J; Variceal Bleeding Study Group: Esophageal balloon tamponade versus esophageal stent in controlling acute refractory variceal bleeding: a multicenter randomized, controlled trial. Hepatology 2016;63:1957–1967.

Complications of Liver Disease

Digestive Diseases

Dig Dis 2017;35:402–410
DOI: 10.1159/000456595

Translating Our Current Understanding of Ascites Management into New Therapies for Patients with Cirrhosis and Fluid Retention

Elisa Pose Andres Cardenas

GI/Liver Unit, Institut de Malalties Digestives i Metabòliques of Hospital Clínic, and University of Barcelona, Barcelona, Spain

Keywords

Cirrhosis · Ascites · Portal hypertension · Sodium retention · Hypervolemic hyponatremia · Hepatorenal syndrome · Spontaneous bacterial peritonitis

Abstract

Ascites is the most common complication associated with cirrhosis resulting in poor quality of life, high risk of development of other complications of cirrhosis, increased morbidity and mortality associated with surgical interventions, and poor long-term outcome. Patients with cirrhosis and a first onset of ascites, have a probability of survival of 85% during the first year and 56% at 5 years without liver transplantation. Ascites is caused due to increased renal sodium retention as a result of increased activity of the renin-angiotensin-aldosterone system in response to marked vasodilation of the splanchnic circulation. The practical management of ascites involves the proper evaluation of a patient with a thorough history and physical exam. In addition, complete laboratory, ascitic fluid, and radiological tests should be performed. One of the most important steps in the initial assessment of patients with ascites is to refer the appropriate candidates for liver transplantation, as it offers a definitive cure for cirrhosis and its complications. While the initial management of uncomplicated ascites with low sodium diet and diuretic treatment is straightforward in a majority of patients, approximately 10% of patients fail to respond to diuretics and become a real therapeutic challenge. The initial treatment of choice in patients with refractory ascites is large-volume paracentesis (LVP) associated with intravenous albumin; some patients also benefit from transjugular intrahepatic portosystemic shunts (TIPS). When repeated LVP or TIPS cannot be performed, other approaches using vasoconstrictors such as midodrine can be considered although data are scarce. A newly designed automated low flow pump system (Alfapump), which is designed to move ascites from the peritoneal cavity to the urinary bladder where it is eliminated spontaneously through diuresis is promising, but the data are also limited and safety is still a matter of concern. This article focuses on the practical aspects of the evaluation and treatment of patients with ascites and cirrhosis and also discusses how to translate our current understanding of ascites pathophysiology into new treatment methods for patients with fluid retention.

Introduction

Ascites is the most common complication in patients with cirrhosis, and approximately 60% of patients with cirrhosis will develop ascites within 10 years this disease is diagnosed [1]. Patients with the first onset of ascites have a probability of survival of 85% during the first year and 56% at 5 years without liver transplantation [2]. The development of ascites occurs only when portal hypertension exists and also only when the portal pressure as mea-

Andres Cardenas, MD, MMSc, PhD, AGAF, FAASLD
Institut de Malalties Digestives i Metaboliques
University of Barcelona
Hospital Clinic – Villarroel 170, Esc 3-2, ES–08036 Barcelona (Spain)
E-Mail acardena@clinic.ub.es or acv69@hotmail.com

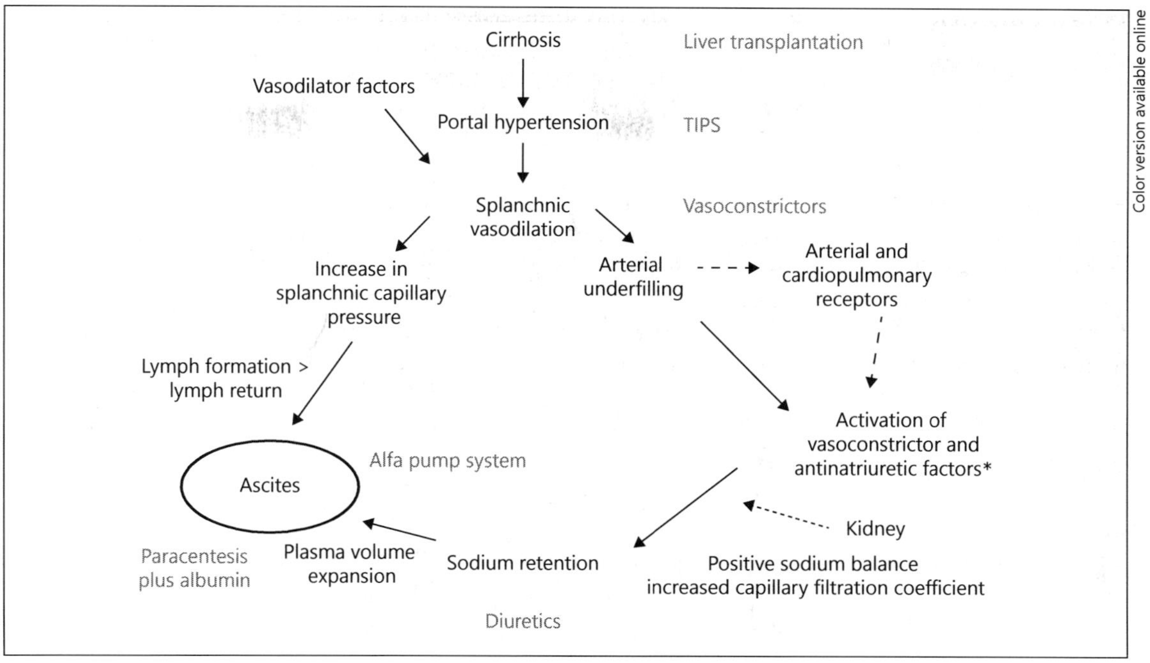

Fig. 1. Pathogenesis of ascites formation in cirrhosis and current therapeutic options for ascites. Portal hypertension is the main factor responsible for the development of splanchnic vasodilation and a decrease in effective arterial blood volume due to vasodilator factors such as nitric oxide. This leads to the activation of antinatriuretic and vasoconstrictor factors (mainly renin-angiotensin–aldosterone system, sympathetic nervous system and argine vasopressin) with subsequent sodium retention. The transjugular intrahepatic portosystemic shunt by reducing portal pressure is an effective treatment of ascites, particularly in patients with refractory ascites. The use of diuretics (spironolactone) that promote natriuresis is the preferred therapy for patients with sodium retention and fluid accumulation. Patients with large-volume ascites should be treated with therapeutic paracentesis and albumin administration followed by diuretics as tolerated. Other options include the use of oral vasocontrictors such as midodrine and also the use of an automated low flow pump system (Alfapump), which is designed to move ascites from the peritoneal cavity to the urinary bladder where it is eliminated spontaneously through dieresis.

sured by hepatic venous pressure gradient is above 12 mm Hg [3]. The major factor contributing to ascites formation is a splanchnic vasodilation secondary to portal hypertension, which results in a decreased effective arterial blood volume [4–6]. Increased hepatic resistance to portal flow due to cirrhosis causes a progressive increase in portal pressure with collateral vein formation with shunting of blood to the systemic circulation. As portal hypertension develops, splanchnic arterial vasodilation occurs due to the enhanced local production of nitric oxide and other vasodilators including carbon monoxide and endogenous cannabinoids as a consequence of endothelial stretching and bacterial translocation [7–10]. In advanced stages of cirrhosis, splanchnic arterial vasodilation is very intense with a markedly reduced effective arterial blood volume that causes arterial pressure to drop [4–6]. As a consequence of the impairment in effective arterial blood volume, there is homeostatic activation of vasoconstrictor and antinatriuretic factors to maintain arterial pressure, resulting in renal sodium and fluid retention. The combination of portal hypertension and splanchnic arterial vasodilation alters the intestinal capillary pressure and permeability, which facilitates the accumulation of the retained fluid in the abdominal cavity. With disease progression, there is a marked impairment in renal solute-free water excretion and renal vasoconstriction, leading to hypervolemic hyponatremia and hepatorenal syndrome respectively. The pathophysiological rationale for the treatment of patients with cirrhosis and ascites is described in Figure 1.

Initial Approach

The initial evaluation of a patient with cirrhosis ascites should always include a meticulous history, physical examination, abdominal ultrasound, upper endoscopy to rule out esophageal varices, and laboratory

Dig Dis 2017;35:402–410
DOI: 10.1159/000456595

Table 1. Management practice points in patients with ascites and cirrhosis

A. Treatment strategy for patients with cirrhosis and moderate volume (grade 2) ascites Start with a low-sodium diet and spironolactone (50–100 mg/day) to reach goal of weight loss: 300–500 mg/day. If needed, doses to be increased every 7 days up to 400 mg/day of spironolactone. Furosemide can be added at a starting dose of 20–40 mg/day and subsequently increased to 160 mg/day if needed
B. Treatment strategy for patients with cirrhosis and large volume (grade 3) ascites Large volume paracentesis plus intravenous albumin (8 g per liter of ascites removed) followed by a low-sodium diet (90 mmol/day) and diuretics if patient tolerated them beforehand
C. Treatment strategy for refractory ascites Large volume paracentesis plus intravenous albumin can be performed as needed. Consider use of transjugular intrahepatic portosystemic shunt in patients with very frequent recurrent ascites very rapid recurrence of ascites and preserved liver function (bilirubin <5 mg/dL, platelet count >75,000, serum sodium level >130 mEq/L, Child–Pugh score <13, Model for End-Stage Liver Disease score <18), aged <70, without hepatic encephalopathy, central or large hepatocellular carcinoma or cardiopulmonary disease

assessment of blood, urine, and ascitic fluid. A urinary sodium level <10–20 mEq/day is indicative of severe sodium retention and indicates poor prognosis. All patients with cirrhosis and ascites should be considered for liver transplantation, given their low 5-year survival. The current classification by the International Ascites Club of Ascites divides patients into 3 groups [11]. In grade 1 ascites, fluid is detected only by ultrasound; in grade 2, ascites is moderate with symmetrical distention of the abdomen and in grade 3, ascites is large or tense with marked abdominal distention. A diagnostic paracentesis should always be performed to exclude causes of ascites other than cirrhosis and rule out spontaneous bacterial peritonitis in cirrhosis. It should be also performed in all patients with new onset of grade 2 or 3 ascites and patients hospitalized for worsening of ascites or any complication related to cirrhosis [12, 13].

Management of Patients with Ascites

General Measures

A low sodium diet of approximately 2–4 g of salt per day (80–120 mmol) (i.e., no added salt and no pre-processed meals) is the cornerstone of management [12–14] and should always be instituted appropriately. Fluid restriction is not necessary unless patients have hypervolemic hyponatremia (defined as a serum sodium less than 130 mEq/L together with ascites and/or edema). An evaluation by a nutritionist is of utmost importance for appropriate education regarding an adequate caloric, protein, and salt intake. Nutritional therapy in cirrhotic patients can improve nutritional status, reduce infection rates, and decrease perioperative morbidity [15]. Another essential measure is alcohol abstinence, as continued use is a cause for continuous ascites recurrence.

Specific Measures

Patients with grade 1 ascites do not require any specific treatment but should avoid foods with large amounts of salt and also stay away from alcohol use. Patients with grade 2 ascites are managed with sodium restriction and diuretics and those with grade 3 ascites with large-volume paracentesis (LVP) plus albumin along with diuretics. Patients with refractory ascites are those who do not respond to high doses of diuretics or develop side effects that preclude their use. The discussion of the management of ascites may therefore be divided into 3 parts: moderate-volume ascites (grade 2 ascites), large-volume ascites (grade 3), and refractory ascites. A summary of recommendations for the management of ascites is included in Table 1.

Grade 2 Ascites

These patients can be treated as outpatients and do not require admission unless they have other complications of cirrhosis. A negative sodium balance is usually obtained with low doses of diuretics that increase renal sodium excretion together with fluid excretion. The diuretics most frequently used in patients with cirrhosis and ascites are aldosterone antagonists, mainly spironolactone, which selectively antagonizes the sodium-retaining effects of aldosterone in the renal collecting tubules, and loop diuretics, especially furosemide, that inhibit the Na^+-K^+–$2Cl^-$ cotransporter in the loop of Henle. Diuretic therapy is effective in nearly 90% of patients with ascites without renal dysfunction [12, 14]. Patients with the first episode of as-

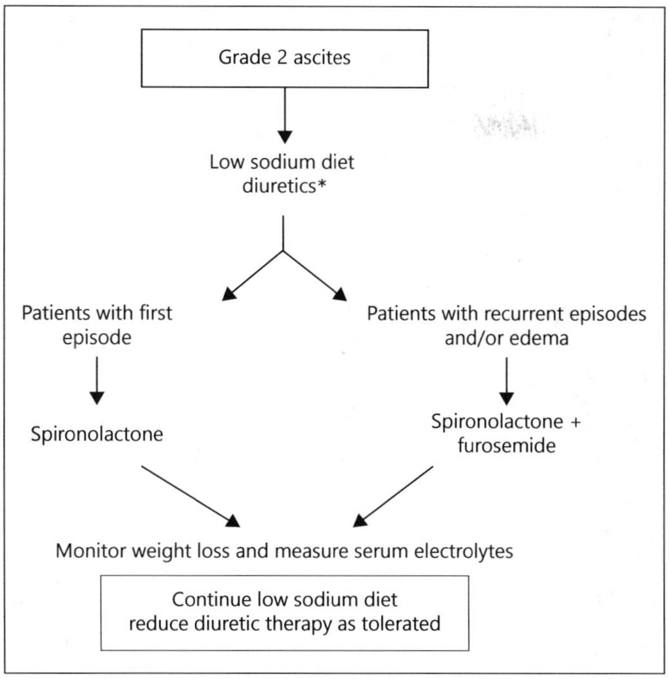

Fig. 2. Treatment strategy for patients with cirrhosis and grade 2 ascites. * Recommended diuretics are described in Table 1.

cites respond well to spironolactone 50–100 mg/day [12]. Those with recurrent episodes of ascites or peripheral edema should receive a combination of spironolactone 100 mg/day with furosemide 40 mg/day [12–14]. If there is no response, compliance with diet and medications should be confirmed and diuretics may then be increased every 7 days by doubling doses (1:1 ratio) to a maximal dose of spironolactone (400 mg/day) and a maximal dose of furosemide (160 mg/day). The goal of treatment is to produce an average weight loss of no more than 500 g/day in patients without peripheral edema and no more than 800–1,000 g/day in those with peripheral edema. In patients who do not respond, compliance with low sodium diet and diuretics should always be assessed. In these cases, a urine sodium measurement provides an accurate assessment of the response to diuretics, which may help in deciding whether there is a need to increase the dose.

Diuretics can cause critical disturbances in fluid and electrolyte balance including hyponatremia, dehydration, renal impairment, hyperkalemia, or hypokalemia. Patients should be closely followed up and serum and urine electrolytes need to be measured within the first 2 weeks after starting or modifying a dose. Diuretics should be stopped or their dose reduced if any of the above-mentioned effects appear. Spironolactone may cause tender gynecomastia and muscle cramps in some patients and in most instances, the dose needs to be reduced or the medication needs to be stopped. Alternative treatments to spironolactone in those patients who require discontinuation are amiloride and eplerenone, but these 2 drugs may be associated with recurrence of ascites. An algorithm explaining the treatment of grade 2 ascites is depicted in Figure 2.

Grade 3 Ascites

A majority of these patients have intense sodium retention (urine sodium frequently lower than 20 mEq/day). Complete removal of ascites with one session of LVP with intravenous albumin (8 g per liter tapped) followed by diuretics is the method of choice to treat large-volume ascites [16, 17]. LVP without plasma expanders is associated with a derangement in circulatory function characterized by the reduction of effective arterial blood volume with subsequent activation of vasoconstrictor and antinatriuretic factors [18, 19]. This post-paracentesis circulatory dysfunction is associated with a high ascites recurrence rate, development of renal failure and/or hyponatremia in 20% of cases, and shortened survival [18, 19]. This disorder can be effectively prevented with the administration of plasma expanders [19–22]. When less than 5 L of ascites are removed, artificial plasma expanders, saline and albumin are equally effective [20–22]. However, if more than 5 L are removed, albumin is recommended. A meta-analysis of 17 trials with a total 1,225 patients showed that albumin reduced morbidity and mortality among patients with tense ascites undergoing LVP, as compared with alternative treatments [23]. Since ascites will invariably recur after paracentesis, patients need to be started or continued on diuretics in order to prevent a positive sodium balance and recurrence of ascites [12]. An algorithm explaining the treatment of grade 3 ascites is depicted in Figure 3.

Refractory Ascites

This occurs in nearly 10% of patients with cirrhosis and ascites [24, 25]. In patients with refractory ascites, sodium excretion cannot be increased with diuretics either because patients do not respond to maximum doses of diuretics or they develop side effects with lower doses that prevent their use (Table 2). These patients in general have Child B or C cirrhosis, have features of advanced liver disease, a high recurrence rate of ascites after LVP, an increased risk of renal failure, and a poorer prognosis. Patients can be treated with either repeated LVP with plasma-expansion or transjugular intrahepatic portosystemic shunts (TIPS). Repeated LVP plus albumin is the recommended initial therapy for refractory ascites by current guidelines [12, 14].

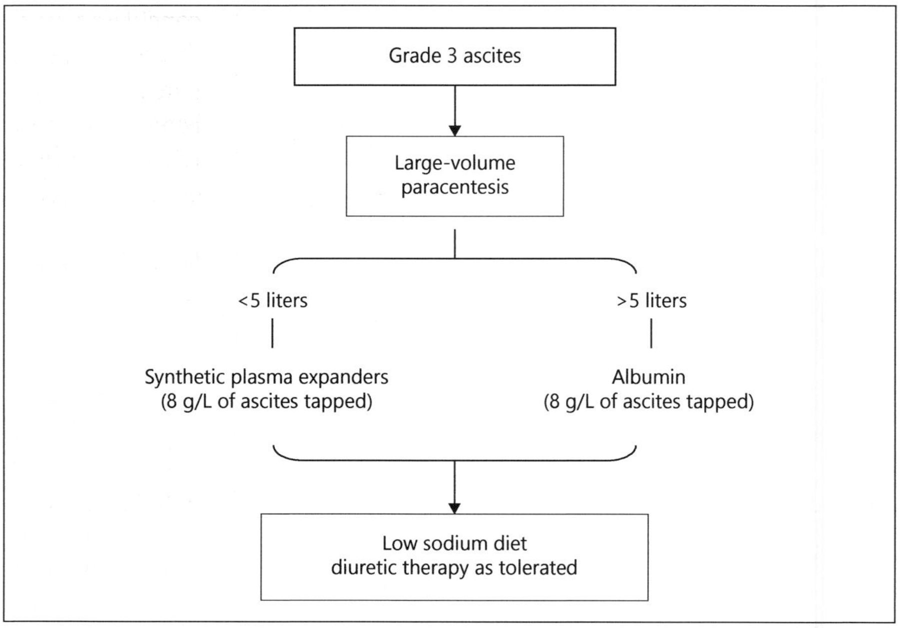

Fig. 3. Treatment strategy for patients with cirrhosis and grade 3 ascites.

Table 2. Definition and diagnostic criteria for refractory ascites in cirrhosis

Diuretic-resistant ascites Ascites that cannot be mobilized or the early recurrence of which cannot be prevented because of lack of response to sodium restriction and diuretic treatment
Diuretic-intractable ascites Ascites that cannot be mobilized or the early recurrence of which cannot be prevented because of the development of diuretic-induced complications that preclude the use of an effective diuretic dosage
Requisites 1. Treatment duration: patients must be on intensive diuretic therapy (spironolactone 400 mg/day and furosemide 160 mg/day) for at least 1 week and on a salt-restricted diet of less than 90 mmol/day.
2. Lack of response: mean weight loss of <0.8 kg over 4 days and urinary sodium output less than the sodium intake.
3. Early ascites recurrence: reappearance of grade 2 or 3 ascites within 4 weeks of initial mobilization.
4. Diuretic-induced complications: diuretic-induced hepatic encephalopathy is the development of encephalopathy in the absence of any other precipitating factor. Diuretic-induced renal impairment is an increase of serum creatinine by >100% to a value >2 mg/dL in patients with ascites responding to treatment. Diuretic-induced hyponatremia is defined as a decrease of serum sodium by >10 mEq/L to a serum sodium of <125 mEq/L. Diuretic induced hypo- or hyperkalemia is defined as a change in serum potassium to <3 or >6 mEq/L despite appropriate measures.

Patients generally require paracentesis every 2–4 weeks, and this can be done in the outpatient setting. The main drawback is early recurrence of ascites and repeated visits to the hospital. In contrast to paracentesis, TIPS, a nonsurgical method of portal decompression that consists of the insertion of an intrahepatic stent between one hepatic vein and the portal vein using a transjugular approach, is effective in preventing ascites recurrence because by reducing portal pressure, ascites disappears in most patients [26]. TIPS is very effective in relieving ascites but can be complicated by stenosis of the prosthesis and/or hepatic encephalopathy [26]. Six randomized clinical trials comparing uncovered TIPS vs. repeated paracentesis demonstrate that TIPS controls ascites effectively and is associated with a lower rate of ascites recurrence [27–32]. Hepatic encephalopathy may occur in approximately 30% of patients.

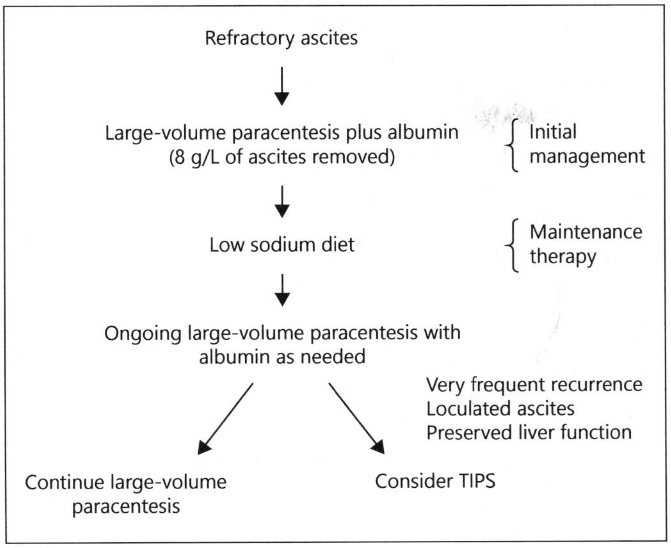

Fig. 4. Treatment strategy for patients with refractory ascites. Consider transjugular intrahepatic portosystemic shunt for those with very rapid recurrence of ascites and preserved liver function (bilirubin <5 mg/dL, platelet count >75,000, serum sodium level >130 mEq/L, Child–Pugh score <13, Model for End-Stage Liver Disease score <18), aged <70, without hepatic encephalopathy, central hepatocellular carcinoma or cardiopulmonary disease.

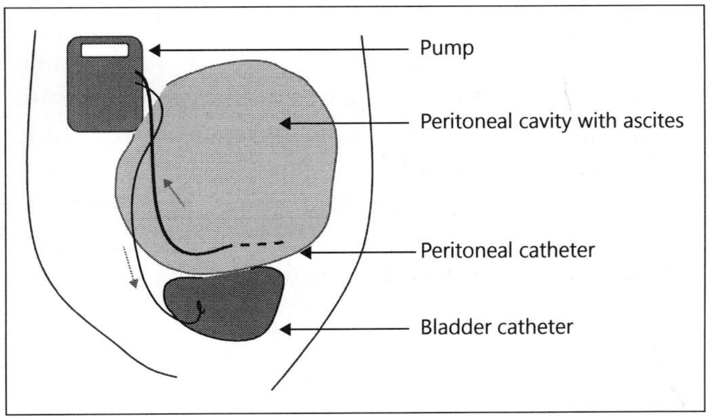

Color version available online

Fig. 5. Automated low flow pump system (Alfapump system). This device is a subcutaneous battery-operated pump that mobilizes ascites from peritoneum to the urinary bladder, where it is eliminated spontaneously through diuresis. Ascites is moved through a peritoneal catheter to another catheter that is implanted in the urinary bladder.

Several meta-analyses of these randomized controlled studies conclude that TIPS is more efficient than other methods at controlling ascites [33–37]. The 2 most recent meta-analyses of these trials indicate that TIPS significantly improves transplant-free survival of cirrhotic patients with refractory ascites [36, 37]. TIPS placement should be considered an option for patients with loculated ascites, those with very rapid recurrence of ascites and preserved liver function (bilirubin <5 mg/dL, Child–Pugh score <13, Model for End-Stage Liver Disease score <18), aged <70, without hepatic encephalopathy, central or large hepatocellular carcinoma or cardiopulmonary disease [24, 26]. An algorithm explaining the treatment of refractory ascites is depicted in Figure 4.

Other Therapies

Automated Low Flow Pump System (Alfapump System)

This device is used for the treatment of refractory ascites. It is a subcutaneous battery-operated pump that was designed to move ascites from peritoneum to the urinary bladder, where it is eliminated spontaneously through diuresis (Fig. 5). Although designed as symptomatic treatment for refractory ascites, it does not correct the underlying cause of the ascites that could help improve the pathogenic mechanisms that lead to the formation of ascites. Ascites is moved through a peritoneal catheter to another catheter that is implanted in the urinary bladder. An initial multicenter study that evaluated the safety and efficacy of this device showed that the pump removed 90% of the ascites and reduced the median number of LVP (3.4 vs. 0.2; $p < 0.01$) per month but with a significant rate of complications mainly due to infections and catheter dislodgement [38]. A small single-center study of 10 patients with refractory ascites showed that the need of paracentesis was reduced to a mean; however, the pump malfunctioned in half of these patients [39]. Finally, the preliminary results of a multicenter randomized controlled study that compared the Alfapump with LVP showed that the number of paracentesis per month were lower (0.2) for the alfapump compared to LVP (1.4) ($p < 0.0001$). There were no differences in survival between groups, and side effects were slightly more common in the Alfapump group [40].

Vaptans

These agents (V2 vasopressin receptor antagonists) act on the kidney and promote solute-free water diuresis can be combined with diuretics in order to improve mobilization of ascites and edema. The effects of V2 receptor antagonists on the distal tubule of the kidney by means of counteracting AVP lead to an increase in the excretion of solute-free water. Thus, these drugs have been evaluated for use in the management of hypervolemic hyponatremia and also ascites in cirrhosis. These drugs are not yet approved for patients with cirrhosis and ascites; however, tolvaptan is approved by the Food and Drug Administration and the European Medication agency for the treatment of hypervolemic and euvolemic hyponatremia. Other V2 receptor antagonists such as satavaptan were evaluated for use in the treatment of ascites in association with diuretics; however, long-term treatment studies in 3 different populations of patients with cirrhosis and ascites demonstrated a lack of efficacy in both ascites management and prevention of its recurrence [41, 42]. Furthermore, use of satavaptan was associated with an increased mortality and the drug was withdrawn from development. Although a number of studies have valuated tolvaptan for the management of refractory ascites in patients with cirrhosis [43–45], a major drawback of this drug is that there is a 23% risk of serious hepatic adverse events occurring with tolvaptan and thus, the FDA placed a black box warning on the drug limiting its use to patients with liver disease [46, 47].

Vasoconstrictors

The use of vasoconstrictor drugs can improve the underlying hemodynamic derangements that lead to ascites formation in cirrhosis, thereby reducing the activity of antinatriuretic factors. Data are available on the use of vasoconstrictors (midodrine and terlipressin) with plasma expansion in patients with cirrhosis and ascites. These drugs improve renal function, urinary sodium excretion, and serum sodium levels and decrease the levels of vasoactive/antinatriuretic systems in patients with advanced cirrhosis and hepatorenal syndrome. Therefore, the use of an oral vasoconstrictor is an attractive approach in the treatment of patients with ascites who do not respond to diuretics. In one study of 39 patients with cirrhosis, oral midodrine (an alpha-1 adrenergic agonist) 10 mg, t.i.d., was given to 11 patients without ascites and 12 with ascites and compared to placebo in 8 patients without ascites and 8 with ascites for 7 days [48]. In the midodrine group, there was a moderate increase in urine sodium excretion in patients with ascites (urinary sodium from 30 ± 15 to 49 ± 16 mEq/L) as well as glomerular filtration rate (from 80 ± 23 to 92 ± 27 mL/min) and urine volume (from 0.98 ± 0.26 to 1.15 ± 0.34 L) and significant decreases in plasma renin activity and aldosterone. Nonetheless, in this study, neither body weight nor abdominal girth as measures of an effect on ascites was recorded. Another study also demonstrated that oral midodrine (7.5 mg every 8 h) plus standard medical therapy (sodium restriction plus diuretics) was significantly superior to standard medical therapy alone in the control of ascites ($p = 0.013$) at 3 months [49]. The mortality rate in the standard medical therapy group was significantly higher than that in the midodrine group ($p < 0.046$). There was no significant difference in the frequency of complications at the end of follow-up. Intravenous terlipressin has also been evaluated as a potential therapy for patients with nonrefractory and refractory ascites. There is very limited information; however, available data indicate that it improves glomerular filtration rate and natriuresis in both types of ascites, but a clinical effect on weight or abdominal girth was not recorded [50, 51]. The use of these drugs in cirrhosis and ascites is limited to a small number of reports; therefore, more controlled studies are needed to evaluate their efficacy and safety in treating patients with ascites.

Clonidine, a centrally acting α_2-agonist and sympatholytic agent, was evaluated as an adjunct treatment in patients with cirrhosis and ascites. In a randomized study, oral clonidine (0.075 mg b.i.d.) led to a more rapid mobilization of ascites with fewer complications than placebo in patients with cirrhosis, ascites, and a plasma norepinephrine level of >300 pg/mL [52]. This medication was also evaluated in a randomized study of clonidine plus diuretics vs. diuretics alone, which showed that the highest efficacy was obtained in patients who had high serum levels of norepinephine and the presence of 2 specific genetic polymorphisms that predicted clonidine response in cirrhotic patients [53]. Although the results are interesting, the study was not a double-blind placebo-controlled trial, the medication was administered only for 3 months, and in practice genetic polymorphisms cannot be easily performed to ensure adequate response. More studies from other centers confirming the efficacy and safety of clonidine need to be carried out before considering this drug a therapeutic agent for patients with refractory ascites.

Disclosure Statement

The authors have nothing to disclose.

References

1 Ginés P, Quintero E, Arroyo V, et al: Compensated cirrhosis: natural history and prognostic factors. Hepatology 1987;7:122–128.

2 Planas R, Montoliu S, Ballesté B, et al: Natural history of patients hospitalized for management of cirrhotic ascites. Clin Gastroenterol Hepatol 2006;4:1385–1394.

3 Ripoll C, Groszmann R, Garcia-Tsao G, et al: Hepatic venous pressure gradient predicts clinical decompensation in patients with compensated cirrhosis. Gastroenterology 2007;133:481–488.

4 Ginès P, Cárdenas A, Solà E, Schrier RW: Liver disease and the kidney; in Schrier RW, Coffman TM, Falk RJ, Molitoris BA, Neilson EG (eds): Schrier's Diseases of the Kidney, ed 9. Philadelphia, Lippincott Williams & Wilkins, 2012, pp 1965–1996.
5 Schrier RW, Arroyo V, Bernardi M, Epstein M, Henriksen JH, Rodés J: Peripheral arterial vasodilation hypothesis: a proposal for the initiation of renal sodium and water retention in cirrhosis. Hepatology 1988;8:1151–1157.
6 Bernardi M, Moreau R, Angeli P, Schnabl B, Arroyo V: Mechanisms of decompensation and organ failure in cirrhosis: from peripheral arterial vasodilation to systemic inflammation hypothesis. J Hepatol 2015;63:1272–1284.
7 Iwakiri Y: Pathophysiology of portal hypertension. Clin Liver Dis 2014;18:281–291.
8 Caraceni P, Domenicali M, Giannone F, Bernardi M: The role of the endocannabinoid system in liver diseases. Best Pract Res Clin Endocrinol Metab 2009;23:65–77.
9 Wiest R, Garcia-Tsao G: Bacterial translocation (BT) in cirrhosis. Hepatology 2005;41:422–433.
10 Riordan SM, Williams R: The intestinal flora and bacterial infection in cirrhosis. J Hepatol 2006;45:744–757.
11 Moore KP, Wong F, Gines P, et al: The management of ascites in cirrhosis: report on the consensus conference of the International Ascites Club. Hepatology 2003;38:258–266.
12 European Association for the Study of the Liver: EASL clinical practice guidelines on the management of ascites, spontaneous bacterial peritonitis, and hepatorenal syndrome in cirrhosis. J Hepatol 2010;53:397–417.
13 Ginès P, Cárdenas A, Arroyo V, Rodés J: Management of cirrhosis and ascites. N Engl J Med 2004;350:1646–1654.
14 Runyon BA; AASLD Practice Guidelines Committee: Management of adult patients with ascites due to cirrhosis: an update. Hepatology 2009;49:2087–2107.
15 McCullough AJ: Nutrition and malnutrition in liver disease; in Wolfe MM, Davis GL, Farraye F, Giannella RA, Malagelada JR, Steer ML (eds): Therapy of Digestive Disorders, ed 2. Saunders, 2006, pp 67–83.
16 Ginés P, Arroyo V, Quintero E, et al: Comparison of paracentesis and diuretics in the treatment of cirrhotics with tense ascites. Results of a randomized study. Gastroenterology 1987;93:234–241.
17 Salerno F, Badalamenti S, Incerti P, et al: Repeated paracentesis and i.v. albumin infusion to treat 'tense' ascites in cirrhotic patients. A safe alternative therapy. J Hepatol 1987;5:102–108.
18 Ruiz-del-Arbol L, Monescillo A, Jimenéz W, et al: Paracentesis-induced circulatory dysfunction: mechanism and effect on hepatic hemodynamics in cirrhosis. Gastroenterology 1997;113:579–586.
19 Ginès P, Tito L, Arroyo V, et al: Randomized comparative study of therapeutic paracentesis with and without intravenous albumin in cirrhosis. Gastroenterology 1988;94:1493–1502.
20 Ginès A, Fernández-Esparrach G, Monescillo A, et al: Randomized trial comparing albumin, dextran 70, and polygeline in cirrhotic patients with ascites treated by paracentesis. Gastroenterology 1996;111:1002–1110.
21 Moreau R, Valla DC, Durand-Zaleski I, et al: Comparison of outcome in patients with cirrhosis and ascites following treatment with albumin or a synthetic colloid: a randomised controlled pilot trail. Liver Int 2006;26:46–54.
22 Sola-Vera J, Miñana J, Ricart E, et al: Randomized trial comparing albumin and saline in the prevention of paracentesis-induced circulatory dysfunction in cirrhotic patients with ascites. Hepatology 2003;37:1147–1153.
23 Bernardi M, Caraceni P, Navickis RJ, Wilkes MM: Albumin infusion in patients undergoing large-volume paracentesis: a meta-analysis of randomized trials. Hepatology 2012;55:1172–1181.
24 Cárdenas A, Ginès P: Management of refractory ascites. Clin Gastroenterol Hepatol 2005;3:1187–1191.
25 Salerno F, Guevara M, Bernardi M, Moreau R, Wong F, Angeli P, Garcia-Tsao G, Lee SS: Refractory ascites: pathogenesis, definition and therapy of a severe complication in patients with cirrhosis. Liver Int 2010;30:937–947.
26 Boyer TD, Haskal ZJ; American Association for the Study of Liver Diseases: The role of transjugular intrahepatic portosystemic shunt (TIPS) in the management of portal hypertension: update 2009. Hepatology 2010;51:306.
27 Lebrec D, Giuily N, Hadengue A, et al: Transjugular intrahepatic portosystemic shunts: comparison with paracentesis in patients with cirrhosis and refractory ascites: a randomized trial. French Group of Clinicians and a Group of Biologists. J Hepatol 1996;25:135–144.
28 Rössle M, Ochs A, Gülberg V, et al: A comparison of paracentesis and transjugular intrahepatic portosystemic shunting in patients with ascites. N Engl J Med 2000;342:1701–1707.
29 Ginès P, Uriz J, Calahorra B, et al: Transjugular intrahepatic portosystemic shunting versus paracentesis plus albumin for refractory ascites in cirrhosis. Gastroenterology 2002;123:1839–1847.
30 Sanyal AJ, Genning C, Reddy KR, et al: The North American study for the treatment of refractory ascites. Gastroenterology 2003;124:634–641.
31 Salerno F, Merli M, Riggio O, et al: Randomized controlled study of TIPS versus paracentesis plus albumin in cirrhosis with severe ascites. Hepatology 2004;40:629–635.
32 Narahara Y, Kanazawa H, Fukuda T, et al: Transjugular intrahepatic portosystemic shunt versus paracentesis plus albumin in patients with refractory ascites who have good hepatic and renal function: a prospective randomized trial. J Gastroenterol 2011;46:78–85.
33 Deltenre P, Mathurin P, Dharancy S, et al: Transjugular intrahepatic portosystemic shunt in refractory ascites: a meta-analysis. Liver Int 2005;25:349–356.
34 Albillos A, Bañares R, González M, et al: A meta-analysis of transjugular intrahepatic portosystemic shunt versus paracentesis for refractory ascites. J Hepatol 2005;43:990–996.
35 D'Amico G, Luca A, Morabito A, et al: Uncovered transjugular intrahepatic portosystemic shunt for refractory ascites: a meta-analysis. Gastroenterology 2005;129:1282–1293.
36 Salerno F, Cammà C, Enea M, et al: Transjugular intrahepatic portosystemic shunt for refractory ascites: a meta-analysis of individual patient data. Gastroenterology 2007;133:825–834.
37 Bai M, Qi XS, Yang ZP, Yang M, Fan DM, Han GH: TIPS improves liver transplantation-free survival in cirrhotic patients with refractory ascites: an updated meta-analysis. World J Gastroenterol 2014;20:2704–2714.
38 Bellot P, Welker MW, Soriano G, et al: Automated low flow pump system for the treatment of refractory ascites: a multi-center safety and efficacy study. J Hepatol 2013;58:922–927.
39 Thomas MN, Sauter GH, Gerbes AL, Stangl M, Schiergens TS, Angele M, Werner J, Guba M: Automated low flow pump system for the treatment of refractory ascites: a single-center experience. Langenbecks Arch Surg 2015;400:979–983.
40 Adebayo D, Bureau C, deRieu MC, et al: Alfapump system versus large volume paracentesis in the treatment of refractory ascites; results from a multicenter randomised controlled study (RCT). J Hepatol 2016;64:GS18A.
41 Wong F, Gines P, Watson H, Horsmans Y, Angeli P, Gow P, Minini P, Bernardi M: Effects of a selective vasopressin V2 receptor antagonist, satavaptan, on ascites recurrence after paracentesis in patients with cirrhosis. J Hepatol 2010;53:283–290.
42 Wong F, Watson H, Gerbes A, Vilstrup H, Badalamenti S, Bernardi M, Ginès P; Satavaptan Investigators Group: Satavaptan for the management of ascites in cirrhosis: efficacy and safety across the spectrum of ascites severity. Gut 2012;61:108–116.
43 Ohki T, Sato K, Yamada T, Yamagami M, Ito D, Kawanishi K, Kojima K, Seki M, Toda N, Tagawa K: Efficacy of tolvaptan in patients with refractory ascites in a clinical setting. World J Hepatol 2015;7:1685–1693.
44 Akiyama S, Ikeda K, Sezaki H, et al: Therapeutic effects of short- and intermediate-term tolvaptan administration for refractory ascites in patients with advanced liver cirrhosis. Hepatol Res 2015;45:1062–1070.
45 Zhang X, Wang SZ, Zheng JF, et al: Clinical efficacy of tolvaptan for treatment of refractory ascites in liver cirrhosis patients. World J Gastroenterol 2014;20:11400–11405.
46 Torres VE, Chapman AB, Devuyst O, et al: Tolvaptan in patients with autosomal dominant polycystic kidney disease. N Engl J Med 2012;367:2407–2418.

47 http://www.fda.gov/Safety/MedWatch/SafetyInformation/SafetyAlertsforHumanMedicalProducts/ucm336669.htm.
48 Kalambokis G, Fotopoulos A, Economou M, et al: Effects of a 7-day treatment with midodrine in non-azotemic cirrhotic patients with and without ascites. J Hepatol 2007;46:213–221.
49 Singh V, Dhungana SP, Singh B, Vijayverghia R, Nain CK, Sharma N, Bhalla A, Gupta PK: Midodrine in patients with cirrhosis and refractory or recurrent ascites: a randomized pilot study. J Hepatol 2012;56:348–354.
50 Krag A, Møller S, Henriksen JH, Holstein-Rathlou NH, Larsen FS, Bendtsen F: Terlipressin improves renal function in patients with cirrhosis and ascites without hepatorenal syndrome. Hepatology 2007;46:1863–1871.
51 Fimiani B, Guardia DD, Puoti C, D'Adamo G, Cioffi O, Pagano A, Tagliamonte MR, Izzi A: The use of terlipressin in cirrhotic patients with refractory ascites and normal renal function: a multicentric study. Eur J Intern Med 2011;22:587–590.
52 Lenaerts A, Codden T, Meunier JC, et al: Effects of clonidine on diuretic response in ascitic patients with cirrhosis and activation of sympathetic nervous system. Hepatology 2006;44:844–849.
53 Yang YY, Lin HC, Lee WP, et al: Association of the G-protein and α2-adrenergic receptor gene and plasma norepinephrine level with clonidine improvement of the effects of diuretics in patients with cirrhosis with refractory ascites: a randomised clinical trial. Gut 2010;59:1545–1553.

Complications of Liver Disease

Digestive Diseases

Dig Dis 2017;35:411–417
DOI: 10.1159/000456596

Nutrition and Liver Health

Alan A. Jackson

NIHR Southampton Biomedical Research Centre, Southampton General Hospital, University of Southampton, Southampton, UK

Keywords

Reductive adaptation · Expansive adaptation · Kupffer cell · Fructose · Copper · Glycine

Abstract

Good clinical practice is based on a secure and accurate diagnosis. Poor nutrition is frequently associated with disorders of the liver, and a specific nutrition diagnosis is needed for providing best care and experiencing successful outcome. There is opportunity for better-structured approaches to making secure and consistent nutritional diagnoses in patients with liver disease. Nutrition is the set of integrated processes by which cells, tissues, organs and the whole body acquire the energy and nutrients to retain normal structure and perform the required functions. At the level of the whole body, this is achieved through dietary supply and the capacity of the body to transform the substrates and cofactors necessary for metabolism. All of these domains (diet, metabolic capacity, activity of the microbiome, body composition and the level of demand for energy and nutrients) are influenced by levels of physical activity and can vary according to physiological and pathological disease states. The liver plays a central role in establishing and maintaining these regulated processes. Its capacity to achieve and maintain these functional capabilities is established during one's early life. When these capabilities are exceeded and the ability to maintain the milieu interieur is compromised, ill-health supervenes. Stress tests that assess flow through gateway pathways can be used to determine the maximal capacity and functional reserve for critical functions. The inability of the liver to reliably integrate body lipid metabolism and the accumulation of abnormal lipid are obvious manifestations of impaired regulation both in situations of weight loss, for example, the fatty liver of severe malnutrition, and in situations of energy excess, as in non-alcoholic fatty liver disease. The use of stable isotopic probes and the more recent definition of the variability in the metabolome in different nutritional and pathological states indicate the great potential for clinical tools that would enable a more precise nutritional diagnosis, but these require systematic investigation and application. For the present, approaches that place emphasis on being able to control the metabolic state without exposing the liver to unnecessary metabolic stress remain the basis for successful nutritional support.

Introduction

As in any other aspect of medicine, the ability to reliably identify problems or make a secure diagnosis sits at the heart of good clinical practice and underpins the application of evidence for improvements in treatment and the delivery of care. The same principle applies to nutrition where there is the need to make a secure nutritional diagnosis for the many problems, which so frequently become a major consideration in patients with hepatic dysfunction. At some stage, the numerous nutrition-related pathophysiological processes, which are disturbed by the disease processes, are likely to come to dominate the clinical picture.

KARGER

E-Mail karger@karger.com
www.karger.com/ddi

Alan A. Jackson
NIHR Southampton Biomedical Research Centre
Southampton General Hospital, Tremona Road
Southampton SO16 6YD (UK)
E-Mail aaj@soton.ac.uk

The liver plays a central role that is critical for the regulation and control of the body's metabolic state. It modulates the delivery of nutrients to all parts of the body. Through these processes, the high energy and nutritional needs of the brain are satisfied. It also supports the balance that has to be found between the potentially competing demands set by all tissues for energy and nutrients. In order to meet the needs of the body, careful integration is required of those nutrients that are made available from the dietary intake, from intermediary metabolism and as a result of the metabolic behaviour of the microbiome [1]. This balance of needs and supply is moderated in a major way by the type and amount of physical activity, which in itself exerts a major influence on the provision provided through the diet, metabolic set and responsiveness and the behaviour of the gastrointestinal tract and its microbiome. Therefore, for the sake of consistency and for arriving at a secure diagnosis, it is desirable that a structured approach is adopted. This approach should adequately consider the range of relevant variables of importance to improve the consistency with which a secure nutritional diagnosis is made in all patients with hepatic problems.

Making a Nutritional Diagnosis

Any secure clinical diagnosis is made on the basis of a good history, the elicitation and interpretation of symptoms and signs and the judicious application of special tests. Frequently, the diagnosis is system based, determined by the effects of environmental challenge such as infection, or the functional state of specific organ systems, such as cardiovascular disease or mental ill-health. It is unusual and oftentimes exceptional to make a primary nutritional diagnosis, although that diagnosis can set the stage for reduced resilience to environmental stressors, or reduced capacity of a tissue or organ to maintain its usual function. Fatty liver disease is often the final common pathway for metabolic perturbations with which the liver is no longer able to cope [1, 2]. In the earliest descriptions of kwashiorkor, it was identified as a notable feature of severe childhood malnutrition [3] and was characterised as the hallmark of the condition described in the Caribbean in 1948 by Waterlow in his seminal MRC monograph, "Fatty Liver Disease in the British West Indies." He saw evident problems of poor nutrition in children. As much as 50% of total body fat was present in the clinically enlarged liver, which could extend to the brim of the pelvis [4]. Based upon the preferred approach to treatment at that time, surprisingly the condition was resistant to dietary treatment with methylotrophs such as choline or methionine [4]. The fatty liver associated with the limited availability of methyl groups tends to primarily influence centrilobular lipid accumulation, which contrasts with that which is seen with other dietary perturbations such as a low protein diet where the periportal area appears to be most affected probably associated with altered glutathione metabolism [5].

To develop an understanding of the pathophysiology of childhood malnutrition, exploration of the underlying pathophysiological processes to determine the limits of the body's capacity to adapt to poor nutrition and cope with environmental stresses was required [1]. What became increasingly clear is that the body has a usual demand for energy and nutrients on an ongoing basis minute by minute. This demand is usually met from the resource within the body, which is intermittently topped up from dietary sources [6, 7]. The dietary sources are supplemented with nutrients made available through the metabolic activity of the colonic microbiome. This clearly shows that achieving nutritional health represents a complex set of interactions beyond simply the dietary intake, but as a point of principle, the demand for energy and nutrients has to be met in order that good health be achieved and maintained. Any failure for the demand to be met, in whole or in part, leads to changes in function and structure, which will lead to the manifestations of ill-health in either the short or long term. The pattern of demands does vary with the physiological state, and in the face of a wide range of stressors, be they biological, behavioural or social [1, 8, 9]. The most straightforward way in which to determine whether there has been a good fit between the matching of the metabolic demands by the supply is to measure body habitus: body shape and size, its dimensions and composition. The characterisation and interpretation of any changes in the composition of the body, whether they are identified in summary as obesity, or wasting or sarcopaenia, are diagnostic of an historical nutritional imbalance, which includes but goes beyond considerations of energy. These same changes can be indicative of future risk [10–12].

For the liver as an organ, its functions present a variable demand for energy and nutrients. Meeting these demands is integrated across complex structural considerations, which embrace a dual blood supply from the portal vein and the hepatic artery and intercellular activity, which involves the complexities of variation in the cellular type and their location within the lobular architecture. These functions are integrated to meet the needs of the liver itself, but also the needs of the body as a whole. A primary objective is to ensure and maintain metabolic homeostasis, remove toxins and xenobiotics, achieve antioxidant balance and protection and integrate and control the systemic response to infection or inflammation. The extent to which these functions might be achieved successfully requires an adequate metabolic capacity. For example, the metabolic capability has to process available nutrients to meet the cerebral demands for energy and neurotransmission and support for the formation of "conditionally essential" nutrients [8, 9, 13]. One sensitive example of this challenge might be the peroxisomal generation of amino acids or very long chain unsaturated essential fatty acids [13–15]. Peroxisomal structure and function may be seriously compromised in malnutrition [16–18]. Any failure to adequately maintain and integrate this range of functions can result in hepatic pathology: metabolic imbalance leads to non-alcoholic fatty liver disease, ingestion of toxins such as alcohol can directly exceed the capacity for their secure processing, and the addition of infection or inflammation leads to fibrosis, cirrhosis and cancer [2].

There are specific nutrient considerations, separately and together, which can be shown to modulate each of these processes and which frequently may determine the overall outcome.

Maintaining Homeostasis: Achieving Balance

The current epidemic of cardiometabolic syndrome with the attendant non-alcoholic fatty liver is an important statement of our limited understanding of the processes through which metabolic control, capability and capacity are assured. Clinically evident disorders show explicitly that the ability to maintain the integrity of the system has been exceeded. These inadequacies may be exposed as a limitation of specific processes, inadequacy of which is expressed as a specific disease phenotype. Abdominal obesity is associated directly with impaired blood lipid profiles, abnormal insulin sensitivity, evidence of systemic inflammation, increased susceptibility to thrombosis and wider endocrine dysfunction. All of these measures can respond beneficially to modest weight loss indicative of an abnormal nutritional state, characterised as expansive adaptation [1]. However, their common or overlapping characteristics invite a more specific nutritional diagnosis and for this a number of important factors need to be taken into account.

There is a diurnal pattern to the balance of metabolic ebb and flow from and to the liver, from and to the periphery. This may be determined in part by food intake, but equally appears to be an intrinsic feature of metabolism, which is of fundamental importance for enabling the achievement of homeostasis and metabolic balance. These rhythms are well described but poorly understood as illustrated by the timing and pattern of protein degradation [19, 20]. The diurnal pattern appears important for the endogenous synthesis of amino acids and fatty acids with major interaction with the functional activity of the microbiome [21–23]. It is through processes of this kind that such fundamental characteristics as the achievement of nitrogen balance and the maintenance of body composition are assured [21–23]. Against an uncertain and variable dietary intake, there is a degree of "energy and nutrient" buffering by the body, with a rebalancing through the integrated activity associated with excretory processes, through the kidneys, lung and gastrointestinal tract. Although the amount and quality of the diet may vary, under most usual circumstances, a healthy liver is capable of handling itself efficiently. The amount of food consumed is to a large extent determined by the energy needs of the body. The energy needed for body function is made available through the oxidation of macronutrients, carbohydrates lipids and amino acids from protein, and in this way, balance is maintained over extended periods of time. The macronutrients also contribute directly to the quality of the diet, which together with minerals, vitamins, trace elements, water, and oxygen determine the extent to which the diet can meet the pattern of needs for the metabolic activity of the body: the goodness of fit [1]. There are 2 major modulators of these relationships: physical activity and exposure to environmental stressors. Any decrease in physical activity reduces the demand for energy and hence requires less food intake. This in turn decreases the intake of all nutrients making it more difficult to achieve a good fit for nutrients on diets of marginal or poor quality. Any stress, infection or inflammation alters the metabolic set of the body to a large extent integrated through the action of inflammatory cytokines and related molecules (see below), with associated increased losses of nutrients from the body. Once again this makes it more problematic to achieve a good nutrient fit on diets of marginal or poor quality. Both of these together, relative inactivity and response to stressors, result in altered needs for energy and nutrients during the acute phase of any illness, but also unbalanced deficits, which have to be made good during any period of convalescence. This may require special intervention, as it can be difficult for the usual diet to adequately meet the unusual needs imposed by acquired deficiencies, especially if the diet is already of marginal quality [24].

Dig Dis 2017;35:411–417
DOI: 10.1159/000456596

Responding to Stress

The systemic response to stress has been well characterised, but the complexities of the specific nutritional implications are still inadequately understood or appreciated [8, 9, 25, 26]. The coordinated response of hormonal axes, which involves a resetting of the glucocorticoid, insulin and catecholamine axes are well described [8, 9]. The specifics of the acute phase response and the local and systemic effects of pro-inflammatory cytokines such as interleukin, 1 and 6, or tumour necrosis alpha released from white cell populations such as macrophages around the body have been characterised [25, 26]. The factors associated with this response fever, loss of appetite, increased nutrient losses, unusual nutrient requirements for tissues, altered delivery of nutrients to tissues and impaired nutrient utilisation may all be a consequence of the reordering of protein metabolism and hence relate directly to the hepatic function [25, 26]. Weight loss and altered body composition, which ultimately result in sarcopaenia, are a consequence of the associated negative nitrogen balance [22, 23]. Importantly, during the ongoing stress response, the degree of negative nitrogen balance appears related to the severity of the stress and is of importance for survival. However, at a later stage, these losses have to be corrected and for successfully making good the loss, it is important to note that the pattern of nutrient losses is more complex than simply a deficit of nitrogen, amino acids or protein [1, 24, 27].

Thus, although the most obvious nutritional problem might most readily be identified as a change in body composition, wasted muscle or inappropriately located fat, these structural changes may simply reflect the final common pathway for a wider range of more complex upstream insults. Thus, perturbations of protein and/or amino acid metabolism might be attributed to any combination of a limitation in dietary energy (much less frequently limiting protein or amino acids themselves); limitation in one or more cofactors such as vitamin, mineral or trace element; an unusual pattern of demand as a feature of the stress or inflammatory response; increased losses either through the usual routes of excretion or abnormal increases associated with diarrhoea, broken skin or fistulae.

More than any other cell population, the macrophage senses the nature of the cellular environment and its response to the character of this environment sets the opportunities for other cell populations [28, 29]. The evidence suggests that because of its physical location the hepatic Kupffer cells may play a special role in this respect [2]. The plasticity of the Kupffer cell across the extremes of its polarised responsiveness as either an M1 or M2 macrophage is indicative of the critical importance of this function [28–30]. The clinical implications of this are yet to be fully developed. For example, Thurman identified the particular importance that the simplest amino acid, glycine [31–33] might have a role to play in these interactions. He demonstrated that a glycine gated chloride channel, which modulated intracellular calcium may protect against septic shock induced by exposure to lipopolysaccharide [34]. This protection may be enabled in part through a TLR4 receptor mechanism [35]. The protective effect of glycine in the responses of the liver to challenge show time and dose-related complex considerations that would be difficult to identify with confidence unless looked for specifically [36]. Indeed, the metabolic roles played by glycine in vivo are so many and fundamental that the systems to ensure its ready availability are well protected and buffered [13]. Hence, they are unlikely to be readily identified and likely involve special attention [37–39]. Special functions of this kind, associated with a simple amino acid that does not need to be taken in the diet, are easily overlooked.

The extent to which glycine might limit Kupffer cell activation is but one example. There is increasing alarm around the substantial increase in the prevalence of obesity across the globe, most notably in children at such early ages. The attention that has been given to dietary factors has had a special focus on high levels of consumption of sucrose across the population but most especially in young people [40]. This has been especially related to the very high levels of consumption of carbonated soft drinks, and this increased consumption of sucrose or fructose in young people is a matter of great concern [41].

The changing patterns of dietary consumption over the past 25 years have been associated with an increasing prevalence of obesity and its attendant comorbidities. These altered patterns are crudely characterised as an increase in the consumption of alcohol and "junk food." It is possible to identify a more specific characterisation of the properties of these diets and the likely metabolic cost of their frequent high level of consumption. For many years, it has been known that consumption of diets with a high level of fructose, leading to excessive fructose intake can be associated with an increased risk of fatty liver disease and impaired integrity of the intestinal barrier [42, 43]. Indeed, the severely malnourished children referred to earlier were identified as "sugar babies" [3, 4]. What is less widely appreciated is that the adverse effects of high fructose intakes may also increase alcohol-associated liver damage [44]. Importantly, it has been known for many years that there is an interaction through which high fructose intake can exacerbate poor copper status and together these may present as disordered lipid metabolism and increased risk of cardiovascular abnormalities [45]. Copper itself has complex metabolic interactions with other divalent cations, such as iron and zinc, which are especially evident during inflammatory states [24, 25]. There may be amelioration of some of these effects with supplemental glycine [36]. Importantly, detoxification or conjugation processes can deplete glycine availability, for example, through excessive consumption of a preservative such as benzoic acid, frequently used as a food preservative, or a high-protein diet [13, 38]. Limitation in the availability of glycine increases the likelihood of impaired antioxidant capacity due to impaired glutathione formation.

This example of complicated nutrient–nutrient interactions could not have been predicted simply by measuring body composition or even a careful assessment of the dietary intake. These possible mechanisms and the nutritional diagnoses that they represent are yet to be investigated in detail. However, in order to make progress, there is the need for a suitable model of a possible or probable disease process against which to ask the critical questions of relevance. The ability of the body to maintain and integrate its metabolic behaviour and support CNS communication is highly dependent on nutrients, which do not have to be taken preformed in the diet, but whose metabolism is absolutely dependent on adequate hepatic function. The availability from muscle of glutamine and glutamate and the putative importance of physical activity; the role they play in assuring the integrity of the gastrointestinal tract and making citrulline available for the renal production of arginine; and the central role played by the liver in assuring adequate and balanced availability of serine, glycine, cysteine and taurine for complex interacting systems indicate the sort of information that is needed and the type of studies that will enable greater understanding and improved prevention and care.

Principles of Care

Against this seemingly infinite complexity, there is the need to organise and structure the care of patients to provide the best opportunity for recovery. This has been achieved for severely malnourished children by developing and adopting a stepped approach, which acknowledges the need to repair the cellular systems of the body and enable them to restore their functional capacity before they are challenged with the need to correct the alterations in body composition that have been used to identify a disorder. At different times, there have been "fashions" around what is the most important aspect for focus in terms of dietary care. This has led to excessive promise for simple single interventions, which is often not realised within a wider context. Adequate energy, an appropriate pattern of macronutrients, and appropriate pattern of minerals, vitamins, trace elements, oxygen, and water are all necessary. None is sufficient alone and the challenge is to determine the most secure balance at the different stages of the journey from treatment to recovery and during the period of convalescence. Inadequate food consumption leads to wasting and greater vulnerability as a consequence of reductive adaptation [1]. This does need to be corrected, but the changes induced by stressors are more likely to be life-threatening in the short term. Therefore, the highest priority has to be given to the correction of specific nutrient losses, the correction of cellular damage and correction of tissues malfunction. These take priority in the short term. Making good tissues deficits such as sarcopaenia can be reliably achieved only against this background of improved cellular function.

When viewed through a nutritional lens, the guidelines offered in the 10-step approach to treatment of severe malnutrition offered by the World Health Organization have been found to capture the necessary principles that are efficacious across a wide range of complex nutritional problems [24, 27]. In many respects, this approach may appear counter-intuitive in relation to usual clinical practice. Notwithstanding this, the highest priority has to be given to the need to enable the systems of the body to gain metabolic control by supporting them in achieving homeostasis for the system as a whole rather than the treatment of any single biochemical measurement [24]. This requires the ability to recognise and manage reductive adaptation by limiting the intake of energy and protein to match the immediate need for cellular support, the treatment of underlying stressors wherever possible, the correction of specific deficiencies (intracellular nutrients) that are not obvious from usual biochemical tests and the treatment of infections that may well be silent. This could be considered phase 1 of treatment during which the objective is to recognise and address the need to repair the cellular damage. During phase 2, the objective is to replete any tissue loss and correct body composition. Phase 2 is much more difficult to achieve unless phase 1 has been adequately addressed, but correction of the tissue deficit will require a more generous intake of energy, protein and nutrients to meet the demands for net tissue deposition.

When applied faithfully, these principles have been found to significantly reduce mortality even in the sickest individuals; however, effective care may often appear counter-intuitive not least because the structure no longer adequately marks function. Certainly in the face of reductive adaptation and with inevitable specific nutrient deficiencies of uncertain pattern and the strong likelihood of silent infections, greater care is required in management of a problem that might readily be upset by the use of standard, available dietary remedies. This indicates an important research agenda to be executed, which should determine which, and in what order, different nutritional constraints might be limiting at the different stages of recovery [46, 47].

Conclusions

Effective care depends upon a secure diagnosis. Given the multiplicity of hepatic functions and its variable response to nutritional challenge and environmental stressors requires the development of suitable special tests. These tests should (a) assess the capacity of critical rate limiting functions, (b) determine the role of specific nutrients in enabling or disabling these functions, and (c) move to the development of clinical tests that are fit for purpose and can be applied in practice either singly or together.

To better characterise and define the range of nutrition-related functions that may be modified or become limiting, thereby leading directly to hepatic disease will require the development and application of appropriate specific probes.

In the meantime, there would be considerable benefit in the establishment of a systematic, structured approach to clinical nutrition care to better enable the sharing of experience and progressive refinement of effective care.

Disclosure Statement

The author declares no conflict of interest.

References

1 Jackson AA, Wootton SA, Wiseman M: Nature, purpose and implications of research in nutrition; in Lovegrove JA, Hodson L, Sharma S, Lanham-New SA (eds): Nutrition Research Methodologies. John Wiley & Sons, Ltd., 2015.
2 Sakaguchi S, Takahashi S, Sasaki T, Kumagai T, Nagata K: Progression of alcoholic and non-alcoholic steatohepatitis: common metabolic aspects of innate immune system and oxidative stress. Drug Metab Pharmacokinet 2011;26:30–46.
3 Wiliams CD: Kwashiorkor a nutritional disease of children associated with a maize diet. Lancet 1935;2:1151–1152.
4 Waterlow JC: Fatty Liver Disease in Infants in the British West Indies. Medical Research Council, Special Report Series 263. London, HMSO, 1948.
5 Jahoor F, Jackson AA: Hepatic function in rats with dietary-induced fatty liver, as measured by the uptake of indocyanine green. Br J Nutr 1982;47:391–397.
6 Kerr DS, Stevens MC, Robinson HM: Fasting metabolism in infants. I. Effect of severe undernutrition on energy and protein utilization. Metabolism 1978;27:411–435.
7 Kerr DS, Stevens MC, Picou DI: Fasting metabolism in infants: II. the effect of severe undernutrition and infusion of alanine on glucose production estimated with U-13C-glucose. Metabolism 1978;27:831–848.
8 Selye H: The Story of the Adaptation Syndrome. Montreal, Acta Inc., 1952.
9 Selye H: Forty years of stress research: principal remaining problems and misconceptions. Can Med Assoc J 1976;115:53–56.
10 Sinclair M, Gow PJ, Grossmann M, Angus PW: Review article: sarcopenia in cirrhosis – aetiology, implications and potential therapeutic interventions. Aliment Pharmacol Ther 2016;43:765–777.
11 Kappus MR, Mendoza MS, Nguyen D, Medici V, McClave SA: Sarcopenia in patients with chronic liver disease: can it be altered by diet and exercise? Curr Gastroenterol Rep 2016; 18:43.
12 Dasarathy S, Merli M: Sarcopenia from mechanism to diagnosis and treatment in liver disease. J Hepatol 2016;65:1232–1244.
13 Jackson AA: The glycine story. Eur J Clin Nutr 1991;45:59–65.
14 Nobili V, Alisi A, Della Corte C, Risé P, Galli C, Agostoni C, Bedogni G: Docosahexaenoic acid for the treatment of fatty liver: randomised controlled trial in children. Nutr Metab Cardiovasc Dis 2013;11:1066–1070.
15 Parker HM, Johnson NA, Burdon CA, et al: Omega-3 supplementation and non-alcoholic fatty liver disease: a systematic review and meta-analysis. J Hepatol 2012;56:944–951.
16 Doherty JF, Golden MH, Brooks SE: Peroxisomes and the fatty liver of malnutrition: an hypothesis. Am J Clin Nutr 1991;54:674–677.
17 Brooks SE, Goldon MH, Taylor E: Hepatic ultrastructure in children with protein-energy malnutrition. West Indian Med J 1992;41: 139–145.
18 Brooks SE, Doherty JF, Golden MH: Peroxisomes and the hepatic pathology of childhood malnutrition. West Indian Med J 1994;43:15–17.
19 Jackson AA, Soares MJ, Grove G, Waterlow JC: Enrichment in urinary ammonia and urea with hourly oral doses of [15N]glycine: evidence for a step function and a circadian rhythm in protein turnover. Clin Sci 1997;93: 265–271.
20 Ohsumi Y: Historical landmarks of autophagy research. Cell Res 2014;24:9–23.
21 Jackson AA: Salvage of urea-nitrogen in the large bowel: functional significance in metabolic control and adaptation. Biochem Soc Trans 1998;26:231–236.
22 Jackson AA: Salvage of urea-nitrogen and protein requirements. Proc Nutr Soc 1995;54: 535–547.
23 Waterlow JC: The mysteries of nitrogen balance. Nutr Res Rev 1999;12:25–54.
24 Jackson AA: Severe malnutrition; in Warrell DA, Cox TM, Firth JD (eds): Oxford Textbook of Medicine, ed 5. Oxford University Press, 2015. www.oxfordmedicine.com.
25 Grimble RF: Nutritional modulation of cytokine biology. Nutrition 1998;14:634–640.

26 Grimble RF: Modification of the inflammatory aspects of immune function by nutrients. Nutrition Research 1998;18:1297–1317.
27 World Health Organization: Management of Severe Malnutrition: A Manual for Physicians and Other Senior Health Workers. Geneva, WHO, 1999. http://whqlibdoc.who.int/hq/1999/a57361.pdf.
28 Sica A, Invernizzi P, Mantovani A: Macrophage plasticity and polarization in liver homeostasis and pathology. Hepatology 2014; 59:2034–2042.
29 Wan J, Benkdane M, Teixeira-Clerc F, Bonnafous S, Louvet A, Lafdil F, Pecker F, Tran A, Gual P, Mallat A, Lotersztajn S, Pavoine C: M2 Kupffer cells promote M1 Kupffer cell apoptosis: a protective mechanism against alcoholic and nonalcoholic fatty liver disease. Hepatology 2014;59:130–142.
30 Wenfeng Z, Yakun W, Di M, Jianping G, Chuanxin W, Chun H: Kupffer cells: increasingly significant role in nonalcoholic fatty liver disease. Ann Hepatol 2014;13:489–495.
31 Thurman RG, Schemmer P, Zhong Z, Bunzendahl H, von Frankenberg M, Lemasters JJ: Kupffer cell-dependent reperfusion injury in liver transplantation: new clinically relevant use of glycine. Langenbecks Arch Chir Suppl Kongressbd 1998;115:185–190.
32 Wheeler MD, Ikejema K, Enomoto N, Stacklewitz RF, Seabra V, Zhong Z, Yin M, Schemmer P, Rose ML, Rusyn I, Bradford B, Thurman RG: Glycine: a new anti-inflammatory immunonutrient. Cell Mol Life Sci 1999;56:843–856.
33 Rose ML, Rusyn I, Bojes HK, Belyea J, Cattley RC, Thurman RG: Role of Kupffer cells and oxidants in signaling peroxisome proliferator-induced hepatocyte proliferation. Mutat Res 2000;448:179–192.
34 Ikejima K, Iimuro Y, Forman DT, Thurman RG: A diet containing glycine improves survival in endotoxin shock in the rat. Am J Physiol 1996;271(1 pt 1):G97–G103.
35 Xu FL, You HB, Li XH, Chen XF, Liu ZJ, Gong JP: Glycine attenuates endotoxin-induced liver injury by downregulating TLR4 signaling in Kupffer cells. Am J Surg 2008; 196:139–148.
36 Petrat F, Boengler K, Schulz R, de Groot H: Glycine, a simple physiological compound protecting by yet puzzling mechanism(s) against ischaemia-reperfusion injury: current knowledge. Br J Pharmacol 2012;165:2059–2072.
37 Jackson AA, Persaud C, Meakins TS, Bundy R: Urinary excretion of 5-L-oxoproline (pyroglutamic acid) is increased in normal adults consuming vegetarian or low protein diets. J Nutr 1996;126:2813–2822.
38 Meakins TS, Persaud C, Jackson AA: Dietary supplementation with L-methionine impairs the utilization of urea-nitrogen and increases 5-L-oxoprolinuria in normal women consuming a low protein diet. J Nutr 1998;128: 720–727.
39 Jackson AA, Phillips G, McClelland I, Jahoor F: Synthesis of hepatic secretory proteins in normal adults consuming a diet marginally adequate in protein. Am J Physiol Gastrointest Liver Physiol 2001;281:G1179–G1187.
40 Scientific Advisory Committee on Nutrition: Carbohydrates and Health. The Stationery Office Limited, 2015.
41 Scientific Advisory Committee on Nutrition: The Nutritional Wellbeing of the British Population. The Stationery Office Limited, 2008.
42 Reiser S, Smith JC Jr, Mertz W, Holbrook JT, Scholfield DJ, Powell AS, Canfield WK, Canary JJ: Indices of copper status in humans consuming a typical American diet containing either fructose or starch. Am J Clin Nutr 1985;42:242–251.
43 Spruss A, Bergheim I: Dietary fructose and intestinal barrier: potential risk factor in the pathogenesis of nonalcoholic fatty liver disease. J Nutr Biochem 2009;20:657–662.
44 Samuel VT: Fructose induced lipogenesis: from sugar to fat to insulin resistance. Trends Endocrinol Metab 2011;22:60–65.
45 Klevay LM: IHD from copper deficiency: a unified theory. Nutr Res Rev 2016;29:172–179.
46 Cave M, Deaciuc I, Mendez C, Song Z, Joshi-Barve S, Barve S, McClain C: Nonalcoholic fatty liver disease: predisposing factors and the role of nutrition. J Nutr Biochem 2007;18: 184–195.
47 Schütte K, Tippelt B, Schulz C, Röhl FW, Feneberg A, Seidensticker R, Arend J, Malfertheiner P: Malnutrition is a prognostic factor in patients with hepatocellular carcinoma (HCC). Clin Nutr 2015;34:1122–1127.

Digestive Diseases

Dig Dis 2017;35:418–420
DOI: 10.1159/000470876

Falk Symposium Series

155. Keppler D, Beuers U, Leuschner U, Stiehl A, Trauner M, Paumgartner G, eds. Bile Acids: Biological Actions and Clinical Relevance. Falk Symposium 155. 2007 ISBN 978-1-4020-6251-3
156. Blum HE, Cox DW, Häussinger D, Jansen PLM, Kullak-Ublick GA, eds. Genetics in Liver Diseases. Falk Symposium 156. 2007 ISBN 978-1-4020-6393-0
157. Diehl AM, Hayashi N, Manns MP, Sauerbruch T, eds. Chronic Hepatitis: Metabolic, Cholestatic, Viral and Autoimmune. Falk Symposium 157. 2007 ISBN 978-1-4020-6522-4
158. Gasche G, Herrerías Gutiérrez JM, Gassull M, Monterio E, eds. Intestinal Inflammation and Colorectal Cancer. Falk Symposium 158. 2007 ISBN 978-1-4020-6825-6
159. Tözün N, Mantzaris G, Dağlı, Schölmerich J, eds. IBD 2007 – Achievements in Research and Clinical Practice. Falk Symposium 159. 2008 ISBN 978-1-4020-6986-4
160. Ferkolj I, Gangl A, Galle PR, Vucelic B, eds. Pathogenesis and Clinical Practice in Gastroenterology. Falk Symposium 160. 2008 ISBN 978-1-4020-8766-0
161. Carey MC, Gabryelewicz A, Díte P, Keim V, Mössner J, eds. Future Perspectives in Gastroenterology. Falk Symposium 161. 2008 ISBN 978-1-4020-8832-2
162. Bosch J, Lammert F, Burroughs AK, Lebrec D, Sauerbruch T, eds. Liver Cirrhosis: From Pathophysiology to Disease Management. Falk Symposium 162. 2008 ISBN 978-1-4020-8655-7
163. Adler G, Fan DM, Jia JD, LaRusso NF, Owyang C, eds. Chronic Inflammation of Liver and Gut. Falk Symposium 163. 2008 ISBN 978-1-4020-9352-4
164. Tulassay Z, Dítě P, Krejs GJ, Schölmerich J, Schultz HJ, eds. Intestinal Disorders. Falk Symposium 164. 2009 ISBN 978-1-4020-9590-0
165. Keppler D, Beuers U, Stiehl A, Trauner M, eds. Bile Acid Biology and Therapeutic Actions. Falk Symposium 165. 2009 ISBN 978-1-4020-9643-3

165A. Lieberman DA, Malfertheiner P, Riemann JF, Spechler SJ, eds. Strategies of Cancer Prevention in Gastroenterology. Falk Workshop. 2009 ISBN 978-90-481-2628-6

166. Ell C, Ponchon T, Riemann JF, Sakai P, Yamamoto H, eds. GI Endoscopy – Standards and Innovations. Falk Symposium 166. 2009 ISBN 978-90-481-2748-1
167. Day CP, Galle PR, Lohse AW, Thorgeirsson SS, eds. Liver under Constant Attack – From Fat to Viruses. Falk Symposium 167. 2009 ISBN 978-90-481-2758-0

KARGER

E-Mail karger@karger.ch
www.karger.com/ddi

168. Rogler G, Gassul M, Levine A, López San Román A, eds. IBD in Different Age Groups. Falk Symposium 168. 2009 ISBN 978-3-8055-9273-4

169. Buhr HJ, Kharchenko NV, Siegmund B, Zacharash MP, Zeitz M, eds. Inflammation in the Intestinal Tract: Pathogenesis and Treatment. Falk Symposium 169. 2009 ISBN 978-3-8055-9282-6

170. Travis SPL, Spiller RC, Colombel JF, Holzer P, eds. IBD and IBS: Novel Mechanisms and Future Practice. Falk Symposium 170. 2009 ISBN 978-3-8055-9420-2

171. Day CP, Diehl AM, Lehnert H, Manns MP, Negro F, eds. Liver and Metabolic Syndrome. Falk Symposium 171. 2009 ISBN 978-3-8055-9446-2

171A. Gershwin ME, Lohse AW, Manns MP, Vergani D, eds. Immunology and Liver Disease. Falk Workshop. 2009 ISBN 978-3-8055-9446-2

172. Rogler G, Sandborn W, eds. The Keys to IBD 2010: Treatment, Diagnosis and Pathophysiology. Falk Symposium 172. 2010 ISBN 978-3-8055-9588-9

173. Dítě P, Krejs GJ, Malfertheiner P, Tulassay Z, eds. From Chronic Inflammation to Cancer. Falk Symposium 173. 2010 ISBN 978-3-8055-9653-4

174. Chen CW, Cheng J, Ginès P, Ouyang Q, Schölmerich J, eds. Gut and Liver. Falk Symposium 174. 2010 ISBN 978-3-8055-9672-5

175. Häussinger D, Beuers U, Stiehl A, Trauner M, eds. Bile Acids as Metabolic Integrators and Therapeutics. Falk Symposium 175. 2010 ISBN 978-3-8055-9804-0

176. Blum HE, Hunt RH, Schölmerich J, eds. Environment and Lifestyle – Effects on Disorders of the Digestive Tract. Falk Symposium 176. 2010 ISBN 978-3-8055-9809-5

WS Singer MV, Dooley S, McClain CJ, Zakhari S, eds. Liver and Pancreatic Diseases: Consequences of Chronic Alcoholic Consumption. Falk Workshop Freiburg. 2010 ISBN 978-3-8055-9732-6

WS Schlitt HJ, Benseler V, Hellerbrand C, Loss M, Weiss TS, Wiest R, eds. Liver and Immunology. Falk Workshop Regensburg. 2011 ISBN 978-3-8055-9845-3

177. Schulz HJ, Rösch T, Siersema PD, eds. Endoscopy Live Berlin 2011-Intestinal Disease Meeting. Falk Symposium 177. 2011 ISBN 978-3-8055-9874-3

178. Kruis W, Spiller RC, Papagigoriadis S, Engel A, Kreis ME, eds. Diverticular Disease: A Fresh Approach to a Neglected Disease. Falk Symposium 178. 2011 ISBN 978-3-8055-9878-8

179. D'Haens G, Dignass A, Vermeire S, eds. Revisiting IBD Management: Dogmas to Be Challenged. Falk Symposium 179. 2012 ISBN 978-3-318-02187-5

WS Tiegs G, Lohse AW, Thimme R, Trautwein C, eds. Inflammation and Cancer. Falk Workshop. 2012 ISBN 978-3-318-02185-1

WS Miehlke S, Munch A, eds. Microscopic Colitis – Creating Awareness for an Underestimated Disease. Falk Workshop Basel. 2012

181. Tilg H, Blumberg RS, Endres S, Kaser A, Manns MP, eds. Innate Immunity in Gastrointestinal Disorder: Basic and Therapeutic Concepts. Falk Symposium 181. 2012 ISBN 978-3-318-02210-0

182. Friess H, Schmid RM, Fried M, van de Velde CJH, eds. Carcinogenesis, Prevention and Treatment of Colorectal Cancer – State of the Art 2012. Falk Symposium 182. 2012 ISBN 978-3-318-02213-1

183. Rogler C, Beglinger C, Colombel J-F, Michetti P, eds. Dealing with Our 'In-Vironment': New Aspects in IBD Pathogenesis and Therapy. Falk Symposium 183. 2012 ISBN 978-3-318-02258-2

184. Häussinger D, Beuers U, Trauner M, eds. XXII International Bile Acid Meeting – Hepatic and Extrahepatic Targets of Bile Acid Signaling. Falk Symposium 184. 2012

Dig Dis 2017;35:418–420
DOI: 10.1159/000470876

185. Ell C, Galle PR, Mössner J, Meyenberger C, Spechler SJ, Yamamoto H, eds. Interfaces and Controversies in Gastroenterology. Falk Symposium 185. 2013 ISBN 978-3-318-02384-8

186. Galle PR, Clavien P-A, Gores GJ, Protzer U, Schuchmann M, eds. Challenges of Liver Cirrhosis and Tumors: Prevent It, Treat It, Manage Consequences. Falk Symposium 186. 2013 ISBN 978-3-318-02384-8

187. Panés J, Ghosh S, Gomollón F, Louis E, eds. Overcoming Challenges in IBD Management. Falk Symposium 187. 2013 ISBN 978-3-318-02468-5

188. Stange EF, Dignass A, Fellermann K, Herrlinger K, eds. Inflammatory Bowel Diseases: Microbiota versus the Barrier. Falk Symposium 188. 2013 ISBN 978-3-318-02538-5

189. Straumann A, Schoepfer A, Simon H-U, eds. Eosinophilic Esophagitis: A Novel Chronic Inflammatory Disease of the GI Tract. Falk Symposium 189. 2013

WS Krejs GJ, Eherer AJ, Pointner R, eds. GERD: Gastroesophageal Reflux Disease. Falk Workshop Graz. 2013 ISBN 978-3-318-02594-1

190. Levine A, Forbes A, Probert C, eds. Challenges in the Care of IBD in Patients of All Ages. Falk Symposium 190. 2013 ISBN 978-3-318-02662-7

191. Chapman RW, Adams DH, Beuers U, Day CP, Manns MP, eds. Liver Diseases in 2013: Advances in Pathogenesis and Treatment. Falk Symposium 191. 2013 ISBN 978-3-318-02665-8

192. Dignass A, Allez M, Danese S, Marteau P, eds. IBD 2014: Thinking Out of the Box. Falk Symposium 192. 2014 ISBN 978-3-318-02806-5

193. Mulder CJJ, Schuppan D, eds. Celiac Disease and Other Small Bowel Disorders. Falk Symposium 193. 2014 ISBN 978-3-318-03014-3

194. Häussinger D, Beuers U, Keitel V, Trauner M, eds. XXIII International Bile Acid Meeting: Bile Acids as a Signal Integrators and Metabolic Modulators. Falk Symposium 194. 2014 ISBN 978-3-318-05436-1

WS Gerbes AL, Jaeschke HW, eds. The Challenge of Drug-Induced Liver Injury (DILI). Falk Workshop Freiburg. 2015

195. Gerbes AL, Bosch J, Pinzani M, Wong F, eds. Challenges and Management of Liver Cirrhosis. Falk Symposium 195. 2015 ISBN 978-3-318-05448-4

196. Dignass A, Danese S, Mantzaris GJ, Sands BE, eds. Critical Evaluation of Current Concepts and Moving to New Horizons in the Management of IBD. Falk Symposium 196. 2015 ISBN 978-3-318-05486-6

197. Ginès P, Beuers U, Cortez-Pinto H, Lohse AW, Parés A, eds. Autoimmune Diseases of the Liver. Falk Symposium 197. 2015 ISBN 978-3-318-05563-4

198. Rogler G, Kamm MA, Ng SC, eds. Inflammatory Bowel Disease: East Meets West. Falk Symposium 198. 2015 ISBN 978-3-318-05827-7

199. Thimme R, Chazouillères O, Llovet JM, Moradpour D, eds. Highlights from Hepatology 2015: From Chronic Hepatitis to Hepatocellular Carcinoma. Falk Symposium 199. 2015 ISBN 978-3-318-05834-5

200. Schölmerich J, Bruno MJ, El-Omar EM, Ginès P, Podolsky DK, eds. Therapeutic Strategies in Diseases of the Digestive Tract – 2015 and Beyond. Falk Symposium 200. 2015 ISBN 978-3-318-05876-5

201. Tilg H, Kaser A, Manns MP, Szabo G, Trauner M, eds. Gut-Liver Interactions: From IBD to NASH. Falk Symposium 201. 2016 ISBN 978-3-318-05879-6

202. Lukas M, Bortlik M, Kruis W, Stange EF, eds. Evolving Therapies in Clinical Practice in IBD. Falk Symposium 202. 2016 ISBN 978-3-318-05900-7

203. Häussinger D, Beuers U, Keitel V, Trauner M, eds. XXIV International Bile Acid Meeting: Bile Acids in Health and Disease. Falk Symposium 203. 2016 ISBN 978-3-318-05923-6

Digestive Diseases

Author Index Vol. 35, No. 4, 2017

E-Mail karger@karger.com
www.karger.com/ddi

Subject Index Vol. 35, No. 4, 2017

Digestive Diseases

KARGER

E-Mail karger@karger.com
www.karger.com/ddi

• Journal Publication

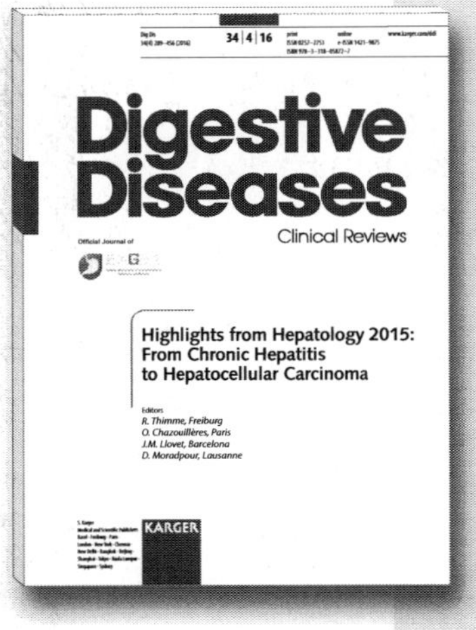

Highlights from Hepatology 2015: From Chronic Hepatitis to Hepatocellular Carcinoma

Editors
R. Thimme
O. Chazouillères
J.M. Llovet
D. Moradpour

Highlights from Hepatology 2015: From Chronic Hepatitis to Hepatocellular Carcinoma
Falk Symposium 199, Freiburg, October 2015: Offical Congress Report
Editors: Thimme, R. (Freiburg); Chazouillères, O. (Paris); Llovet, J.M. (Barcelona); Moradpour, D. (Lausanne)
II + 168 p., 34 fig., 29 tab., 2016
CHF 43.00 / EUR 40.00 / USD 51.00
Soft cover or online prices for personal customers
Prices subject to change, VAT not included
EUR price for eurozone countries,
USD price for USA and Latin America only
ISBN 978–3–318–05872–7
e-ISBN 978–3–318–05873–4

Special Topic Issue
Digestive Diseases
Vol. 34, No. 4 (2016)
Included in subscription

Listed in Journal Citation Reports, PubMed/MEDLINE, Embase

Contents

Dear Librarian

I have reviewed this publication and would like to recommend it for our library.

Recommended by:

Department:

Date:

Signature:

Orders may be placed with any bookshop, subscription agency, directly with the publisher or through a Karger distributor.

The easiest way to order: **www.karger.com/ddi**

Karger – Medical and Scientific Publishers
CH–4009 Basel, Switzerland
orders@karger.com, f: +41 61 306 12 34
www.karger.com

KI16364

KARGER